A Step-by-Step Guide to

STOP
BLOATING
&
HEAL YOUR GUT

Aliki Economides, MS, RDN and Irini Hadjisavva, PhD

A Step-by-Step Guide to

STOP BLOATING
&
HEAL YOUR GUT

CLEAN LOW FODMAP DIET

101 Clean, Unprocessed, Super Healthy
Mediterranean-Inspired, Gluten-Free Recipes

CYPRUS 2021

The photos that do not bear the name of a photographer come from Shutterstock.

Series: VARIOUS TOPICS
Title: A STEP-BY-STEP GUIDE TO STOP BLOATING & HEAL YOUR GUT
Authors: ALIKI ECONOMIDES, MS, RDN AND IRINI HADJISAVVA, PHD
Photography: KYRIAKI LEVENTI – Photochromata Ltd

Copyright © 2021:
LIVANI PUBLISHING ORGANIZATION S.A.
98, Solonos St. – 106 80 Athens. Tel.: 210 3661200, Fax: 210 3617791
http://www.livanis.gr

Production: Livani Publishing Organization

ISBN 978-960-3542-8

Praise for

A Step-by-Step Guide to Stop Bloating and Heal your Gut is a great resource for those suffering with painful bloating and IBS. The book features a great primer on the digestive process, as well as an in-depth review of gastrointestinal and labora-tory tests to help the reader navigate this complex topic. The low FODMAP diet is reviewed in detail from the elimination to the reintroduction phase. I personally love the variety of healthy low FODMAP recipes (101 recipes included) such as delicious smoothies, muffins, main dishes and more!

Kate Scarlata, MPH, RDN
US-based Low FODMAP Diet and Gut Health Expert
Coauthor of The New York Times bestselling *21 Day Tummy Diet, The Real Food for Real People* and *The Low-FODMAP Diet Step by Step: A Personalized Plan to Relieve the Symptoms of IBS and Other Digestive Disorders*, and Author of *The Complete Idiot's Guide to Eating Well with IBS*

If you suffer from abdominal bloating or IBS, you've come to the right place. This well-researched and thorough book will be your trusted guide. The authors, experienced dietitians and scientists, provide accurate food lists, creative menu ideas, and delicious recipes to help yourself by trying a low-FODMAP diet. Beyond FODMAPs, the book covers important points about probiotics, dietary supplements, exercise, and more. I highly recommend *A Step-by-Step Guide to Stop Bloating and Heal Your Gut.*

Patsy Catsos, MS, RDN, LD
Author of *The IBS Elimination Diet and Cookbook*

I have thoroughly read through the book and have tried a few of the recipes. The information was easy to follow and detail oriented. Recipes were easy to follow and quite delicious! Gastrointestinal symptoms and challenges are quite common complaints that require a medical professional diagnosis and registered dietitian follow-up. This professional written and published material will definitely provide sound, accurate knowledge and success in overcoming the challenges experienced by patients and clients.

Susan M. Hazarvartian, MS, RDN, LDN
Adjunct Professor, Simmons University, Boston, USA
Private Practice and Contract Registered Dietitian

Introduction

All people suffering from tummy troubles have their own story to tell. While not unique, these stories are highly personal and serve as daily reminders of the impact that gastrointestinal disease has on their lives.

As the founders of the Digestive Nutrition Clinic and the authors of this book you hold in your hands, we too have experienced the difficulties presented by irritable bowel syndrome (IBS) and other gastrointestinal ailments.

Therefore, before we even get started on this journey, here are our stories, which we look forward to sharing with you and which present a bright light at the end of the tunnel.

"My struggle with bloating started years back when I was living in Boston. I was in graduate school, wrapping up my master's degree. I had just had a baby and was applying for a very competitive dietetic internship when I was diagnosed with functional bloating. The bloating and the pain were having negative effects on my life, and despite trying various dietary approaches, I only received the answer many years later with the low FODMAP diet, which once and for all transformed my life. Since then, I have been on a mission to spread this good news and add my own professional expertise as a nutrition expert, patient and recipe developer in helping patients manage their digestive symptoms and use food as medicine to heal their gut and optimize their health."

- Aliki Economides, MS, RDN

"I was diagnosed with IBS at the age of twenty-seven. I visited a gastroenterologist at George Washington University Hospital in the USA after a rough few months of bloating, intestinal pain, diarrhea and weight loss. During a high-stress period in my life writing my PhD thesis, it seemed that all of my symptoms, which I used to have from childhood, had worsened and were inhibiting me from having a normal life.

"I was convinced garlic was the root of my problem, but my theory was not well received. After running a number of tests and eliminating more serious conditions, IBS was identified as the culprit of my suffering. I was instructed to remove the usual suspects from my diet: dairy products, broccoli, nuts and everything I had noticed bothering me. I practically went through the next ten years eliminating and adding foods, going through bouts of diarrhea, and being bloated and in pain—without exaggerating—three to four times a week."

"I reached a point in my life at which I couldn't handle the discomforts any longer and decided it was time to make a drastic change. I took the plunge and started the low FODMAP diet, and as soon as a month later, the improvements were dramatic. I must admit that this decision has changed my life for the best."

- Irini Hadjisavva, PhD

Every day, we hear similar stories from people in the clinic and witness how gastrointestinal problems such as bloating, abdominal pain, diarrhea and constipation hinder people's lives.

We fully understand that this struggle is real and that sufferers like us deserve support. Likewise, we acknowledge that this pain from which we all suffer is not a figment of our imaginations; it is palpable and can be a true detriment to our day-to-day lives.

However, from our own personal experiences with the low FODMAP diet, it is clear that you do not have to live forever with this pain. Although this approach may not be everyone's cup of tea, between 50% and 80% of patients who have tried it have responded positively to the low FODMAP diet. So read on, delve deeper into the topic, and consider giving the diet a try.

Our Mission

A a team of digestive health professionals, we are on a mission to spread the word on the low FODMAP diet and its positive effects on digestive health for sufferers of bloating and IBS like us. After many years, we can confidently say that we have a solution to control our bloating, manage our digestive symptoms, heal our gut, and optimize our digestive health.

The discovery and further examination of the low FODMAP diet has been one of the most gratifying experiences in our professional lives, as this science-backed dietary plan has helped both us and most of the Digestive Nutrition Clinic's patients to use foods as a straightforward way of combating gastrointestinal symptoms.

How to Use This Book

Section 1
Chapters 1, 2 and 3 will walk you through the various causes of abdominal bloating and distention. All the information is evidence-based and backed by science. Use this book to facilitate your communication with your doctor and dietician, as it will equip you with ample knowledge on various possible causes, mechanisms, tests and procedures.

Section 2
In this section, we will help you connect the dots between an imbalanced gut microbiome and its impact on your health and understand the link between a low-fiber, processed diet and an increased risk of certain diseases. We will demonstrate that a diet high in fiber is one of the most important tools you have to control your garden of gut microorganisms and improve your overall health. We will help you assess your current fiber intake, walk you through different types of fibers, and offer a number of specific fiber recommendations. Via the careful design of a low FODMAP diet, our ultimate aim is to guide you so that you maximize your fiber consumption while minimizing abdominal symptoms.

More specifically, this section of the book will help you with the following tasks:

- Implement the elimination phase of the low FODMAP diet, a scientifically proven way to control bloating and manage digestive symptoms
- Carry out the reintroduction phase of the diet
- Learn about our own clean low FODMAP diet that focuses on unprocessed, healthy and high-fiber ingredients, mainly from the Mediterranean region
- Identify your daily fiber intake
- Familiarize yourself with different types of fibers and their role in the gastrointestinal tract
- Learn about specific daily fiber recommendations for soluble and insoluble fibers, prebiotics and resistant starch

- Maximize fiber intake while maintaining control of symptoms
- Set up a longer, highly personalized and clean low FODMAP diet plan that will offer you the flexibility to plan your own meals that are rich in a large variety of foods while managing your symptoms
- Incorporate probiotics into your daily diet

Section 3

In this final section, you will find a tested and popular meal plan, menu ideas, and 101 of our healthy, gut-friendly, Mediterranean-influenced low FODMAP recipes.

With the aim of maintaining a healthy gut microbiome, our own clean low FODMAP approach relies on unprocessed, healthy and high-fiber Mediterranean ingredients prepared in a pure manner. As mentioned above, a high-fiber diet has tremendous benefits for the maintenance of healthy gut microorganisms. Additionally, the low FODMAP diet has been shown to reduce bloating and other related gastrointestinal symptoms.

Although the clean low FODMAP diet is not a gluten-free diet, all of our recipes are gluten-free, as many of the gluten-containing grains are also high in FODMAPs and have therefore been removed from the diet during the elimination phase. Furthermore, because our clean low FODMAP plan is based on whole grains, we have not used any refined grains in our recipes.

Cheers to a happy belly!

> **!** *The information provided in this book is not intended as a substitute for the advice and care of your healthcare provider. You should always consult your physician or health care provider if you notice any red flags or if you will be making changes to your diet, medication or current treatment. It is recommended that the low FODMAP diet is followed under the guidance and supervision of a registered dietitian. Nutritional needs and tolerances vary for each individual.*

Contents

Section 2

Section 3

Chapter 11

Section 1

Chapter 1:
Ruling out a primary cause or an underlying organic disease

The basics of digestion

To be able to dive into all the digestive woes that trouble us, we first need to understand and appreciate how our digestive system works.

Our digestive (gastrointestinal) tract is a continuous tube that begins in the mouth and ends in the anus. Food enters the mouth and travels along a path through the esophagus, stomach, small intestine and large intestine. Digestion begins in the mouth, initially via chewing, whereby the teeth cut the food into small pieces that are then mixed with saliva containing digestive enzymes, thus beginning the digestion process. It is therefore important to chew food slowly to allow the food to be properly broken down into small pieces and to allow time for the digestive enzymes to begin their work in the mouth.

When we swallow the food, rhythmical contractions (called peristalsis) of the gut wall help the food move down the esophagus and into the stomach. The food mixes with gastric juices, and the churning of the stomach turns the food into a liquid mush called chyme. Then, other digestive enzymes continue the breakdown of food into simpler molecules. Finally, digestion finishes in the upper part of the small intestine. Bile that is produced by the liver and kept in the gallbladder is also secreted into the small intestine to facilitate digestion. The same process applies to digestive enzymes released by the pancreas, which find their way to the small intestine to complete the process of digestion.

Then, the nutrients are absorbed from the gut into the bloodstream to travel to all the parts of our body to provide us with energy and take part in other reactions and bodily processes. Any undigested food particles then move to the colon. Water is absorbed into the bloodstream.

Many of the nutrients that we do not digest are broken down by the millions of bacteria (microbiota) that live in our colons. They ferment on these nutrients and provide our body with plenty of vitamins and other nutrients that are important for our body. Whatever remains undigested is ultimately removed from our bodies as feces when we go to the bathroom.

Abdominal bloating and distention are not a pretty picture!

Patients often cannot describe exactly what abdominal bloating is, but it usually refers to a person's sensation of abdominal fullness or, as often described, an inflated balloon in the abdomen. Some patients experience distension, and others simply feel uncomfortably full without distension. The severity varies from mild to severe, and both symptoms cause discomfort and sometimes pain, both of which can affect the quality of life of the patients.

> **Bloating** refers to a person's sensation of abdominal fullness.
> **Distention** refers to measurable increase in abdominal girth.

> The term **"disease"** describes a state in which the pathology is visible, i.e., something can be seen on an X-ray or endoscopy or is quantifiably measurable in a blood test or other diagnostic test.
> **"Illness"** is simply when the patient does not feel well.
> When the illness is due to a disease that is visible, i.e., a certain pathology or change in the physiology (biochemistry) of the body, then this is called **structural/primary cause or underlying organic disease**. When the patient suffers and has symptoms but no apparent signs of disease, then this is called **functional**.

Visit your physician to establish a diagnosis

Unfortunately, a number of serious conditions can cause abdominal bloating, and these conditions should never be neglected or ignored. You should always consult a physician for further evaluation and to establish a diagnosis when any of the following red flag symptoms are present:

- **Onset of symptoms under the age of 50**
- **A family history of colorectal cancer**
- **Celiac disease**
- **Inflammatory bowel disease**
- **Rectal bleeding/blood in the stool**
- **Dark stool**
- **Anemia**
- **Waking up at night for a bowel movement**
- **Fever**
- **Daily diarrhea**
- **Recurrent vomiting**
- **Symptoms that keep getting worse**
- **Sudden unintentional weight loss**

Some conditions that may be the culprit for such symptoms are as follows:

- Cancer (colon, ovarian or uterine), kidney failure, congestive heart failure or liver disease, which produces fluid that drains and collects in the abdomen
- Crohn's and ulcerative colitis (inflammatory bowel disease)
- Endometriosis
- Endocrine disorders
- Damage of the gastrointestinal (GI) tract, which would allow gas, bacteria and other substances to enter the abdominal area, causing irritation or infections
- Pancreatic insufficiency, which could inhibit the release of important pancreatic digestive enzymes into the gut, thus resulting in inadequate food digestion and the accumulation of food products and gas production in the gut

Colorectal Cancer

Colorectal cancer is cancer that initiates in the colon or rectum. This type of cancer can also be individually termed colon cancer and rectal cancer to make a distinction between its starting location. However, the two share many characteristics in common and tend to be grouped together.

Most frequently, colorectal cancer begins as a growth on the inner lining of the large intestine's wall. This growth is called a polyp. Many of these polyps that develop in the large intestine are benign and never change to become cancerous. However, some types of polyps can develop into cancer over time. It is estimated that this requires approximately 10 years.

There are two types of polyps: adenomatous and hyperplastic or inflammatory polyps. Adenomatous polyps, also called adenomas, indicate a precancerous state, and these polyps can sometimes become cancer. Generally, hyperplastic or inflammatory polyps do not become cancer.

Do not ignore the alarm symptoms

Early colorectal cancer often has no symptoms, which is why preventative screening is so important. As a tumor grows, it may bleed or obstruct the intestine, leading to the following serious symptoms:

Do not ignore the alarm symptoms

- A persistent change in bowel habits, such as diarrhea, constipation, or narrowing of the stool
- A feeling that you need to have a bowel movement, which is not relieved by doing so
- Bleeding from the rectum
- Dark-colored stools or blood in the stool
- Cramping or abdominal pain
- Weakness, fatigue or anemia (low iron levels)
- Unintentional weight loss

Colorectal cancer symptoms can be mimicked by conditions that are not related to cancer, including irritable bowel syndrome (IBS), irritable bowel disease (IBD), hemorrhoids and infection. However, it is of the utmost importance to seek medical advice if these symptoms are present to determine the cause of the symptoms and to rule out serious disease.

Diagnosis

If any of the above symptoms are present or any suspicious findings are found upon a general screening, the doctor will want to follow-up with some tests and exams.

The first step will involve the doctor taking a family and medical history to determine any risk factors. This step will be followed with a physical exam to examine the abdomen and the rest of the body. The doctor will also order blood and stool testing, the purpose of which is to observe whether any cancer markers or other specific chemicals in the blood or stool are abnormally high. Finally, a colonoscopy, biopsy, digital rectal exam, CT scan, ultrasound or MRI of the colon or rectum might be used in cases in which the doctor considers it appropriate to assess whether cancer or another problem exists.

Screening and Early Detection: Why Is Early Detection Important?

Screening is the search for cancer or the presence of polyps before the patient has symptoms. The idea is that if cancer is found in its initial stages before it has metastasized, it will be easier to treat, and survival rates will be much higher. The current guidelines for people with an average risk for colorectal cancer are to start screening at the age of 45 and to continue with regular screening until the age of 75. Screening could involve either a stool-based test or a colonoscopy. However, studies show that colonoscopy is currently the most sensitive screening method.

Talk to your medical provider about any family history or risk factors that they should know. Accordingly, the doctor may recommend starting the screening even earlier.

Celiac Disease

Celiac disease is a genetic disease in which the consumption of gluten, a protein primarily found in wheat, rye and barley, initiates an autoimmune response in the patient. The body's immune system attacks and destroys cells in the small intestine, and as a result, the body cannot properly absorb food. More specifically, the inflammation damages the villi, small fingerlike projections that line the small intestine and increase the surface area through which the absorption of nutrients would take place. In celiac disease, the damage makes the villi small and ultimately even flat, thus negatively affecting the absorption of food. As a result, the patient cannot receive sufficient nutrients to grow well and be healthy.

Some of the symptoms of celiac disease are as follows:

- Bloating
- Abdominal pain
- Gas
- Chronic diarrhea
- Constipation
- Pale, foul-smelling stool
- Vomiting
- Loss of weight
- Fatigue
- Insufficient growth
- Itchy blistering skin rash (dermatitis herpetiformis)
- Mood changes

How common is celiac disease?

Celiac disease affects 1 in 100 people in the general population. It is a genetic disease that involves the human leukocyte antigen (HLA) gene system, so it can run in families. Therefore, the presence of the disease in a sibling, parent or child increases your risk to 1 in 10, but it most certainly does not guarantee that you will 100% develop the condition. A combination of environmental factors and gene variations is generally required for the development of celiac disease.

Celiac disease affects women and men equally and is present both in children and the adult population, as it can begin at any age. Unfortunately, it is estimated that approximately 83% of celiac disease cases are not diagnosed, either because the patient has no symptoms or because the symptoms resemble many other conditions, so celiac disease is not suspected. It is observed that digestive symptoms are more prominent in children than in adults.

Is celiac disease serious?

Celiac disease is serious, and the patient needs to make sure they eliminate 100% of the gluten from their diet to stay healthy. It is a genetic condition, and the autoimmune reaction that occurs upon the ingestion of gluten remains in the person forever. Even tiny quantities of gluten, such as in breadcrumbs or from cutting your bread on a board where gluten-containing bread was cut, can have devastating effects on the patient. If celiac disease remains undetected and intestinal damage continues, it can lead to serious conditions, such as the following:

- **Anemia (due to iron deficiency)**
- **Vitamin and mineral deficiencies**
- **Osteoporosis**
- **Infertility and miscarriage**
- **Lactose intolerance**
- **Depression or anxiety**
- **Thyroid disease**
- **Other autoimmune disorders, such as type 1 diabetes and autoimmune hepatitis**
- **Pancreatic malfunction**
- **Stunted growth**
- **Some cancers of the gastrointestinal tract**
- **Migraines**
- **Seizures**
- **Dementia**

How is celiac disease diagnosed?

For celiac disease to be detected, a person must be including gluten in their diet to prevent false negative results. The doctor will diagnose the condition by examining family history, conducting a series of blood tests and performing a biopsy.

It is generally recommended that the following individuals be screened:

- Children older than 3 years old and adults who are experiencing any of the aforementioned symptoms of celiac disease

- Anybody who has a parent, sibling or child who has celiac disease
- Anybody who has one of the following conditions: a linked autoimmune disorder, such as diabetes 1 mellitus, autoimmune thyroid disease, or autoimmune liver disease; Down syndrome; Turner syndrome; Williams syndrome; and selective immunoglobulin A (IgA) deficiency

There are specific blood tests that help doctors diagnose celiac disease. These tests detect elevated levels of antibodies that the body makes specifically in response to gluten. However, these tests are only accurate and valid if the person is on a gluten-containing diet.

Blood tests

 (a) *IgA class Tissue transglutaminase antibody (IgA-tTG)*

This is the first and most commonly ordered test for celiac disease.

In celiac disease, the immune system mistakenly considers gluten a foreign invader and attacks it. Specifically, it makes antibodies that attack an enzyme in the intestines called tissue transglutaminase (tTG). This blood test measures the levels of these anti-tTG antibodies (IgA-tTG) in the blood.

This test is 98% sensitive (i.e., the test is positive in 98% of people with celiac disease) and 95% specific (i.e., the test is negative in 95% of healthy people without the disease).

It should be noted that the results of the tTG-IgA test may be dependent on the degree of intestinal damage, so it may be less sensitive for people who have milder cases of celiac disease.

 (b) *Quantitative immunoglobulin A (IgA) test*

This test is carried out to rule out a deficiency of IgA, which appears in 2-3% of patients with celiac disease. Such a deficiency can lead to false-negative results with regard to IgA class antibody measurements, so it is important to be certain that such a deficiency does not exist. In the case of an IgA deficiency, the IgG class of tTG antibodies can be measured.

(c) *Deamidated gliadin peptide antibody test (DGP IgA and IgG)*

This test measures the amount of anti-deamidated gliadin peptide antibody in the blood. This test should be part of the testing of young children who are suspected to have celiac disease, as well as of adults screened for celiac disease who tested negative for tTg or EMA antibodies or who are IgA deficient.

 (d) *IgA Endomysial antibody (EMA)*

This test measures the levels of anti-endomysial IgA antibodies and is usually performed on difficult-to-diagnose patients. It cannot, however, be used in the case of IgA deficiency.

It is 90-95% sensitive (i.e., the test is positive in 90-95% of people with celiac disease) and 99% specific (i.e., the test is negative in healthy people without the disease).

A false-positive test is not very likely but possible; that is, people who do not have celiac disease may show a positive test result. This is especially true for patients with other associated autoimmune disorders.

False-negative results are rare but also possible. If your serology test results are negative but symptoms continue, we recommended that you talk to your doctor. The most accurate way to confirm a diagnosis is via a small intestinal biopsy.

1.   Biopsy of the small intestine (distal duodenum)

This test remains the gold standard and is the most accurate way to confirm the presence of celiac disease. It can also help diagnose patients who are negative for elevated antibodies in the blood. This procedure is performed via endoscopy, and it recognizes damage in the small intestine. However, it is expensive, time consuming and unpleasant for patients.

2.   Gene testing to diagnose celiac disease

The genetic test identifies whether the person tested carries the HLA-DQ2 and/ or HLA-DQ8 genes. This test does not confirm that the person has celiac disease but instead shows if the individual carries the HLA-DQ2 and/or HLA-DQ8 genes. In fact, these alleles are present in 25-35% of the general population. The DQ alleles are genes that predispose individuals to celiac disease; when they are present, they increase the risk of developing celiac disease from 1% to 3%. The HLA gene test does not provide a clear diagnostic result and is in fact only useful if negative. A negative gene test excludes the likelihood of developing celiac disease by 99%. Celiac disease very rarely occurs in patients negative for the DQ-predisposing markers.

One might consider the test if he or she follows a gluten-free diet or if other test results are inconclusive (especially in children under the age of 3). Additionally, it is recommended that people (and especially children) with a first-degree family member (parent, sibling or child) diagnosed with celiac disease also have gene testing. This will prevent any unnecessary screening for celiac disease in the future. Since a negative gene test excludes the likelihood of developing celiac disease by 99%, this information can be quite useful for first-degree relatives of patients with celiac disease.

In the case that one of your first-degree family members tests positive for celiac disease, it is recommended that you carry out the gene testing, as there is a 40% chance of developing celiac disease. Finally, gene-positive first-degree relatives should be screened every 3-5 years or immediately if symptoms of celiac disease appear.

Don't forget the gluten!

Once people who have celiac disease go gluten-free, their blood antibodies to gluten disappear and their intestinal damage heals, meaning the tests will probably not show anything conclusive or worrisome. Therefore, serology and biopsy testing are only accurate if the person tested is on a diet that includes gluten, as these tests are based on the body's reaction to gluten.

The gluten challenge!

If you follow a gluten-free diet but want to get tested serologically or via biopsy for celiac disease, your dietitian or doctor may propose that you go on a gluten challenge. This will trigger your body to produce antibodies against gluten if you have celiac disease.

The duration of this challenge is usually 6-8 weeks and should always be done under the supervision and guidance of your physician. The recommended amount of gluten is 3-10 grams per day (1 slice of bread contains approximately 2 grams).

 Beware that you should not undergo a gluten challenge if you are pregnant.

> Approximately one in twenty people diagnosed with IBS also have celiac disease. The American College of Gastroenterology Task Force recommends that those with IBS-D or IBS-M be screened for celiac disease.

What is the treatment for celiac disease?

There is no treatment or cure for celiac disease. To eliminate symptoms of the disease, the patient needs to follow a strict 100% gluten-free diet. A dietitian can help you develop a suitable diet that you can abide by. Currently, there are many alternatives to gluten-containing grains, as well as several gluten-free products available in the market. The avoidance of gluten should allow your intestines to heal over time.

Furthermore, the patient needs to be monitored by a physician for any nutritional deficiencies and the development of any accompanying autoimmune or other disorders.

Asymptomatic or Silent Celiac Disease

There are many patients with celiac disease who remain undiagnosed because they do not present with any of the typical symptoms of celiac disease or because they present with no symptoms at all. Such cases are referred to as asymptomatic or silent celiac disease. Patients could present with signs of iron-deficiency anemia but have no GI symptoms that would signal celiac disease. However, even if symptoms are initially silent, upon the consumption of gluten, there is consequent destruction of the intestinal villi, and over time, it would lead to manifestation of celiac disease.

Because there may be an absence of the typical previously described digestive symptoms associated with celiac disease, patients with silent celiac disease can often go unnoticed. It is currently known that celiac disease can cause both weight gain and weight loss, and healthcare professionals will frequently not suspect overweight patients to have celiac disease, so those patients will be underdiagnosed. Furthermore, even though both tTG and EMA tests are very specific and sensitive, they both detect immunoglobulin A (IgA) antibodies, which can be a problem for a small proportion of the population with celiac disease (2-5%) who have an IgA deficiency. Such patients who are tested for celiac disease show false-negative results. Indeed, there have been cases in which people with a negative IgA test and negative biopsies later tested positive for celiac disease. Subtle cues that might indicate silent celiac disease are symptoms of IBS in a patient who is also anemic and shows signs of infertility. Additionally, asymptomatic celiac disease might appear in a patient who has thyroid disease or who has other members of their family with celiac disease.

Studies have shown that people with asymptomatic celiac disease tend to normalize or ignore subtle symptoms and only notice the symptoms once they follow a gluten-free diet and their symptoms improve.

Check for the following celiac disease symptoms if silent celiac disease is suspected.

- Anemia
- Behavioral changes
- Bloating
- Gas
- Abdominal pain
- Bones that break easily
- Bone or joint pain
- Bruising
- Chronic fatigue
- Stunted or delayed growth as a child/failure to thrive
- Depression or irritability
- Diarrhea or constipation
- Discolored teeth and problems with the enamel
- Dry eyes
- Swelling, especially in hands and feet
- Epstein-Barr infection
- Recurrent infections
- Hard-to-flush stools
- Difficulty losing weight
- Indigestion and acid reflux
- Infertility
- Irritability
- Lactose intolerance

- Learning difficulties
- Memory difficulties
- Menstrual problems
- Migraines
- Mouth sores and ulcers (canker sores)
- Vitamin and mineral deficiencies (such as iron, calcium, or vitamins A, D, E, and K)
- Seizures
- Short stature
- Rashes
- Tingling or numbness in hands and feet
- Unexplained weight gain (and difficulty losing weight)
- Unexplained weight loss

Inflammatory Bowel Disease (IBD)

This is a serious disease that affects one's quality of life and can lead to life-threatening conditions. The exact cause of IBD remains unknown. Stress and diet can aggravate IBD but do not cause it. The two major categories of IBD are **Crohn's disease (CD)** and **ulcerative colitis (UC)**. These chronic diseases tend to run in families and affect males and females equally. However, it is important to note that most people with IBD do not have a family history.

In IBD, an abnormal response by the body's immune system results in an attack of and damage to the person's GI tract. Normally, the immune system detects and tries to destroy foreign intruders such as bacteria and viruses, but in this case, the abnormal response also results in the attack of the body's own digestive tract cells. In ulcerative colitis, there is inflammation and sores (ulcers) in the inner-most lining of the colon, also known as the mucosa layer, which faces the lumen of the large intestine and the rectum. In Crohn's disease, there is inflammation of the lining of the digestive tract (can be in any part of the digestive tract from the mouth to the anus). Inflammation can present at any of the layers of the gut wall and not only the mucosa, and it is often observed deeply spread throughout the tissue.

Symptoms of IBD (shared between Crohn's disease and ulcerative colitis)

The following are symptoms of the inflammation of the gastrointestinal tract:

- Diarrhea
- Rectal bleeding
- Urgent need to move bowels
- Abdominal pain and cramping
- Feeling of incomplete evacuation
- Constipation (which can also lead to bowel obstruction)

Other symptoms associated with IBD are as follows:

- Fever
- Loss of appetite
- Weight loss
- Fatigue
- Night sweats
- Loss of normal menstrual cycles

IBD is a chronic condition, but the patient may be in remission with occasional flare ups with IBS-like symptoms. Rates of IBD have been rising worldwide, possibly as a result of the Westernization of diets and lifestyles around the globe.

There is no single test that confirms the diagnosis of IBD. The diagnosis is based on a physical examination, patient history and various tests, which include the following:

- Blood tests
- Endoscopies (colonoscopy, sigmoidoscopy, gastroscopy, proctoscopy, double balloon enteroscopy, capsule endoscopy)
- Stool tests to determine levels of calprotectin; fecal calprotectin acts as a measure of inflammation and is produced by the specific white blood cells and macrophages that are always present where intestinal infection and/or inflammation occur
- Scans (MRI, CT scan, small-bowel imaging, ultrasound, X-rays)

Gastro-esophageal reflux (GERD)

People with GERD feel a burning sensation in their throats (heartburn) due to acid from the stomach coming back into the esophagus. This might be due to one of two reasons: (i) the sphincter (valve) between the stomach and the esophagus does not close properly to allow stomach acid to flow back into the esophagus, or (ii) a part of the stomach is found above the diaphragm, which is a condition called hiatal hernia.

People can have mild acid reflux occasionally, and this event is not a major concern. GERD occurs when mild acid reflux occurs at least twice a week or when moderate to severe acid reflux appears at least once a week.

Be aware of the following common symptoms of GERD:

- **Burning sensation in the chest, usually after eating**
- **Regurgitation of fluid or food into mouth or throat**
- **Chest pain**
- **Difficulty swallowing**
- **A feeling of a lump in your throat**

Symptoms usually get worse during the night or after eating a meal, bending over, lying down, or participating in certain physical activities. If you have reflux at nighttime, you could also experience other symptoms, such as the following:

- **Chronic cough**
- **Laryngitis**
- **Disrupted sleep**
- **Newly developed asthma or worsening of asthma**

Long-lasting GERD can have some serious complications, such as narrowing of the esophagus (**esophageal stricture**), esophageal ulcers and bleeding, voice changes, and **precancerous changes to the esophagus (Barrett's esophagus).**

Smoking, eating large meals or eating late at night, eating fatty or fried foods, eating acidic fruits and spicy foods or drinking coffee and alcohol can exacerbate the symptoms of acid reflux. Generally, the condition can be kept under control with lifestyle and dietary changes as well as mild, over-the-counter medication.

The FODMAP fructans have also been linked to reflux, so the low FODMAP diet may be able to help alleviate some of the symptoms of GERD (see section 2 in the book). However, if GERD is very serious, people may need stronger prescription medications or even surgery.

Bile Acid Malabsorption (BAM) or Bile Acid Diarrhea (BAD)

This is a chronic condition resulting from excess bile acids in the colon. Bile acids are produced to solubilize lipids and help the body absorb them efficiently. After they perform their function, bile acids are reabsorbed from the colon into the blood so that they can be reused. If excess bile acids accumulate in the colon, they prevent stools from forming properly, leading to a painful condition with the following symptoms:

- **Multiple bouts of watery, urgent or explosive diarrhea**
- **Fecal incontinence**
- **Foul-smelling diarrhea that is usually yellow in color (or looks greasy)**
- **Gas**
- **Painful stomach cramps**
- **Bloating**

Studies have shown that BAM is found in ⅓ of patients with IBS-D and up to ½ of patients with functional diarrhea.

Treatment involves the use of special medication called bile acid sequestrants (BAS), which bind to bile acids in the small intestine and prevent them from affecting the colon. A low-fat diet also helps reduce symptoms.

There are different tests for BAM. The most definitive test for BAM detects an increase in bile acid in the stool. However, this requires 48 hours of fecal collection, and this procedure proves to be difficult and impractical and therefore is not frequently used. There are some blood tests that measure blood biomarkers such as 7a-OH-4-cholesten-3-one (C4); however, this test requires very specialized laboratories and is not readily available worldwide. Finally, the SeHCAT (75Se-homocholic acid taurine) test can also be used, but it is also not readily available worldwide.

Endometriosis

Endometriosis is an often-painful medical condition in women in which the lining of the uterus (the endometrium) grows outside the uterus, usually in the fallopian tubes, ovaries or along the pelvis. This tissue continues to act as a normal endometrium, so it thickens and sheds every month due to hormonal fluctuations. The tissue has no way of being removed from those areas; however, it builds up, causing irritation and scar tissue, which can lead to organs sticking together. Approximately 10% of women of reproductive age have endometriosis.

GI symptoms are common among women with endometriosis. A number of studies have shown that IBS may be more common among women with endometriosis; however, it is not clear how the two conditions are related.

Common symptoms of endometriosis include the following:

- **Painful periods**
- **Pelvic pain that is not related to menstruation**
- **Infertility**
- **Painful during intercourse**
- **Back pain**
- **Pain on defecation**
- **Abdominal bloating and discomfort**
- **Nausea**
- **Altered bowel movements (constipation and/or diarrhea)**

The following are key symptoms of endometriosis that overlap with those of IBS:

- **Visceral hypersensitivity (greater-than-normal pain within the organs)**
- **Bloating**
- **Diarrhea or constipation**
- **Pain on defecation**
- **Nausea**
- **Reduced quality of life**

Endometriosis can often be confused with IBS. To rule out endometriosis, it is important to talk to your doctor about your symptoms. **Laparoscopy is the only definitive way to diagnose endometriosis.**

A retrospective study by Monash University showed that women with IBS and endometriosis show a distinct symptom profile, and a diet low in FODMAPs appears to be effective in managing GI symptoms in these women. Patients with IBS and endometriosis responded more favorably to a low FODMAP diet than did patients with IBS alone.

Gut Infections

Parasites are organisms that live in or on another organism or host. Some parasites do not affect their hosts; others can make their hosts sick, resulting in a parasitic infection. Parasitic infections can cause symptoms similar to IBS symptoms, and it is possible that patients with parasitic infections are misdiagnosed with IBS.

Recent studies have proposed a possible role of protozoan parasites, such as Blastocystis hominis (B. hominis) and Dientamoeba fragilis, in the development of IBS. The role of B. hominis in IBS is inconclusive due to contradictory reports and due to the controversy surrounding whether B. hominis is a human pathogen. Entamoeba histolytica infections arise mostly in developing countries, and symptoms mimic IBS symptoms. Infection with Giardia intestinalis can yield symptoms that vary from none to diarrhea, gas, upset stomach, greasy stools and abdominal pain. These IBS-like symptoms can be continuous, intermittent, sporadic or recurrent.

It is suggested that all patients with IBS consider routine parasitological investigations to rule out the presence of protozoan parasites. These tests involve stool tests that can provide information on what may be happening in the stomach, intestines or other parts of the gastrointestinal tract. These tests can be important for a variety of conditions, such as the following:

- Allergies and inflammation
- Infections by bacteria, viruses and parasites
- Nutrient, fat and sugar absorption
- Intestinal bleeding

Tests to rule out diseases and infections

What is tested in the stool?

The **hemoccult** test can detect blood in the stool. The presence of blood could be due to allergies, peptic ulcers, inflammation, bacterial infections, viruses, parasites or polyps.

The **calprotectin** test provides a measure of inflammation in the intestines. Calprotectin is a protein of the white blood cells and macrophages, which are always present when there is infection and/or inflammation. The presence of the protein can therefore indicate a bacterial infection, the start of IBD or a flareup of existing Crohn's disease or ulcerative colitis.

Culture tests confirm the presence of different infection-causing bacteria in the intestines. These tests can be ordered if you have diarrhea and/or bloody stool for several days. A stool culture can check for the presence of *Salmonella, Shigella, Yersinia, Campylobacter* and a specific form of *Escherichia coli (E. coli)*.

The *Clostridium difficile* test checks for the presence of a specific strain of *Clostridium* bacteria in the colon. These bacteria are often found in the stool and are usually harmless. However, certain strains can produce toxins that cause diarrhea.

The *Helicobacter pylori* **stool antigens** test examines the stool for foreign proteins (antigens) produced by H. pylori bacteria. These bacteria cause peptic ulcers in the esophagus, stomach and small intestine, as well as cancer of the stomach.

PCR (polymerase chain reaction) of stool is the analysis of the stool using a molecular technique that increases the quantity of genetic material (DNA) found in the stool and therefore allows for the creation of a genetic fingerprint and the identification of a wide range of parasites and other pathogens that may be present in the stool. This is a far more sensitive test than the old-fashioned technique of examination through a microscope and allows for an exact species diagnosis.

Tests to rule out diseases

Celiac Disease

Serology: tTg + lgA or tTg + DGPlgG, EMA.

Small intestinal biopsy if the patient's antibody blood tests are high. This is the most accurate and most conclusive diagnostic test for celiac disease.

HLA-DQ2/DQ8 genetic test (only useful if negative)

Keep the following points in mind:
1. Gluten consumption must reach satisfactory levels before celiac serology and biopsy to avoid false negative results.
2. IgA deficiency presents in 2-3% of people with celiac disease. Always check that total IgA levels are normal.

Inflammatory bowel disease (IBD) (e.g., Crohn's disease and ulcerative colitis)

Physical examination, patient history and blood tests, stool examination, endoscopy, biopsies, and imaging studies.

Fecal calprotectin screening.

Diverticular disease

Barium enema or endoscopy (flexible sigmoidoscopy or colonoscopy).

Clinical examination during an acute attack is required and disease is generally confirmed with a CT scan.

Ovarian or Bowel Cancer

Recording of family and medical history and physical examination.

Blood and stool tests to identify the presence of any cancer markers or abnormally elevated chemicals in the blood or any blood present in the stool.

A colonoscopy, biopsy, digital rectal exam, CT scan, ultrasound or MRI of the colon or rectum might also be carried out.

Pelvic floor disorders

Medical history and physical examination.

Anorectal manometry.

Endometriosis

Laparoscopy to diagnose the presence of endometriosis.

Endocrine disorders (e.g., hyperthyroidism/hypothyroidism)

Medical history and physical examination.

Blood tests to determine blood thyroxine levels.

Pancreatic exocrine insufficiency

Fecal elastase-1 screening (as well as other indirect tests).

Observation of symptom improvement when the patient receives pancreatic enzyme replacement.

Bile acid malabsorption

Fecal bile acid measurement.

An increase in fecal bile acid is the most conclusive method to detect bile acid malabsorption. (A 48-hour collection of feces is required, and as a result, this test is not used very often.)

SeHCAT (75Se-homocholic acid taurine) test

7a-OH-4-cholesten-3-one (C4) blood test

Food Allergy vs Food intolerance

Food hypersensitivity is a label for all adverse reactions to food.

However, there are major differences between a food allergy and a food intolerance.

A food allergy is an immediate (i.e., within minutes) reaction to ingested food and is mediated by IgE antibodies produced by the body's immune system against a specific protein in the food. The reaction can be severe and life-threatening, and symptoms can include the following:

- **Breathing problems**
- **Throat tightness**
- **Hoarseness**
- **Coughing**
- **Vomiting**
- **Abdominal pain**
- **Hives**
- **Swelling**
- **Itching**
- **Dizziness**
- **Drop in blood pressure**
- **Anaphylaxis**
- **Loss of consciousness**

The most common food allergies are milk, eggs, fish, shellfish, peanuts, tree nuts, soybeans and wheat.

A detailed clinical history and conventional allergy testing are important in the diagnosis of an IgE-mediated food allergy. This involves specific IgE testing using either skin or blood tests and based on the patient's clinical history.

> **Other non-IgE mediated food allergies** exist, in which components of the immune system other than IgE antibodies are involved. In these cases, the reaction to the food is generally delayed (may take hours or days) and involve symptoms such as vomiting, bloating and diarrhea. The mechanism of non-IgE-mediated food allergies is not well understood, and allergy testing is not useful given that no IgE antibodies are produced. Examples of such non-IgE mediated allergies are eosinophilic esophagitis (EoE), food protein-induced enterocolitis syndrome (FPIES) and proctocolitis.

Non-allergic food hypersensitivity is also known as food intolerance or food sensitivity. This condition does not involve the immune system. The symptoms emerge more slowly, often hours after the ingestion of certain foods. Usually, this condition involves reasonable amounts of the food, unlike an allergy, in which mere traces can trigger the allergic reaction. Here, the patient develops GI symptoms, such as gas, bloating, diarrhea, constipation, nausea, abdominal pain, and cramping, and non-GI symptoms, such as brain fog, depression, joint pain and skin rash, after the ingestion of certain foods.

- Nausea
- Gas
- Cramps
- Abdominal pain
- Diarrhea
- Bloating
- Constipation
- Reflux
- Mouth ulcers
- Irritability
- Nervousness
- Headaches
- Rashes
- Eczema
- Hives
- Sinus
- Asthma
- Fatigue
- Flulike aches and pains
- Moodiness

These intolerances are usually due to the absence of the right enzyme for the digestion of a particular food, reactions to food additives or preservatives, sensitivities to naturally occurring sugars such as FODMAPs, or sensitivities to chemicals. The typical list includes the following:

- **Dairy products**
- **Gluten**
- **Sensitivities to sugars, such as FODMAPs**
- **Sucrose or maltose** (these sugars need to be broken down into simple sugars by specific enzymes to be able to be absorbed)
- **Natural food chemicals**
  1. **Salicylates** are naturally occurring organic chemicals found in many fruits, vegetables, herbs and nuts. Salicylates are the defense systems of plants against pathogens and environmental stress.
  2. **Amines** are the product of protein breakdown. Foods increase in amines as they age, mature, ripen or ferment. (Biogenic amines include histamine and tyramine)
  3. **Glutamates** can exist in two different forms in foods: as free amino acids or as a part of a protein. When they are in their free form, they enhance the flavor of food. Foods rich in natural glutamates are cheese, tomato, mushrooms and meat and yeast extract. MSG (Monosodium glutamate) is used as a food additive to enhance flavor.
- **Chocolate (due to phenylethylamine, which can cause migraines)**
- **Eggs (particularly egg whites)**
- **Food additives**
  1. **Preservatives** (sulfites, benzoates, butylhydroxyanisol (BHA), butylhydroxytoluene (BHT))
  2. **MSG**
  3. **Artificial colors/food dyes** (i.e., tartazine)
  4. **Emulsifiers**
- **Caffeine**
- **Yeast**
- **Alcohol**
- **Artificial sweeteners**
- **Toxins, viruses, bacteria or parasites that have contaminated food**

Diagnostic tests for food intolerances

Because the immune system is not involved, there are no reliable diagnostic tests, and the only way to know for sure if a food is triggering your symptoms is through a strict elimination and structured rechallenge process. This process can be difficult, and there are many factors that could mislead the results, so this process is best conducted under the guidance of a dietitian with expertise in food intolerances.

Nutrition and food intolerances are very complicated subjects and can occur in isolation or in any other combination, including FODMAPs, food or chemical intolerance, celiac, nonceliac gluten sensitivity and allergies.

Histamine Intolerance

Histamine is released by mast cells in the body but can also be found in fermented foods, such as cheese, fermented soy products, wine, vinegar and sauerkraut, as well as in fish that has spoiled. Eggplant, spinach and certain other foods also contain naturally high quantities of histamine.

Symptoms of histamine intolerance may be induced even by small amounts of dietary histamine intake and can include the following: dilation of blood vessels, flushing of the skin, fast heart rate, hives, digestive problems, headaches, drop in blood pressure or asthma. Such sensitivity to histamine from foods may arise from a genetic deficiency in the enzyme that breaks down histamine or due to an interaction between the histamine with the medication a person is taking. A diet that is low in histamine could minimize the symptoms.

Scombroid poisoning occurs after the ingestion of fresh, canned or smoked fish with high histamine levels because the fish was not processed or kept properly. The symptoms mimic those of an allergic reaction.

Tyramine Intolerance

Tyramine is a biogenic amine. Aged cheeses (specifically Camembert and Cheddar), aged or pickled or smoked meats or fish, pickles, sauerkraut, liver, vinegar, red wine, beer, yeast extracts, avocado, bananas, raspberries, eggplant, tomato and red plums can all contain tyramine.

An intolerance to tyramine (you may have also heard it referred to as a cheese reaction) may be due to a genetic predisposition or a reaction between a group of antidepressants called monoamine oxidase inhibitors (MAOIs) and the tyramine found in the food. This reaction can result in symptoms such as high blood pressure, increased heart rate, hyperthermia, tremors and seizures within 15-90 minutes after the consumption of the food.

Other possible causes of symptoms to consider

> **Don't forget: You need a diagnosis before adopting nutritional changes.**

Nonceliac gluten sensitivity (NCGS) or Nonceliac wheat sensitivity (NCWS)

Nonceliac gluten sensitivity (NCGS), or more recently called nonceliac wheat sensitivity (NCWS), is a condition that involves both GI and non-GI symptoms upon wheat or gluten consumption in patients in whom celiac disease or a wheat allergy have been excluded. GI symptoms may imitate those in IBS, but patients also show a prevalence of non-GI symptoms such as **headache, foggy mind, joint pain and numbness in the legs, arms or fingers.** Symptoms typically appear hours or days after the consumption of gluten. However, the typical changes observed in celiac disease are absent. There is no damage to the mucosal lining of the intestines, no elevations in tissue-transglutaminase or deamidated gliadin antibodies and no increased mucosal permeability. It is not considered an immune condition. It is also not a gluten allergy because it is not IgE-antibody mediated and does not cause vomiting, itching, swelling of the throat, shortness of breath, or other symptoms associated with an allergic reaction, which would happen quickly after the consumption of wheat.

NCGS or NCWS is thought to be a non-IgE-mediated allergy that triggers the immune system in other ways. Allesio Fasano, MD, proposes that gluten sensitivity may have a spectrum and that individuals may show varying levels of sensitivity to gluten. How frequently the condition occurs is unknown; however, it is estimated to affect 0.5-13% of the population.

There is currently no diagnostic test for NCGS/NCWS because there are no known or measurable biomarkers. Its symptoms resemble those of other functional gastrointestinal disorders, most specifically those of IBS, so with any identifiable biomarkers being absent, it is difficult to pinpoint the condition. Evidence from studies shows that in patients with gluten sensitivity, the elimination of gluten from the diet might decrease or eliminate symptoms; however, this process should be performed under the guidance of a clinical dietitian.

Currently, there is considerable debate over whether NCGS/NCWS is caused by gluten or other wheat components. It has been suggested by new research that gluten alone may not be responsible for the symptoms. Recent findings show that it may in fact be the fructans (FODMAPs) of wheat, barley and rye that may be associated with this condition, and the elimination of gluten-containing foods also eliminates this FODMAP group, thus resulting in a reduction of symptoms.

Moreover, the latest research has focused on the role of amylase-trypsin inhibitors (ATIs) from wheat in gastrointestinal inflammation and their possible role in NCGS/NWGS. Although gluten is the most prevalent protein in grains such as wheat, barley or rye, ATIs make up to 4% of the protein content and are important for one to consider as a culprit. Researchers posit that ATIs activate an innate immune response (the body's first line of defense to an invading foreign substance) and can induce intestinal infiltration and the release of inflammatory chemicals in the gut. The amounts of immune-activating ATIs have increased significantly in the more recent varieties of wheat, barley and rye. These ATIs do not undergo breakdown in the intestines, and baking (heating) or processing does not appear to significantly decrease the ATI content or their effects in stimulating the immune system. Thus, ATIs could play a role in the enhancement and worsening of symptoms observed in some patients with NCGS/NWGS.

Sucrase-Isomaltase Deficiency

Sucrase-isomaltase deficiency is also called sucrose intolerance and is the result of decreased activity of the glucosidase enzyme. This enzyme is involved in the breakdown of starches and sugars, particularly sucrose (table sugar) and maltose (found in grains). Sucrose is broken down into glucose and fructose, and maltose is broken down into two glucose molecules. As a result of this enzyme deficiency, carbohydrates, and mainly sucrose molecules, are malabsorbed and build up in the intestines. They draw in water by osmosis and are fermented by bacteria in the colon, triggering symptoms that resemble those of IBS-D: stomach cramps, bloating, excess gas production, and diarrhea.

There are two types of sucrase-isomaltase deficiency: congenital and secondary or acquired.

Congenital sucrase-isomaltase deficiency appears to affect 2-9% of people of North American and European origin. This deficiency arises due to mutations in the sucrase isomaltase (SI) gene, which codes for the production of the enzymes. As a result of mutations in this gene, the structure, function or production of the enzyme may be affected. Symptoms of congenital deficiency appear early in a baby, usually after grains, fruit and juices are introduced in their diets, but as children get older, they seem to process sucrose and maltose more easily and with fewer symptoms. However, deficiencies can lead to decreased weight gain and decreased growth (failure to thrive) and malnutrition.

This congenital deficiency is thought to be underrecognized. However, it is not yet established whether it is involved in the development of symptoms in patients with functional gastrointestinal disorders.

Secondary or acquired sucrase-isomaltase deficiency may also exist, but it is thought to be mainly temporary. For example, animal studies have shown that the degeneration of the intestinal villi in celiac disease can lead to sucrase-isomaltase deficiency for a certain period of time and revert once villous atrophy is overcome.

Testing for sucrase-isomaltase deficiency is generally performed in children, and there is little scientific evidence to date that testing is useful for adults. The deficiency can be identified in children with duodenal or jejunal biopsies, which allow for a measurement of the activity of sucrase, lactase, isomaltase and maltase enzymes. This technique is difficult and may result in mistakes. A sucrose breath test measuring hydrogen gas can also be performed, but doing so in children is difficult, and the test itself has many inaccuracies. Finally, genetic testing can be performed to identify mutations, but these results should be combined with clinical data for assessment.

Candida

Candida is a fungus, specifically, a type of yeast that is part of our natural flora and exists on our skin and in the mouth, intestines and vagina. Although there are several different strains of Candida, the most common is Candida albicans.

Generally, in the bodies of healthy individuals, Candida occurs in balanced numbers and does not cause any problems. Its numbers are kept in check by our immune system and the bacteria that live in the same places and compete with the Candida for food and space.

When candidiasis occurs, there is overgrowth and infection caused by Candida, and treatment requires either oral or topical antifungal medications. However, this condition generally appears in immunocompromised individuals, people with diabetes or those who wear dentures. The presence of candidiasis in non-immunocompromised people is actually greatly disputed.

There have been suggestions that an overgrowth of Candida may be associated with IBS symptoms; however, no research findings have been able to show such a correlation, so it still remains a hypothesis by some. Yeast overgrowth in the gut is not thought to be an infection or candidiasis, and with the exception of one review that indicated some possible correlation between Candida overgrowth and IBS symptoms and theories as to how the two may be related, no other findings show this association. Recent research involves the testing of ways in which blood, breath and urine samples can be used to determine if increased numbers of yeast exist. Thus far, the testing has issues with sensitivity and reliability.

To date, no scientific results indicate that a specific change in diet could stop Candida overgrowth in the gut or other parts of the body and in turn help relieve IBS symptoms.

A Leaky Gut

The leaky gut is a scientifically disputed matter. A leaky gut refers to the single layer of cells that line the intestinal tract, becoming, in some cases, leaky or more permeable than they should be. This layer is what forms a barrier between your gut and the rest of the body, and it normally functions to allow the absorption of nutrients but prevent the movement of large molecules and bacteria from the intestines into the blood. If it temporarily becomes more leaky, it can allow such substances to move into the blood and then potentially travel to the rest of the body.

Increased intestinal permeability can be observed by gastroenterologists in some cases. People with Crohn's disease, patients with celiac disease consuming gluten and patients receiving chemotherapy can have a leaky gut. The same applies after the overconsumption of alcohol or the consumption of aspirin and nonsteroidal anti-inflammatory drugs (NSAIDs), which can irritate the gut. These substances can affect the connections between the intestinal cells and allow some of the larger molecules and germs to enter the blood. Stress has also been shown to make the gut leaky. However, all these cases are transient. Gastroenterologists believe that these irritants cause inflammation at the specific site, but the gut is eventually able to heal and return to normal.

A leaky gut gastrointestinal diagnosis that would require a specific treatment is scientifically questionable. It has been proposed that leaky guts caused by conditions such as yeast or bacteria overgrowth, a poor diet or overuse of antibiotics can trigger an immune response and more prevalent body inflammation that can be responsible for several conditions, such as food allergies, asthma, multiple sclerosis, tiredness and chronic fatigue syndrome, among others; however, there is currently no scientific evidence to support this hypothesis. There is no real evidence to suggest that a specific diet plan, the use of probiotics or the use of herbal preparations can target and cure leaky gut syndrome.

Do mast cells play a role in gastrointestinal problems?

Mast cells have recently received much scientific attention due to their role in GI problems. They are cells of the immune system that, when activated, produce histamine. In healthy individuals, histamine and other mast cell-produced chemicals are produced to initiate a protective response against foreign body intruders and to heal the body. These chemicals are also involved in allergies and anaphylaxis, and in the gut, they have important roles in food allergies as well as in defending against and getting rid of parasites.

There exists a spectrum of mast cell disorders, which present with inappropriate activation of the mast cells and/or an increased number of mast cells. For example, the condition of mastocytosis involves an increased number of mast cells as well as an abnormal activation of mast cells. In the case of mast cell activation syndrome (MCAS), however, the number of mast cells remains stable, but the cells are over-activated or easily activated and can produce chemicals that affect the body in negative ways. Mast cell activation syndrome may be initiated by a number of different foods, chemicals, fragrances, exercise, and stress.

Why are we addressing mast cells in this book? There are various digestive conditions, including IBS, that can mimic mast cell disorders, including adverse reactions to food, eosinophilic esophagitis, eosinophilic gastroenteritis, gastroenteritis, gastroesophageal reflux disease, gluten enteropathy, and irritable bowel syndrome.

Mast cell diseases can have gastrointestinal symptoms that mimic IBS, such as the following:

• Diarrhea
• Nausea
• Vomiting
• Abdominal pain
• Bloating

Additionally, there is a possible emerging role of mast cells in IBS. Specifically, mast cell activation leads to visceral hypersensitivity because it increases the response of the nerves to stimulation. Therefore, these nerves will react more strongly, giving a sensation of increased pain. This process is tightly linked to IBS, in which patients also show increased visceral hypersensitivity.

Stress releases corticotropin-releasing factor, which activates mast cells to produce a response. Stress is also a factor that exacerbates IBS symptoms.

If mast cell activation syndrome is suspected, the health care provider will recommend measurements of **serum tryptase** and a **24-hour urine test for n-methyl histamine and ll-beta prostaglandin F2 alpha**.

Treatment of mast cell activation aims to either stabilize the cells so they do not overproduce histamine or to stop the effects of histamine using anti-histamine treatments. Such medications would include the following: mast cell stabilizers; H1 blockers, which suppress histamine-mediated effects; and H2 blockers, which block the action of histamine in the stomach. It should be clarified, however, that none of these treatments is currently prescribed as IBS treatment.

Reducing stress via stress management techniques is also very important, as stress activates mast cells.

Finally, a change in diet that would involve a reduction in histamine-containing foods might help reduce symptoms. This approach has been shown to work for some patients but not for all of them. This change should always be implemented under the guidance of a clinical dietitian, as such diets are very personal and because records of histamine food content are generally outdated.

Chapter 2:
Bloating and Functional Gastrointestinal Disorders (FGIDs)

Functional Gastrointestinal Disorders (FGIDs)

Abdominal bloating can result from a *primary cause* or *underlying organic disease*; however, most people complain about bloating when they suffer from a *functional gastrointestinal disorder (FGID)*.

As we have explored in chapter 1 of this book, there are many possible primary organic causes of abdominal bloating and distension. If a primary cause or organic disease cannot be found and conditions such as anorexia nervosa, bulimia, or somatization disorder (also known as Briquet's syndrome) have been ruled out, then bloating is usually considered functional and part of the FGID spectrum.

Functional abdominal bloating is never constant or ongoing. It usually comes and goes in one or two patterns: shortly after meals or towards the end of the day. Patients usually awaken with a flat belly, and the bloating then develops and worsens over the course of the day.

The severity of abdominal bloating can vary from mild discomfort to severe pain and can affect people's everyday lives, from their family and social life to their workplace and finances, often resulting in absenteeism from work and recurrent visits to the doctor in pursuit of a solution to the problem. People admit to trying different medications and techniques but feel helpless and desperate most of the time.

Functional gastrointestinal (GI) and motility disorders are the most common GI disorders in the general population. Although statistics can vary, it has been assessed that approximately 1 in 4 people (or even more) have one of these disorders. Such conditions are the cause of approximately 40% of the GI problems doctors and therapists see.

? Why do we suffer from functional bloating?

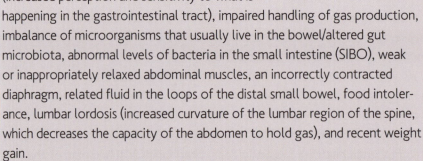

The cause of functional bloating remains unclear, and while several different explanations have been proposed, there is no conclusive answer. Due to our insufficient understanding of these mechanisms, the available therapeutic options are limited.

Potential mechanisms are gut hypersensitivity (increased perception and sensitivity to what is happening in the gastrointestinal tract), impaired handling of gas production, imbalance of microorganisms that usually live in the bowel/altered gut microbiota, abnormal levels of bacteria in the small intestine (SIBO), weak or inappropriately relaxed abdominal muscles, an incorrectly contracted diaphragm, related fluid in the loops of the distal small bowel, food intolerance, lumbar lordosis (increased curvature of the lumbar region of the spine, which decreases the capacity of the abdomen to hold gas), and recent weight gain.

Even though bloating is such a frequently occurring symptom, health care providers often dismiss it as a bothersome but non-life-threatening condition. Thus, more often than not, bloating is not measured even though it is so prevalent, bothersome and important to consider in FGIDs.

There are three fundamental characteristics that are disturbed in FGIDs, the technical names of which are as follows: motility, sensation, and brain-gut dysfunction.

- **Motility** describes the muscular movement of the GI tract. Normal motility is a methodical sequence of muscular contractions from the top to the bottom of the tract (peristalsis). In FGIDs, there are abnormal muscle spasms and pain. If the spasms are too fast, it leads to diarrhea, and if the spasms are too slow, it can lead to constipation.
- **Sensation** describes how the nerves of the GI tract perceive and respond to stimuli such as the digestion of food. In FGIDs, the nerves are sometimes so sensitive that even normal contractions can induce pain or discomfort, which is visceral sensitivity (an enhanced perception of sensations). As a

result of this sensitivity, even small changes in volume (stretching) and movement in the gut seem large to the patient, and patients feel bloated even though there are no visible signs of distension. Nerves that respond to stimuli (i.e., digesting a meal) are very sensitive to pain and discomfort, while in other people who do not have FGIDs, these sensations would be perceived as normal.

- **Brain-gut dysfunction.** The brain and gut communicate with each other in a bidirectional manner. In FGIDs, there is a dysfunction in the way in which the two organs communicate, which gives the perception of increased pain and bowel difficulties. Stress tends to make this interaction worse.

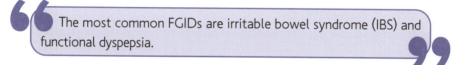

The most common FGIDs are irritable bowel syndrome (IBS) and functional dyspepsia.

- **Irritable bowel syndrome** (IBS) patients suffer from abdominal pain linked to defecation or changed bowel habits.
- **Functional dyspepsia** is a feeling of indigestion, uncomfortable fullness in the stomach and nausea after a meal that may inhibit individuals from eating a normal meal. There may also be pain or discomfort in the upper GI area and/or bloating for many hours after a meal. There is no symptom relief after going to the bathroom.
- **Functional abdominal bloating/distension** involves fullness and/or distension of the abdomen that is not associated with changes in bowel movements.
- **Aerophagia** is air swallowing that can cause bloating.
- **Functional diarrhea** is characterized by continuous or recurrent loose (mushy) or watery stools but without any abdominal pain.
- **Functional constipation** constitutes a group of functional disorders. The most commonly sustained feature is persistent, difficult, infrequent or an apparent incomplete defecation, and it is more frequently seen in women and as people age.
- **Unspecified functional bowel disease** involves functional bowel symptoms that do not meet the criteria defined for functional diarrhea, functional constipation, functional abdominal bloating or IBS.
- With respect to **opioid-induced constipation**, studies have shown that 40-80% of patients who take opioids for pain management frequently

suffer from constipation as a side effect. This can be accompanied by abdominal cramping, bloating and abdominal pain.

Irritable Bowel Syndrome (IBS)

The definition for IBS is that patients suffer from abdominal pain linked to defecation or changed bowel habits.

There are four types of IBS:
- IBS with constipation (IBS-C)
- IBS with diarrhea (IBS-D)
- Mixed IBS (IBS-M) with mixed bowel habits involving both constipation and diarrhea
- Unclassified IBS (IBS-U), which cannot be categorized in any of the other IBS groups

Why is it called Irritable Bowel Syndrome (IBS) and how common is it?

People with IBS have very sensitive nerve endings in the bowel wall. Normal activities, such as eating a meal, experiencing stress at work or menstruating, are perceived differently in the intestines, thus creating a flare-up of symptoms including diarrhea, bloating, pain and discomfort.

IBS affects 10 to 20% of the population and is the most common functional gastrointestinal disorder. IBS is not a serious disease, and there are no long-term organic complications associated with it. There is no greater need for preventive checkups than for other people. Women are twice as likely to be affected than men, and the disease is more common in young people under the age of 45. Up to 75% of IBS patients report bloating as a symptom. In a survey, 60% of patients with IBS said bloating was their most troublesome symptom, while 29% said abdominal pain was their most troublesome symptom.

However, the severity of the pain can vary from mild to severe, both from person to person and from time to time. The impact of IBS can range from mild inconvenience to severe debilitation, affecting a person's emotional, social and professional life. Approximately 50% of IBS patients do not let their family or circle of friends know that they suffer from the disease. They may feel embarrassed to discuss their problem (which always involves some sort of bowel issue) and feel misunderstood and isolated. Patients' constant feelings can lead to further isolation, low self-image, absenteeism from work and avoidance of social events and fun outdoor activities. As a consequence, these experiences can negatively affect health outcomes.

A study published in 2018 revealed some sad statistics. Of the 513 IBS-D patients questioned, the following results were found:

- 25% reported that **"IBS stops them from enjoying life"**
- 11% agreed with the statement that **"when my IBS is bad, I wish I was dead"**
- More than 33% of the patients said that they **"constantly worry about whether and when their IBS symptoms will return"**
- 20% said that **"their symptoms negatively affect their life at work".**

One other study highlighted that people with irritable bowel syndrome (IBS) would give up 25% of their remaining lifetime to experience relief from their gut symptoms!

Patients with IBS report that they feel they have no control over their lives, as illustrated in the following statements: "IBS is controlling my life" and "I never know if a specific food or situation will trigger an episode... there is no rhyme or reason in regard to IBS".

How is IBS diagnosed?

There is no single test to diagnose IBS. Several gastrointestinal conditions produce similar symptoms. A medical history, physical examination and selected tests are used to rule out other more serious gastrointestinal conditions. Then, the diagnosis will be made based on symptom criteria.

The American College of Gastroenterology does not recommend lab tests or diagnostic imaging in people younger than 50 years old unless they are accompanied by red-flag symptoms, such as weight loss, anemia, or a family history of celiac disease, IBD or colorectal cancer.

A formal set of diagnostic criteria known as the Rome IV criteria are used to establish a diagnosis.

Rome IV criteria for IBS

Recurrent abdominal pain for an average of at least 1 day a week in the last 3 months with two or more of the following characteristics:
1. Related to defecation
2. Associated with a change in the frequency of stool
3. Associated with a change in the form (consistency) of stool

Symptoms must have started at least 6 months ago.

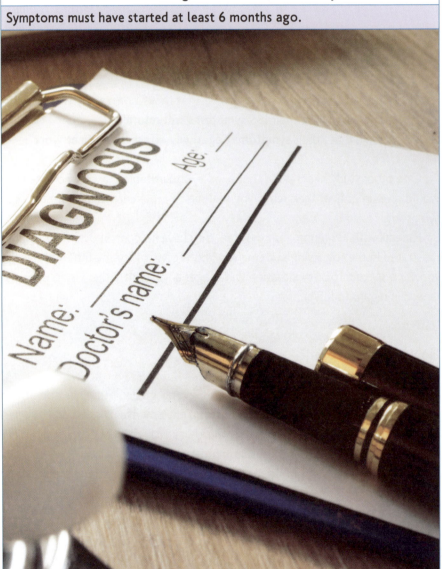

Beware of these possible causes of IBS

Even though the cause of IBS still remains unclear, there are a few theories:

- One of the possible mechanisms for IBS is **abnormal motility** of the colon. Slow motility can lead to constipation, and fast motility can lead to diarrhea. Nevertheless, motility issues do not validate IBS in all patients, and it is still uncertain whether motility issues are the cause of IBS or a symptom of the condition.
- **Severe gastrointestinal infection** (e.g., Salmonella or Campylobacter or viruses) can trigger the development of IBS but is not seen in all IBS patients. It is worth noting, however, that the risk of developing IBS is thought to be 4-6 times higher after a stomach intestinal infection caused by parasitic bacteria. This is called postinfectious IBS.
- **Stress, anxiety and mental health state** could play a role in IBS. Evidence shows that stress and anxiety exacerbate IBS symptoms; however, these factors are most likely not the cause.
- **Food intolerances, food sensitivities or allergies** are other mechanisms that are being studied.
- **Visceral hypersensitivity** is an enhanced perception of sensations. As a result of this sensitivity, even small changes in the volume (stretching) and movement in the gut seem larger to patients, and they may feel bloated even though there are no visible signs of distension.
- **Small Intestinal Bacterial Overgrowth (SIBO)** may lead to IBS. This involves a change in the number of bacteria in the small intestine, where normally very few bacteria reside.
- **Genetic role**. The effect of genes and heredity in IBS is unclear; however, some studies have shown that IBS occurs more frequently in people with a family history of IBS.
- Changes in the levels of **chemicals, neurotransmitters, gastrointestinal and reproductive hormones** could play a role in IBS.

" Stress does not cause IBS but stress can worsen or trigger symptoms. This is the reason that we encourage people with IBS to address stress and consider relaxation therapies. "

Another issue with which IBS patients must struggle is a lack of support from their main healthcare providers. There is an underlying belief by IBS sufferers that doctors do not adequately diagnose or treat their symptoms, often dismissing such symptoms as simply being in their heads. According to a recent National Institutes of Health (NIH) survey, 40% of IBS patients have expressed their complete dissatisfaction with their primary care provider's treatment of their symptoms, while only approximately 30% have been happy with their doctors. Furthermore, a similar written exercise showed that over 50% of IBS patients have had a "negative" experience with their health care provider, citing a lack of empathy from the doctor, an absence of trust in the doctor, and a failure to treat the symptoms as the main reasons behind their answers. Additionally, another study showed that gastroenterologists consider IBS patients to be less serious, reasonable and disabling than those suffering from "organic" disease. IBS patients were asked to write about their experience with health care providers, and these were some of the responses: "My health care provider (HCP) thinks I am crazy" and "Nothing my HCP does helps my IBS". From this survey, only 17% said that "My HCP has been helpful and reassuring". The patients were asked to make a wish list, and these lists featured the following responses: "Believe in my symptoms", "listen, understand and take me seriously" and "do not tell me to live with it".

On the other hand, another study that involved physicians' perspectives indicated that many health care providers feel frustrated with uncertain diagnoses and the absence of a cure for IBS. Gastroenterologists appear to be more judgmental towards IBS patients than are primary care practitioners and think that calls made by patients with functional GI disorders are not as serious and concerning as patients with organic disease symptoms.

Overall, there tends to be an underestimation of the burden of IBS on many of its patients, which requires attention and dedicated efforts towards the alleviation of symptoms and the improvement of the quality of life of these patients.

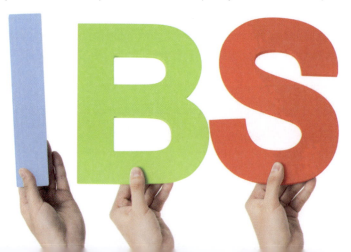

Chapter 3:
The Beautiful and Complex World of The Gut Microbiome

There are trillions of bacteria living in our gut.
What is the consequence when these bacteria are disturbed?

We all grow up hearing, "Don't touch that, it's dirty," or "Go wash your hands, you'll get sick," and we fear bacteria like they are our worst enemy. However, not all bacteria are created equal.

We have bacteria that are harmful and others that are beneficial. A large number of bacteria live in or on our body, and we coexist in harmony. To put things in perspective, there are more microorganisms living on our hands than there are people living on Earth.

More than 95% of the microorganisms that live in our body actually live in our gut. Collectively, these microorganisms are called our gut microbiota, and they have recently received much scientific attention. Also called the guardians of the gut, the 100 trillion microorganisms that live in our digestive tract are composed of bacteria, fungi, viruses, archaea and eukaryotes. In fact, we have more bacterial cells than human cells in our body. Most of them are found in the distal bowel and the colon and can weigh up to 2 kg. There are approximately 2000 different species of bacteria present in the gut, and each person's microbiome composition is unique, similar to a fingerprint. Approximately 93.5% of the species are from four dominant phyla: Firmicutes, Bacteroidetes, Proteobacteria, and Actinobacteria.

The microbiota genome (all the sets of genes in these organisms) is called the gut microbiome, and while the human genome has approximately 23,000 genes, the microbiome has more than three million genes that produce a myriad of metabolic products in our bodies.

The importance of the microbiome is increasingly appreciated, with animal and human studies showing their link and role in both how our mind works and our health and disease conditions, i.e., cancer, cardiometabolic diseases, allergies and obesity.

How Does Our Unique Microbiome "Fingerprint" Develop?

The most critical and major bacterial colonization of the gut occurs during the first two to three years of a person's life. Interestingly, before a baby is born, the gut is thought to be mostly sterile or contain very few microbes.

The first major interaction with bacteria occurs during vaginal birth, when the baby comes into contact with vaginal bacteria while moving through the birth canal. During this interaction, a large number of bacteria move into the baby's gut. Following that, changes in the microbiome are observed to correlate with changes in feeding, starting with breastfeeding and then moving to simple and then more complex solid foods. Studies show the microbiome to differ based on the type of birth (vaginal or C-section) and type of food given to a baby. Birth by C-section, the use of antibiotics before or immediately after birth and formula feeding have been shown to affect the microbiota in different ways, with some studies linking them to a higher risk of metabolic and immune diseases.

By the age of two to three years, the diversity of the microbiota and their numbers become relatively stable but continue to change until we become adults. After that, excluding major changes that would affect the gut microbiota, the composition and numbers remain relatively stable and predictable. We each end up with our own "fingerprint" with respect to the types and numbers of gut bacteria.

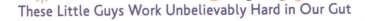

These Little Guys Work Unbelievably Hard in Our Gut

Some of the important functions of the gut microbiota are as follows:

- Gut microbiota protect from harmful pathogens by outcompeting them for food and space.
- They work hard to produce essential and nonessential amino acids and some vitamins (great examples are folate and biotin, which regulate the production of colon epithelial cells).
- They form short-chain fatty acids, which are 2- to 6-carbon fatty acids produced by the bacterial fermentation of fiber that have high anti-inflammatory properties.
- They help in the metabolism of nondigestible carbohydrates, such as resistant starches, cellulose, hemicellulose, pectin and gums, any smaller

carbohydrates that were not properly digested, and sugars and alcohols that have not been absorbed. All of this activity produces energy and important metabolic products that are absorbed in the body as well. Additionally, these processes produce energy and nutrients that enable the bacteria to grow and maintain their diversity and healthy numbers.

- They have a role in cholesterol synthesis.
- They affect hormone production and can regulate appetite.
- They influence digestive enzyme activity.
- They communicate with the epithelial cells of the intestine and can affect the thickness of the muscle wall of the intestines.
- They are involved in the production of the mood-affecting chemical serotonin. Although serotonin affects the brain, evidence shows that 90% of our body's serotonin actually occurs in the gut. The serotonin made in the gut is principally produced by endocrine cells called enterochromaffin cells (EC cells) and some types of immune cells and neurons. Research has shown that EC cells depend on the gut microbiota to be able to make a large proportion of the serotonin.
- Finally, gut microbiota enhance the normal development and function of our gut immune system, both early on in our development and later in life. The bugs are extremely important in assisting the immune system in responding and releasing peptides, cytokines and white blood cells to fight off intruders. This activity can have immense benefits for three reasons. First, it may protect the normal gut flora (bacteria that normally reside in our gut). Second, it can initiate an attack on pathogenic organisms that enter the body. Third, it can even trigger the death of the host cells, for example, the death of cancerous colon cells.

Microbiota Disturbances are Implicated in a Number of Diseases

Keeping our microbiome undisturbed and stable is extremely important!

Reduced gut bacterial diversity has been repeatedly observed in people with inflammatory bowel disease (IBD), type 1 and type 2 diabetes, celiac disease, psoriatic arthritis, atopic eczema, obesity, and arterial stiffness compared to healthy controls.

The microbiome has also been implicated in the development of some cancers, Parkinson's disease, and depression, and research in mice has demonstrated a link between the gut microbiome and anxiety. The composition of the microbiome has even been linked to one's response to chemotherapy and immunotherapy.

In the case of IBD, it makes sense that alterations in the gut microbiome in either direction (major reduction or significant increase of some species) could maintain or affect the inflammation observed in the disease. Studies of both animal models and patients have shown that antibiotics can decrease or prevent inflammation, indicating a role of the gut microbiota in IBD.

An increasing number of research findings lately support the involvement of the gut microbiota in the development of IBS. This is very obvious from studies that show that the risk of IBS increases sevenfold in patients who previously had infectious gastroenteritis. Furthermore, there is evidence that the dysregulation of serotonin production in the gut is also linked to IBS.

Finally, gut bacteria may play a role in the inhibition of allergy development. Studies have shown that the gut microbiota makeup of infants and children with allergies is different from that of infants and children without allergies.

What Affects Our Microbiome and What Can We Do to Help?

The health of our microbiome is extremely important, and we need to put our utmost efforts toward repopulating it and keeping it healthy. Evidence indicates that our environmental exposures, such as lifestyle, diet and drugs, affect our microbiome more than genetics do. The ultra-processed foods we consume, which contain additives and emulsifiers, have a negative impact on the bugs that live and work hard in our gut. Research in mice has shown that a diet consisting of low concentrations of two popular emulsifiers, carboxymeth-ylcellulose and polysorbate 80, decreased the numbers of health-promoting Bacteroidales and Verrucomicrobia, while the number of Proteobacteria, which promote inflammation, increased relative to that in control mice that were not given emulsifiers.

The use of antibiotics, while often life-saving, kills or affects the growth of not only the bad bacteria but also the beneficial bacteria in our bodies. Antibiotic use has continuously been on the rise, not only affecting our microbiome that we depend on but also leading to serious antibiotic resistance.

Adding to that is our obsession with using antiseptics and hand sanitizers and with bleaching and sterilizing our homes, thinking that we need to rid our homes of all microbes. Remember when we used to play with dirt when we were children?

Research has shown that stress influences the gut microbiota. Stress can affect the gut epithelium and change peristalsis, gut secretions and mucin formation. As a result, the living environment of the gut microbiota changes, with a subsequent effect on bacterial composition and/or their growth and metabolism.

Have you heard of the hot topic of Fecal Microbiota Transplantation (FMT)?

Fecal microbiota transplantation (FMT) is a relatively new trend with promising potential. The process involves exactly what the name implies: taking stool from a healthy individual, processing it and making it into a liquid to then transfer it to the colon of the recipient patient in order to "directly change the recipient's microbial composition and confer a health benefit". For the time being, FMT is only approved for the treatment of Clostridium difficile (C. diff.) infection that has appeared at least three times even following antibiotic treatment. There is currently no supporting scientific evidence for use of FMT for IBS treatment. However, much research is currently being conducted on the usefulness of FMT in various areas of disease, and even though we are a long way from clinical approval, there might be potential to this procedure in relieving gut symptoms as well.

Microbiota imbalances and celiac disease: the story of the Finnish-Russian border, Karelia

We know that genetics and eating the protein gluten found in wheat and other grains are responsible for the development of celiac disease. Nearly everyone with the disease has at least one of two versions of gene variations that increase their immune response to gluten. One-third of the general population carries HDL susceptibility genes, but only 2-5% of people with these genes develop celiac disease. Some of the possible reasons for the onset of the disease are the amount and quality of gluten, the type of infant feeding (possibly a lower risk with breastfeeding) and the age at which gluten is introduced into the diet.

Genes and gluten are not the only factors affecting the development of celiac disease. New evidence points to a dysbiosis or imbalance in the microbial communities as a factor leading to celiac disease and other autoimmune disorders. As we previously mentioned, our microorganisms colonizing our gut play an important role in immune system development and function by providing a protective response against harmful microorganisms. Under normal conditions, the microorganisms are in a balanced state, which supports the immune system. When this balance is disturbed, there is a risk for various immune-mediated diseases. Our gut microorganisms may have a protective role against or contribute to the development of celiac disease by regulating the interaction of genetics and environmental factors.

A study at the Finnish-Russian border, Karelia, suggests a possible microbial role in the development of celiac disease. This study was unique and very interesting because Karelia was historically a single province, with the two study populations (Finnish and Russian) sharing partly the same ancestry and eating similar grain products but living in very different socioeconomic circumstances. These qualities make this setting ideal for the study of gene-environmental interactions in the pathogenesis of celiac disease.

This study, which involved 3654 children from Finland and 1988 children from Russia in Karelia, showed a celiac disease prevalence of 1 in 496 among Russian children but 1 in 107 among Finnish children (using equal diagnostics). Celiac disease was not the only difference between the two groups. Finland ranks first in the world for type 1 diabetes, which was six times more frequently occurring than in Russian Karelian children. Allergies are also one-fourth as common in Russian Karelians. Because both populations share the same ancestry (and therefore similar genes), it can be suggested that differences in celiac disease rates are associated with a protective environment in which the Russian Karelian children are raised. Lower prosperity and hygiene standards in Russian Karelia create a microbial wealth in the body that may have a protective effect from autoimmune and allergic diseases by strengthening the immune system.

Small Intestinal Bacterial Overgrowth (SIBO)

As the name suggests, small intestinal bacterial overgrowth (SIBO) exists when an excessive number of bacteria is observed in the small intestine and where the environment should be almost otherwise sterile. Normally, fewer than 10^3 organisms/mL are found in the upper small intestine and are generally of specific types. When the numbers increase severely to more than 10^5-10^6 organisms/mL or when the type of microbe present changes, this can signal overgrowth and SIBO.

Food is digested in the mouth, stomach and small intestine, and soluble nutrients are absorbed from the small intestine into the blood. There is no need for bacteria to be present in the small intestine to aid digestion, as our body generally has all the enzymes it needs for digestion. Whatever material is not absorbed will move to the colon, where water is reabsorbed and the remnants form the feces that will be removed from the body. In the colon, bacteria exist as a natural flora and play a significant role in our well-being, as we have previously mentioned.

In SIBO patients, the excess bacteria in the small intestine ferment malab-sorbed food and produced gas. This gas and accompanied distension, abnormal pain and/or effects on bowel movement are all symptoms of SIBO. Unfortu-nately, to date, much remains unknown about SIBO. An apparent increase in the prevalence of the condition is being observed and is partly due to the availability of higher-quality tools to detect it. However, the condition is still thought to be frequently undiagnosed.

How exactly does SIBO develop?

SIBO develops when the normal homeostatic mechanisms that control enteric bacterial populations are disrupted. The two processes that most commonly predispose to bacterial overgrowth are diminished gastric acid secretion and small intestine dysmotility. Disturbances in gut immune function and anatomical abnormalities of the GI tract also increase the likelihood of developing SIBO. Once present, bacterial overgrowth may induce an inflammatory response in the intestinal mucosa, further exacerbating the typical symptoms of SIBO.

A decrease in the production of hydrochloric acid from acid-suppressing drugs, antibiotic use, damage of the intestine by alcohol, and partial bowel obstruc-tion or motility disorders affect how quickly things move through the intestine leading to stasis and bacterial overgrowth. Other conditions that appear to increase the risk of SIBO include the following: diabetes; scleroderma; hypothy-roidism; immune deficiency syndrome; chronic renal disease; IBS; gastroparesis; colonic inertia; celiac disease that remains untreated; Crohn's disease; chronic pancreatitis; Ehlers-Danlos syndrome (EDS), which is a genetic connective tissue disorder; surgery, such as gastric bypass, small bowl resection or ileocecal valve removal; and diverticulosis in the small intestine leading to infoldings of the large intestinal wall-forming pockets that could trap food and bacteria.

Mark Pimentel, MD, states that "probably 70-80% of patients who visit him with bacterial overgrowth have some sort of neuropathy or motility disturbance of the intestinal tract due to food poisoning". The disturbance seems to slow down the movement in the intestines or cause stasis, which allows the bacteria to start building up in large numbers.

Some of the symptoms observed in SIBO are as follows:

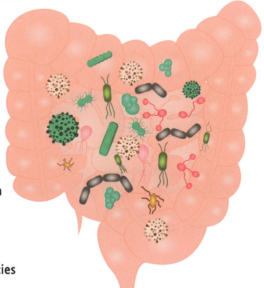

- **Bloating**
- **Gas**
- **Distension**
- **Abdominal pain**
- **Diarrhea**
- **Irregularity in bowel movement**
- **Constipation**
- **Indigestion and heartburn**
- **Fatigue**
- **Depression**
- **Weight loss**
- **Certain nutrient deficiencies**
- **Rashes**

Many of these symptoms may appear soon after eating, as the bacteria start fermenting the food right away in the small intestine.

Symptoms observed in SIBO patients are similar to those in IBS patients. In fact, most case-control studies have shown that SIBO occurs more commonly in IBS sufferers than in control groups, thus suggesting an association between SIBO and IBS. The most frequent and significant association is between SIBO and IBS with diarrhea (IBS-D).

It is worth noting that Parkinson's disease, restless leg syndrome, fibromyalgia and rosacea coincide with SIBO presentation. Moreover, evidence shows that with SIBO management, these conditions also appear to improve.

How is SIBO diagnosed?

There is substantial disagreement in the literature regarding which test is the most appropriate in either the clinical or research setting. Two tests are commonly employed: bacterial culture and breath tests.

(a) Small intestine aspirates and bacterial culture

Although quantitative culture of the upper gut aspirate has traditionally been used as the gold standard for the diagnosis of SIBO, its limitations include difficulty, invasiveness, cost, contamination by oropharyngeal flora, and the inability to culture as much as 70% of the bacteria colonizing the gut. Moreover, the distribution of bacterial overgrowth may be patchy, and upper gut aspirate may not be able to detect bacterial overgrowth in the distal gut. Therefore, it does not offer a very valuable tool.

(b) Using breath tests for hydrogen and methane

There is a lactulose breath test and a glucose breath test, in which the patient swallows a sugar solution and then breathes into foil bags every 15 minutes for two hours to collect the gas. Generally, 80% of gases such as hydrogen and methane are eliminated with the flatus, but approximately 20% are exhaled when breathing out. Methane measurements tend to be more accurate in the case of SIBO. However, both methods are plagued by false-positive or false-negative results due to the lack of specificity or sensitivity. Furthermore, each testing center has different criteria for SIBO diagnosis, making detection and validity more confusing.

Recent findings show a link between hydrogen sulfide gas and diarrhea. It

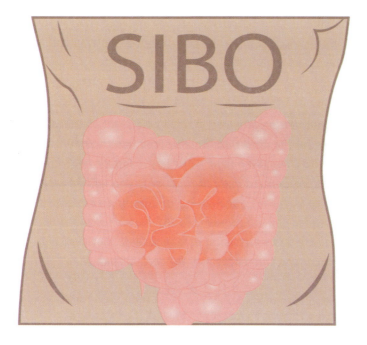

has been suggested by Mark Pimentel's group that new breath tests will include hydrogen sulfide detection for SIBO and IBS-D.

How is SIBO treated?

For the time being, the most commonly used and most successful treatment for SIBO is antibiotics. In particular, the best antibiotic for SIBO is rifaximin, which is non-absorbable and works well in the gut without having major overall effects on the body. Antibiotics aim to kill or stop the growth of bacteria that are present in large numbers in SIBO patients and to help improve the inflammation that exists in the intestine. However, various courses of antibiotics often make people feel worse, so more exploration and experimentation are still needed in this field.

Often, the low FODMAP diet, low-fermentable diet, low- or no-starch diet, or the specific carbohydrate (SAPS) diet or Paleo diet is prescribed in conjunction with antibiotics to patients receiving treatment for SIBO. Such diets reduce carbohydrate intake. Because the bacteria act on malabsorbed, fermentable carbohydrates that enter the intestine, reducing carbohydrate intake would reduce SIBO symptoms and eventually halt or reduce bacterial overgrowth because bacteria would not have food on which to feed. However, the body of literature that exists is small, and there is no concrete evidence that these diets work for SIBO patients. More controlled studies are required to show the efficacy of such diets in treating SIBO. For the time being, the answer is that we do not know which one is best for SIBO.

> **!** *The information provided in this book is not intended as a substitute for the advice and care of your healthcare provider. You should always consult your physician or health care provider if you notice any red flags or if you will be making changes to your diet, medication or current treatment. It is recommended that the low FODMAP diet is followed under the guidance and supervision of a registered dietitian. Nutritional needs and tolerances vary for each individual.*

Section 2

Chapter 4:
The low FODMAP diet

What are FODMAPs?

How many times have you been at a restaurant and ordered French onion soup to only then feel completely miserable hours later?

Do you dream about a few cold slices of watermelon by the seaside on a hot summer day but know that it will make you run straight to the bathroom afterwards?

Do you wish you could have a bowl of vegetarian bean chili for lunch at work and not worry about all the bloating, gas and pain?

Well, here's why this happens.

These foods and many more contain what are known as FODMAPs, which are guilty of causing symptoms of bloating, gas, abdominal pain, diarrhea and/or constipation when consumed by people with a sensitive gut.

Lucky for us sufferers, Monash University in Melbourne, Australia, has developed an innovative and evidence-based diet via the elimination of high FODMAP-containing foods. This diet plan is the first scientifically proven program to manage gastrointestinal symptoms and could be your ticket to gastrointestinal bliss, considering that 50 to 80% of patients respond positively to it.

However, first, let's get to the science behind FODMAPs and the low FODMAP diet.

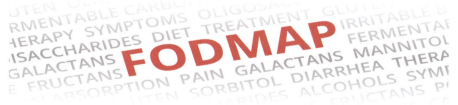

FODMAPs are a group of small chain carbohydrates (sugars and fibers) found naturally in foods. The acronym FODMAP represents the following:

F ERMENTABLE
O LIGOSACCHARIDES
D ISACCHARIDES
M ONOSACCHARIDES
A ND
P OLYOLS

What do these names mean?

Fermentable means easily broken down by bacteria found in the gut. This process produces gases as biproducts.

Oligosaccharides are two categories of sugars: **fructo-oligosaccharides (FOS or fructants)** and **galacto-oligosaccharides (GOS or galactans).** Fructans are chains of fructose with a glucose unit attached at the end, while galactans are galactose chains with a fructose molecule attached at the end.

Disaccharides are molecules that consist of two sugar units joined together. In this case, the culprit disaccharide is **lactose**, a molecule composed of the two digestible sugars glucose and galactose.

Monosaccharides are single sugar units that require no digestion. These sugar units are glucose, fructose and galactose. In the case of FODMAPs, **fructose** poses a problem but only when present in excess of glucose, meaning in larger quantities than glucose when ingested. This is a problem because fructose absorption into the gut occurs efficiently and effectively only when glucose exists in equal or larger proportions. Glucose is absorbed across the intestinal wall efficiently and appears to carry fructose along with it. When there is excess fructose, however, another absorption method is required to carry the extra fructose across. This pathway is often compromised in some individuals, leading to the excess fructose being malabsorbed (not absorbed properly into the bloodstream).

Polyols are sugar alcohols, which are basically sugar molecules with an alcohol group attached. Polyols include isomalt, maltitol, mannitol, polydextrose, sorbitol and xylitol.

What are some examples of foods containing FODMAPs?

High in FRUCTANTS	High in GALACTANS	High in LACTOSE	Excess FRUCTOSE	High in POLYOLS
Wheat	Pulses	Whole, reduced fat or skimmed (cow, goat or sheep) milk	Apples	Apples
Barley	Legumes	Evaporated milk	Cherries	Pears
Rye	Cashews	Sweetened, condensed milk	Figs	Apricots
Nectarines	Pistachios	Ice Cream	Mangoes	Peaches
Watermelon		Cow's or goat's yoghurt	Pears	Plums
Garlic		Cream cheese	Dried fruit	Prunes
Onion		Cottage cheese	Asparagus	Blackberries
Cashews		Ricotta cheese	Artichokes	Watermelon
Pistachios		Fresh Cream	Agave syrup	Cauliflower
Chamomile tea			Honey	Items with artificial sweeteners i.e. gums, mints, desserts, etc.
Fennel tea			High-fructose corn syrup	
			Fruit juices	

What happens to FODMAPs when they are ingested?

These molecules enter the body when food is ingested but do not get absorbed into the bloodstream and instead build up in the small intestine for a number of reasons. Upon consumption, fructants and galactans are undigested because humans lack the enzymes to break them down, so they remain in the intestine instead of being absorbed into the bloodstream. Lactose builds up in the intestine because many IBS or other GI sufferers do not have the enzymes (or enough enzymes) to break it down. Fructose is a molecule that is readily absorbed in the intestine; however, it needs to be accompanied by glucose. If fructose is ingested in excess of glucose, then malabsorption results, and fructose builds up in the intestine. Lastly, the sugar alcohols—polyols—are absorbed by the body but only partially and in a very slow manner. Thus, they tend to accumulate in the small intestine in large quantities.

What happens to FODMAPs when they are not absorbed?

FODMAP molecules are small and soluble and therefore osmotically active, meaning that they draw water towards them. In this case, they draw water into the small intestine. This excess water, along with the malabsorbed FODMAPs, passes to the colon. There, the molecules are broken down (fermented) by bacteria (microbiota) living in the colon, a process that releases methane and hydrogen gas. The accumulation of gas, along with the presence of excess water, causes swelling and distension in the intestines. This leads to bloating, pain, diarrhea and/or constipation.

In addition, patients with functional gastrointestinal disorders (FGIDs), particularly IBS, often suffer from visceral hypersensitivity, which is a heightened sensitivity to pain in the inner organs, in this case the gastrointestinal tract. It appears that the neurons in the gut are more sensitized and therefore overreactive, sending amplified messages to the brain and resulting in a magnified sensation of pain. Therefore, the bloating, pain and urgency due to the accumulation of ill-absorbed FODMAPs in the gut are exaggerated due to visceral hypersensitivity, resulting in a feeling of more pain and discomfort.

How Effective is the low FODMAP diet?

The low FODMAP diet has a positive impact on IBS, and there is much scientific evidence to support it. Based on a 2018 published review, to date, there are at least 10 randomized controlled or randomized comparative trials of the low FODMAP diet. These studies are the high-quality, controlled trials that we should be looking for! The majority of these studies show that the low FODMAP diet has had positive outcomes in 50 to 80% of the participating IBS patients.

Research studies have found a low FODMAP diet to improve gut symptoms, quality of life and abdominal pain in people with IBS. Evidence has shown that a low FODMAP diet increases the quality of life of patients twofold compared to those following standard dietary recommendations for IBS. More specifically, patients following this diet saw more significant improvements in their overall quality of life, levels of anxiety and ability to be active than those with the standard dietary recommendations for IBS.

Success of the low FODMAP diet is mostly shown in studies for IBS-D or IBS-mixed patients. There is much less information on how the diet works in patients suffering from IBS-C. However, the fact that studies show that the FODMAP diet can help up to ¾ of people with IBS is very encouraging. Interestingly, a recent national survey of over 1500 gastroenterologists in the US showed that over half of the healthcare providers recommend diet therapy to more than 75% of their IBS patients, with the low FODMAP diet being the one most commonly recommended.

Other possibilities for the potential use of the low FODMAP diet in gastrointestinal disorders have been identified. However, more research and follow-up studies are needed to make full recommendations.

For instance, studies show that the low FODMAP diet helps reduce functional gastrointestinal symptoms of quiescent (inactive) IBD, which are IBS-like, and helps improve quality of life in patients.

The results published in 2018 from a randomized clinical trial showed that a reduced intake of dietary FODMAPs among breastfeeding mothers is associated with a greater improvement in the symptoms of infantile colic than those among mothers on a typical diet.

Functional gastrointestinal disorders in children are thought to be the reason for 50% of visits to pediatric gastroenterologists. It has been proposed that up to 20% of children in the USA suffer from IBS and that usually a decrease in one or a few of the triggers, such as lactose, sorbitol or fructose, appears to have positive and adequate results in minimizing symptoms. A double-blind random-ized controlled trial of children with IBS aged 7 to 17 years was carried out in 2015. Thirty-three children completed a crossover study. When consuming a low FODMAP diet, the children had a lower severity and number of abdominal pain incidences than when they consumed a diet typical of American children. However, this finding is only an indication; many more studies with longer interventions are necessary before the low FODMAP diet can be recommended as dietary therapy in children with IBS. If children are to follow a restricted diet such as the low FODMAP diet, it should only be done under the supervision of a specialized pediatric dietitian, as restricted diets can have negative consequences, such as food fears, nutritional inadequacies and possible eating disorders in growing children.

Lastly, the low FODMAP diet could be useful in the management of symptoms of SIBO; however, there is not enough evidence at the present time to apply this diet as a primary treatment option.

Chapter 5:
Fibers and Bloating

First, what is dietary fiber?

In this book, you will notice that we place great emphasis on the consumption of fiber. Dietary fiber, as we will see, has tremendous benefits for the maintenance of a healthy gut microbiome, gut health and overall body health. A meal high in fiber can be more filling and satisfying, and regular fiber consumption can decrease cholesterol levels and decrease blood glucose and/or insulin levels (after a meal). Dietary fiber can help with digestion and bowel movements, but it can also exacerbate symptoms of bloating, abdominal pain and flatulence in IBS sufferers.

Our aim is to guide you in maximizing your fiber consumption to the recommended amount per day but also minimizing possible abdominal symptoms. Even though the topic of fibers is a complicated one, we make sure to break it down for you so you can navigate through the topic of dietary fiber as easily as possible.

In Chapter 9 you will see that we make a number of fiber recommendations we think you will find useful. We help you assess your current fiber intake, introduce means by which you can increase your fiber intake with the low FODMAP diet and make specific fiber recommendations for IBS. Therefore, let's dive into the world of fibers.

Dietary fiber refers to carbohydrates from plants that cannot be digested or absorbed in the small intestine. In turn, these carbohydrates are either completely or partially fermented (broken down by bacteria) in the large intestine. The term includes a wide range of different substances and can be further classified based on the following: size (short-chain and long-chain); solubility, meaning the ability to dissolve in water; and fermentation characteristics. Fermentation refers to the rate and extent to which fibers are broken down in the large intestine by bacteria. Fermentation in turn produces energy for gut microorganisms and other products, such as short-chain fatty acids and gases.

To elaborate further, fibers that accumulate in the colon can have a vast number of effects:

- Fibers increase bacterial numbers and abundance because bacteria feed on fibers and grow.
- The fermentation of fibers produces short-chain fatty acids, which are large regulatory molecules with a high number of health benefits, including proper immune system function.
- The fermentation of fibers in the colon also produces gases that can increase bloating, flatulence and pain in IBS.
- Fibers have gel-forming properties that can affect stool consistency. Fibers can soften hard stool in constipation and firm up loose stool in diarrhea.
- Fibers can increase stool bulk.
- Fibers can increase the amount of water that is absorbed by the stool.
- Fibers can decrease the amount of time the stool remains in the colon (shorten colonic transit time) by increasing the amount of water that goes in the stool and by causing more peristalsis (contractions of the intestinal wall that will push the stool along).

There are different types of fibers. What are they?

The topic becomes complicated with respect to different types of fibers. As we have said, generally speaking, fiber refers to a group of materials and not only one, and many debates exist regarding the most proper way to define fiber.

First, let us examine the solubility and fermentation levels of fibers. Fibers are generally categorized based on their solubility and fermentation level in the small intestine. Therefore, we have **soluble and insoluble fibers** but **also highly fermentable, intermediate and nonfermentable fibers.**

Soluble Fibers

Soluble fiber dissolves in water and forms a thick layer in our digestive tract. This gel slows down the time food molecules need to move through the intestines and attracts water like a sponge, thus making the stool softer.

Soluble fibers are more readily fermented than insoluble fibers, and fermentation is a key trigger for functional gastrointestinal disorders. We classified soluble fibers into **highly and quickly fermentable, highly fermentable and intermediate fermentable.**

Fermentation Characteristic	Food Source of This Fiber
Highly and quickly fermentable e.g., FOS, GOS	Vegetables (onion, garlic) Grains (wheat, rye, pulses)
Highly fermentable e.g., resistant starch (starch that functions like a soluble fiber) Pectin, inulin, partially hydro-lyzed guar gum	Vegetables (cooked and cooled potato and corn) Fruits Grains Pulses

Intermediate Soluble Fibers

Fermentation Characteristic	Food Source of This Fiber
Intermediate fermentable	Grains (oats, psyllium husks)

Insoluble Fibers

Insoluble fibers do not dissolve in water and pass through the digestive system mostly intact. Such fiber adds bulk to the stool and helps the stool to move effectively through the intestine. We classified insoluble fibers as **moderately-highly fermentable and nonfermentable,** such as cellulose, hemicelluloses and lignin.

Insoluble fiber can create mechanical stimulation in the bowel. This can trigger motility and help constipation but can also make symptoms worse in people with sensitive guts.

Fermentation Characteristic	Food Source of This Fiber
Moderately-highly fermentable	Vegetables Fruit Bread and grains Seeds
Nonfermentable Derived from plant cell wall, such as cellulose, hemicellulose and lignin	Vegetables (celery, green leafy vegetables) Fruits (peels/skins of fruits) Nuts Seeds

What are Prebiotics and why do we care about them?

Soluble fibers from plant foods have prebiotic properties. Based on the consensus of the International Scientific Association for Probiotics and Prebiotics (ISAPP), the term prebiotic is defined as **"a substrate that is selectively utilized by host microorganisms conferring a health benefit"**. We definitely know that eating prebiotic foods promotes the growth of beneficial bacteria in the gut. Prebiotics are indigestible parts of food that are fermentable and that are not affected by gastric acidity. Such foods include many fruits and vegetables, particularly those that have complex carbohydrates, such as resistant starch and fiber. Our bodies are not able to digest such complex carbohydrates, so they pass through our digestive system and end up in the colon, where they are broken down by bacteria and other microorganisms in the process of fermentation. Therefore, prebiotics are very important for the maintenance of a healthy gut microbiome, which we all know plays a significant role in our well-being.

Fructo-oligosaccharides (FOS), galacto-oligosaccharides (GOS), inulin, and possibly other soluble fibers are prebiotics and can stimulate the preferential growth of lactobacilli, bifidobacteria and other health-promoting bacteria in the colon. Many of these prebiotic foods fall in the category of high FODMAPS and in many people with functional gastrointestinal disorders, they result in symptoms such as bloating, flatulence and abdominal discomfort and pain upon consumption. For this reason, a low FODMAP elimination diet tends to restrict many of these offenders, for example, garlic and onion. It is therefore extremely important to gradually reintroduce high FODMAP prebiotic foods in our diet during the reintroduction phase to ensure that we promote the growth of good bacteria in our gut.

Even during the elimination phase of the diet, however, it is fundamental to consume a variety of prebiotic foods in their small, safe low FODMAP serving sizes. It is also important to remember that the elimination phase—carried under the guidance of a registered clinical dietitian—lasts only for a short period of time of 2-6 weeks.

Resistant starches (RS) are highly fermentable soluble carbohydrates that function similarly to a soluble fiber. They are also classified as a "prebiotic" because they act as food for beneficial bacteria. Importantly, RS are slowly fermented by gut bacteria and result in a more steady and controllable production of gas compared to FODMAPs, which makes resistant starch less likely to contribute to gastrointestinal discomfort and makes it a more suitable choice for people with functional gastrointestinal disorders.

There are four types of resistant starch. RS1, found in partially milled grains and legumes, is inaccessible to enzymes for digestion. RS2, found in unripe bananas and starches high in amylose content, manages to avoid being digested. RS3 types are found in the following: bread; tortillas; and potatoes, rice and pasta that have been cooked and then cooled; these resistant starches form when foods are cooked and then cooled. Finally, RS4 is a starch type that is chemically modified.

Fancy Some MACs? Microbiota Accessible Carbohydrates (MACs)

Because the term fiber commonly refers to indigestible carbohydrates, it tends to be slightly confusing, as some of these fibers are used by gut bacteria, while others are not. For example, cellulose is not used by gut bacteria, while resistant starches (which are readily fermentable carbohydrates but do not fall in the category of fibers) are used by microbiota. For this reason, a recently proposed term, microbiota accessible carbohydrates or MACs, was given to all the carbohydrates that are available and used by gut microbiota. Both **prebiotic fibers** and **resistant starch** are types of MACs.

How much fiber do we need to consume each day and how does that translate to good health?

People who eat more fiber have a reduced risk of death. Studies show that the greatest benefit of fiber is indirect: it feeds our microbes, which in turn keep us healthy.

A high-fiber diet with whole foods is associated with the following well-established physiological effects:

- A decrease in blood total and/or low-density lipoprotein (LDL) cholesterol
- A decrease in blood glucose and/or insulin levels (after a meal)

Additionally, a high fiber diet may have probable links with the following physiological effects; however, more scientific evidence is required:

- A decrease in blood pressure
- Weight loss
- Positive changes in the microbiota of the colon
- Increased satiety

In regard to fiber consumption, the Institute of Medicine, which provides science-based advice on matters of medicine and health, provides the following daily recommendations for adults.

	Age 50 or younger	Age 51 or older
Men	38 grams	30 grams
Women	25 grams	21 grams

The fiber we consume ends up in the colon completely untouched. The colon is also where most of our microbes live, so fiber becomes fuel for our microbes. They use fiber as food and energy, and the more food they have, the better, as they are more likely to thrive and reproduce.

At this point, we do not quite understand all the mechanisms through which our microbes work to enhance our health and immune function. We know that they produce nutrients for our body, including short-chain fatty acids such as butyrate, that help our body stay healthy. In chapter 3, we present all of the functions of the gut microbiome in our body. Therefore, we want to keep the gut microbiota happy and provide them with fiber for fermentation. Animal studies have demonstrated that an extremely low-fiber diet can shrink the microbes in our colon tenfold.

Fiber consumption can influence the types of microbiota present in our gut, change the gut environment for the microbiota that live there and promote the overall growth of beneficial bacteria. Specifically, many fiber types with prebiotic properties, such as oligosaccharides and inulin, fall into the MAC category of fibers and promote the growth of beneficial bacteria, such as lactobacilli and bifidobacterial.

As we have previously observed, changes in the gut microbiome are associated with various conditions, such as irritable bowel syndrome, obesity, cardiovascular disease and asthma, so it is important to clearly define the specific role that fibers play in gut microbiome alterations. MACs have been shown to control inflammation and serve as markers of metabolic syndrome, which is significant.

Generally, a greater consumption of dietary fiber has been linked with a reduced risk of various chronic diseases, including cardiovascular disease and diabetes, and it may reduce the risk of all-cause mortality.

Fiber recommendations for Functional Gastrointestinal Disorders (IFFGD)
The International Foundation for Functional Gastrointestinal Disorders (IFFGD) suggests that IBS patients aim to consume the same amount of fiber recommended for the general population. Incorporating more fiber into one's diet can improve bowel function and lessen GI symptoms. Keep in mind, however, that some fiber-rich foods, such as bran, can lead to more gassiness and bloating.

Nonfiber food components that have prebiotic properties

Recent research into prebiotics has recognized food molecules other than fibers to have prebiotic properties. One of these types of molecules receiving attention lately for its participation in improving gut health is polyphenols. These molecules are naturally occurring phytochemicals with antioxidant properties that appear to be appreciated by the beneficial bacteria in our gut. Studies using animals showed that polyphenol consumption increased good bacteria in the gut. Research demonstrates that the consumption of polyphenols favored an increase in the beneficial microbiota in the gut and a decrease in the bad bacteria. Polyphenol-rich foods include red wine, coffee, tea, dark chocolate, virgin olive oil, cocoa powder, ginger, cumin, and capers, among others, as well as several vegetables and fruits.

The impact of dietary fats, such as omega-3 fatty acids, on the gut microbiota has not been extensively studied; however, these fatty acids have recently received attention as possible prebiotics. Omega-3 PUFAs (Polyunsaturated Fatty Acids) can have a positive effect by changing the microbiota composition in gastrointestinal diseases and increasing the levels of anti-inflammatory molecules, such as short-chain fatty acids. Additionally, this relationship between the gut microbiota, omega-3 fatty acids and immunity helps to maintain a healthy intestinal wall as well as play a role in immunity. Finally, recent work with human and animal models shows that omega-3 PUFAs can influence the communication between the gut and the brain (gut-brain axis) through means guided by the gut microbiota.

Therefore, because omega-3 fatty acids might be possible prebiotics and also have other important health benefits, we recommend their consumption. The three main omega-3 fatty acids are alpha-linolenic acid (ALA), eicosapentaenoic acid (EPA), and docosahexaenoic acid (DHA). Foods that contain these fatty acids include the following:

- Fish and other seafood (especially salmon, mackerel, tuna, herring, and sardines)
- Nuts and seeds (flaxseed, chia seeds, and walnuts)
- Plant oils (flaxseed oil, soybean oil, and canola oil)
- Omega-3 fortified foods (as stated on their packaging) such as eggs, yogurt, juices, milk, and soy beverages.

Chapter 6:
Probiotics
Complementing the low FODMAP diet with probiotics
What are They and are They Useful?

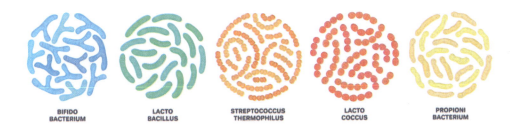

BIFIDO
BACTERIUM

LACTO
BACILLUS

STREPTOCOCCUS
THERMOPHILUS

LACTO
COCCUS

PROPIONI
BACTERIUM

Probiotics

Probiotics are live microorganisms that, when administered in adequate amounts, confer health benefits upon the host. There are more than 300 clinical studies involving 50,000 people in which researchers have investigated the health benefits of probiotics or placebo in various health conditions. Many of these studies have demonstrated effectiveness.

Despite this fact, research in this area is incomplete, and we do not have enough scientific evidence to make solid recommendations; it is unclear what strains of bacteria, what doses and what routes of administration are safe and effective for specific patients. The reason for lack of clarity is the tremendous variation among studies in terms of the species, strains, forms, dosages and scores for the measurement of symptoms.

At this point, we do not know the precise mechanism of action for various probiotics in gastrointestinal diseases, but the theory is that probiotics can replace missing strains or exclude unfavorable strains of bacteria in the gut. They can promote an anti-inflammatory response, improve visceral hypersensitivity (sensitivity to pain), change gut motility (movement of the gut) and intestinal permeability (leaky gut), and fix the dysfunction of the gut-brain axis.

Several lines of evidence indicate a role of bacteria in the biological causes of functional bowel disorders. For instance, many people with irritable bowel syndrome (IBS) report the onset of symptoms following an enteric infection. Microbiota differences have been observed in people with or without IBS. People with IBS have lower amounts of *Lactobacillus* and *Bifidobacterium* in their guts. Additionally, people with IBS have higher levels of harmful *Streptococcus, E. coli* and *Clostridium.* Studies in mice show that healthy mice that receive microbiota from mice with IBS develop IBS-like symptoms. Additionally, gut microbiota may influence IBS symptoms; people with a lower number of bifidobacteria are associated with higher pain scores in IBS.

Finally, recent research findings from Kings College, London, showed that the incorporation of probiotics into the low FODMAP diet helps offset the microbiota changes observed during the elimination phase of the diet.

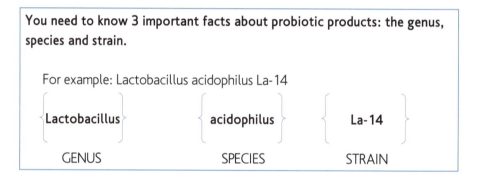

You need to know 3 important facts about probiotic products: the genus, species and strain.

For example: Lactobacillus acidophilus La-14

Lactobacillus	**acidophilus**	**La-14**
GENUS	SPECIES	STRAIN

One cannot assume that research published on one strain of probiotic applies to another strain or even to strains of the same species. Documentation of the type of bacteria, genus, species and strain, as well as the potency (number of viable bacteria per dose) and purity (presence of contaminating or ineffective bacteria), is very important to consider.

Checklist of what to look out for when choosing a probiotic:

- **Talk** with your doctor before taking a probiotic supplement.
- **Probiotics should be avoided in patients with** chronic medical conditions, patients receiving treatment for acute or chronic infections, patients who are immunocompromised, patients with indwelling intravenous catheters, patients suffering from infections of the gastrointestinal

tract, or patients who are sick enough to require hospitalization in an intensive care unit.

- **Check the label if you have specific dietary needs.**
- **Choose** a product that has been scientifically shown to provide a benefit in a condition you want to target.
- **Avoid** products that contain prebiotic additives such as inulin, chicory root or FOS if you cannot tolerate them.
- **Check** viability, which means the date that the bacteria are guaranteed to still be active. Avoid products for which the labels note the bacteria count "*at time of manufacture*" because the viability of the product cannot be guaranteed at the time of sale.
- **Look** at the number of bacteria or CFUs (*colony-forming units*). The number of viable bacteria in the product is sometimes called "*live cultures*".
- **Always consider** the suggested dose.
- **Check** proper storage conditions for the product.

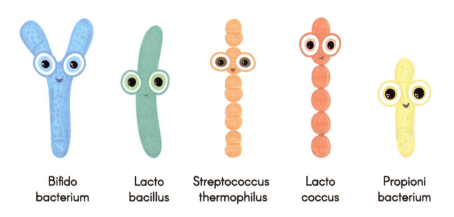

| Bifido bacterium | Lacto bacillus | Streptococcus thermophilus | Lacto coccus | Propioni bacterium |

Probiotics may have a beneficial effect on various GI symptoms and conditions

At this point, probiotics may have a beneficial effect on various GI symptoms and conditions. However, sufficient evidence has not quite yet been established to allow for the development of general recommendations and clinical guidelines. The global market for probiotics was valued at US $32.06 billion in 2013, and finding the suitable product on the market is a daunting task. Remember that dietary supplements are not tested by the U.S. Food and Drug Administration, and various products on the market may not be suitable or specific for the condition you are looking to treat. The best advice is to work with a registered dietitian or your physician to find the product that is suitable for you based on the clinical data available.

Several studies have suggested that the daily intake of probiotics could improve IBS symptoms. Specifically, reductions in abdominal bloating, flatulence, pain and global relief have been noted in studies. However, the results have been inconsistent, and most strains have only one small study behind them. Comparison among studies is often difficult because many of these studies use different combinations of strains of bacteria. Further research is therefore required for more conclusive evidence.

Probiotic species shown to be effective in irritable bowel syndrome (based on evidence from at least one properly designed randomized trial) include the following:

- *Bifidobacterium (animalis) lactis CNCM* **(fermented milk products)**
- *Bifidobacterium longum 35624* **(supplement)**
- *Lactobacillus plantarum 299v* **(supplement, capsule or drink)**

Probiotic species shown to be effective in constipation (based on evidence from at least one properly designed randomized trial) include the following:

- *Bifidobacterium (animalis) lactis CNCM* **(fermented milk products)**
- *Lactobacillus reuteri DSM 17938* **(supplement)**
- *Lactobacillus casei Shirota* **(fermented milk products)**

Probiotic species shown to be effective in functional abdominal pain include the following:

- *Bacillus coagulant GB1-30, 6086* **(supplement)**

It is important to note that while probiotic use for the treatment of infectious diarrhea is well documented, probiotics to **treat diarrhea in IBS** have not been shown to be particularly effective.

Additional products (supplements) for relief in overall IBS symptoms include the following:

- *Bifidobacterium bifidum MIMBb 75, B. longum subsp. Infantis 35624*
- *Escherichia coli Dsm17252*
- *Lactobacillus rhamnosus GG, L. rhamnosus Lc705, Propionibacterium freudenreichii subsp. shermanii JS and Bifidobacterium breve Bb99*
- *Bifidobacterium bifidum BGN4, B. animalis subsp. lactis AD011, Lactobacillus acidophilus AD031 and L. paracasei subsp. paracasei BS041*
- *Lactobacillus rhamnosus GG, L. rhamnosus Lc705, Propionibacterium freudenreichii subsp. shermanii JS*
- *Lactobacillus acidophilus (CUL60 and CUL21), Bifidobacterium animalis subsp. lactis CUL34 and B. bifidum CUL20*
- *L. rhamnosus, E. faecium, L. acidophilus and L. plantarum.*

Are probiotics safe to use?

Probiotics are usually considered safe for healthy people. Side effects may include mild gas and bloating. Despite this belief, potential side effects may be greater because probiotic use has not been systematically observed for its long-term impact. Risks are greater in people who are immunocompromised, have certain bowel problems or have other health problems. A recent review (2018) found inadequate or missing reporting of side effects. In fact, only 9 of 384 trials appropriately reported side effects according to the guidelines. Most of our knowledge about safety comes from studies of *Lactobacillus* and *Bifidobacterium*; less is known about other probiotics. Information on the long-term safety of probiotics is limited, and safety may differ from one type of probiotic to another.

Some recent evidence has been causing concern regarding the use of probiotic supplements. Two recent studies (2018) published in Cell have raised some questions on the benefits of using probiotic supplements. The first study emphasized individual variation in response to probiotic use and that more studies are needed to tailor specific strains based on individual responses to specific medical problems. The second study found that probiotic supplements (11 strains, including *Lactobacillus* and *Bifidobacterium*) taken after a course of antibiotic therapy actually delayed the restoration of normal bacteria balance in the gut for as long as five months. While results from such studies are significant to bear in mind, these were small studies that had tested a single probiotic product and were limited due to a lack of clinical endpoints because they were assessing microbiome changes but were not reflected in symptom changes. The studies have raised concerns; however, more work is needed to assess how microbiome changes affect symptoms. Nonetheless, there are plenty of trials that have shown that some (but not all) probiotics work well on some conditions, so work is needed to further evaluate probiotic use.

Probiotic Resources

- WGO Practice Guideline on Probiotics and Prebiotics

http://www.worldgastroenterology.org

- The International Scientific Association for Probiotics and Prebiotics (ISAPP) is a non-profit organization dedicated to promoting the science behind **probiotics** and **prebiotics**.

http://isappscience.org

- European Society of Primary Care Gastroenterology Consensus Guidelines on Probiotics

http://espcg.eu/wpcontent/uploads/2013/09/ENGLISHLEAFLET-ESPCG-2013

- Clinical Guide to Probiotic Supplements Available in the United States and Canada

http://usprobioticguide.com

http://www.probioticchart.ca

Chapter 7:
The Health Benefits of Fermented Foods

Fermented Foods: Should You Believe the Hype?

Fermented foods have been receiving much well-deserved attention lately.

Fermentation is the process by which microorganisms, such as bacteria and yeast, convert sugars in the absence of oxygen into acids, alcohol and carbon dioxide. Fermented foods have a reduced risk of contamination because the acids and alcohol produced from the fermentation process have antimicrobial properties. This process has been used for thousands of years as a biological way to preserve foods.

Many types of bacteria, including *Lactobacillus, Strepto-coccus, Enterococcus, Lactococcus* and *Bifidobacterium,* are called lactic acid bacteria (LAB) because they convert sugar or other carbohydrates to lactic acid. The lactic acid produced gives a sour taste to foods such as pickled cucumbers, kimchi and yogurt.

Furthermore, yeast fermentation produces alcohol and carbon dioxide. Different strains of saccharomyces cerevisiae yeast are used to produce alcohol in wine and beer, as well as to make bread dough rise as carbon dioxide gas is formed in the dough. This combination of bacteria and yeast is used in the production of many fermented foods, such as wine, sour beer and kombucha. Because there are thousands of possible microorganism combinations, many different types of fermented products can be made.

The health benefits of fermented foods are immense. Fermented foods can promote health due to beneficial changes to the original food, the synthesis of important metabolites and proteins, and the delivery of important living microorganisms to the gut.

Clinical studies have shown that consuming fermented foods helps with weight maintenance and reduces the risk of cardiovascular disease and type 2 diabetes. Furthermore, eating yogurt has been linked with reduced total mortality, while consuming fermented milk has led to improved glucose metabolism and reduced muscle soreness. Additionally, studies have determined that kimchi possesses anti-diabetes and anti-obesity benefits.

Fermented foods may also help with autoimmune conditions and alter mood and brain activity. However, ample clinical data on these findings are not available at this point.

In terms of the role of fermented foods and gastrointestinal health, one study found that the consumption of fermented milk improved IBS symptoms, possibly due to the beneficial changes in gut bacteria facilitated by the fermented foods. Furthermore, these types of foods helped relieve diarrhea and restore gastrointestinal balance, particularly in people taking antibiotics.

The most important benefit of fermented foods comes from the delivery of probiotics to the gastrointestinal tract. A fully hygienic modern diet and lifestyle can have a negative effect on our gut microorganisms. This imbalance between good and bad organisms can lead to various health problems. Fermented foods can fill in the gap by replenishing gut microorganisms and recalibrating your gut.

Although the greatest benefits of fermented foods come from delivering live microorganisms into the gastrointestinal tract, there are other ways in which these foods may benefit individuals. The process of fermentation has the following benefits:

- It boosts the nutritional value of certain foods by allowing nutrients to be better absorbed and used by the body, by producing many health-promoting active compounds, and by producing a variety of B vitamins in foods. For example, by eating fermented foods, vegetarians can obtain vitamin B12, which is otherwise absent from plant foods.
- It resynthesizes some of the folate destroyed by heat during milk pasteurization and makes milk products more digestible as microbes digest lactose and break down milk proteins.
- It degrades part of the gluten protein complex due to the combination of sourdough bacteria and enzymes.
- It produces bioactive compounds with potential benefits against inflammation and for an immune or glycemic response.

- It converts unsaturated fatty acids to conjugated linoleic acid, which has anti-inflammatory and antioxidant properties.
- It improves the polyphenol and vitamin content and decreases the amount of caffeine in tea.
- It removes or reduces toxic chemicals or antinutrients, such as phytic acid, in foods.
- It produces the neurotransmitter gamma-aminobutyric acid (GABA), which may help reduce anxiety.
- It enhances the extraction of antioxidant phenolic compounds from grapes in winemaking. It also improves shelf life and enhances food safety by inhibiting the growth of foodborne pathogens and degrading toxins, such as aflatoxin.
- It creates desirable tastes and textures in food and converts inedible products into edible products, as in the case of olives, in which the bitter tasting phenolic compounds are removed in fermentation.

Furthermore, an interesting study using mice showed a decrease in colitis in those fed on milk with *Lactobacillus casei BL23* bacteria versus mice fed on the same strain of bacteria but incubated in nonnutritive buffer. Lastly, the probiotic properties of fermented foods can maintain gut barrier function and produce organic acids that nourish the cells of the colon and improve gut health.

Are fermented foods the same as probiotics?

For fermented foods to be considered probiotic, they need to still maintain adequate levels of live microbes, which have been shown to have a health benefit. Not all fermented foods can meet those criteria, and not all fermented foods have live cultures. For instance, although cheese is fermented, it is not the same as yogurt. Cheese typically does not have live cultures.

Fermented foods such as yogurt, sauerkraut, kimchi, and kefir can have live bacteria in the numbers of 1 million to 1 billion cells/gram or millimeter of food, and interestingly enough, even after the food is consumed, a large amount of those bacteria manage to survive going through the gut. The ingestion of fermented foods could potentially increase the microbiota in the gut by up to 1000 times and may be able to offset the negative impact of the modern diet on the microbiota.

Be aware of the following to ensure that fermented foods contain live cultures:

- Consume foods that were fermented using natural processes.

- Avoid jars of pickles that were pickled using vinegar and not by the natural fermentation process of using live organisms. These products do not contain probiotics.

- Look for the words "naturally fermented" on the label.

- Look for bubbles in the liquid, which indicates that live organisms are present producing gas that forms the bubbles.

It appears that the health benefits of specific probiotic cultures can be allotted to a species rather than to a strain, or that this principle at least applies to some species of lactobacillus. For example, organisms in sauerkraut, kimchi and other fermented foods are often closely related, even to the species level, to organisms that have been reported to have probiotic functions. However, certain clinical benefits, such as a particular immune effect, may be more strain-specific.

Are there any worries about consuming fermented foods? Weighing benefits versus risks

The dietary importance of fermented foods on health has been noted in various studies. For the time being, however, we need more randomized controlled trials on fermented foods to better understand the health benefits associated with their consumption and to show a clear cause and effect between eating fermented foods and improved health.

More studies are also required to show any side effects and any risks involved with the consumption of fermented foods. For example, certain microorganisms associated with pickled foods can convert nitrates and nitrites to N-nitroso compounds (NOCs), which may be carcinogenic; however, more experimental work is needed to establish a strong effect.

Important Probiotic Species in Yummy Fermented Foods

> ### *Yogurt*
> - *Bifidobacterium infantis*
> - *Bifidobacterium bifidum*
> - *Lactobacillus acidophilus*
> - *Lactobacillus bulgaricus*
> - *Streptococcus thermophilus*
> - *Lactobacillus helveticus (in certain yogurts)*
> - *Bifidobacterium longum (in certain yogurts)*
> - *Lactobacillus casei*
> - *Lactobacillus delbrueckii ssp. bulgaricus*

> ### Nondairy yogurt
> - *Lactobacillus casei*

> ### Fermented milks
> - *Lactobacillus delbrueckii ssp. bulgaricus*
> - *Streptococcus thermophilus*
> - *Lactobacillus casei*
> - *Lactobacillus acidophilus*
> - *Lactobacillus rhamnosus*
> - *Lactobacillus johnsonii*

> ### Low-fat cheddar cheese
> - *Lactobacillus casei*

> ### Cheese (Mesophilic starter)
> - *Lactobacillus lactis ssp. lactis*
> - *Lactobacillus lactis ssp. cremoris*
> - *Lactobacillus lactis ssp. lactis var. diacetylactis*
> - *Leuconostoc mesenteroides ssp. cremoris*

> ### Cheese (Thermophilic starter)
> - *Streptococcus thermoplillus*

- *Lactobacillus delbrueckii ssp. Bulgaricus*
- *Lactobacillus helveticus*
- *Lactobacillus delbrueckii ssp. lactis*

Cheeses (Mixed starter)

- *Lactobacillus lactis ssp. lactis*
- *Lactobacillus lactis ssp. cremoris*
- *Streptococcus thermoplillus*

Kefir

- *Lactobacillus helveticus*
- *Bifidobacterium longum*
- *Lactobacillus rhamnosus GG*
- *Lactobacillus casei*
- *Bifidobacterium bifidum*
- *Lactobacillus kefir*
- *Lactobacillus kefiranofacies*
- *Lactobacillus brevis*
- *Lactobacillus plantarum*
- *Lactobacillus paracasei spp. paracasei*
- *Lactobacillus lactis spp. lactis*
- *Leuconostoc mesenteroides*

Green olives

- *Lactobacillus plantarum*

Pickled olives

- *Lactobacillus brevis*
- *Lactobacillus plantarum*
- *Lactobacillus pentosus*

Pickles

- *Bifidobacterium bifidum*

Pickled cucumber

- *Lactobacillus brevis*
- *Lactobacillus plantarum*
- *Lactobacillus pentosus*
- *Lactobacillus acidophilus*
- *Lactobacillus fermentum*
- *Leuconostoc mesenteroides*

Sauerkraut (fermented cabbage)

- *Lactobacillus brevis*
- *Lactobacillus fermentum*
- *Lactobacillus plantarum*
- *Leuconostoc mesenteroides*

Fermented vegetables

- *Lactobacillus plantarum*
- *Lactobacillus reuteri*

Sourdough

- *Lactobacillus sanfransiscensis*
- *Lactobacillus farcimini*
- *Lactobacillus fermentum*
- *Lactobacillus brevis*
- *Lactobacillus plantarum*
- *Lactobacillus amylovorus*
- *Lactobacillus reuteri*
- *Lactobacillus pontis*
- *Lactobacillus panis*
- *Lactobacillus alimentarius*
- *Weissella cibaria*

Kimchi

- *Bifidobacterium bifidum*
- *Leuconostoc mesenteroides*
- *Lactobacillus plantarum*

- *W. kimchii sp. nov*
- *Lactobacillus kimchi*
- *Lactobacillus sakei*
- *Weissella koreensis*

Miso

- *Lactobacillus acidophilus*
- *Bifidobacterium bifidum*

Tempeh

- *Lactobacillus acidophilus*
- *Bifidobacterium bifidum*

Some wines and vinegars

- *Bifidobacterium bifidum*

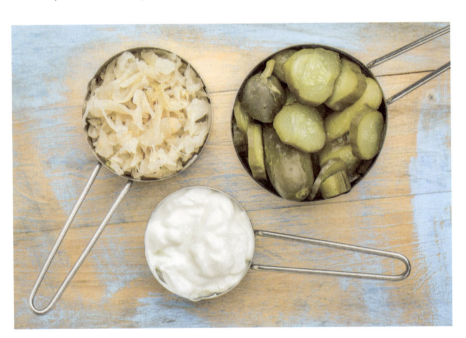

Chapter 8:
Other Natural Ways to Help Alleviate Symptoms

Digestive Enzyme Supplements

As you saw in section 1 of this book, people who lack specific digestive enzymes cannot digest their food properly, have issues with malabsorption and therefore suffer from consequential symptoms such as bloating, abdominal pain, gas, diarrhea or constipation. Digestive enzyme supplements that would take over the job of the missing enzymes could be useful for people suffering from digestive disorders. Although there have been studies on digestive enzyme supplements, it should be noted that more evidence is still required on how effective such supplements can be.

It is recommended that digestive enzyme supplements are not consumed during the elimination phase of the low FODMAP diet. Furthermore, during the reintroduction phase of the diet, we need to know which FODMAPs result in symptoms when consumed and in which doses they can be tolerated. Therefore, the use of enzyme supplements during that time could eliminate symptoms and would not allow us to gather the full picture of which FODMAP groups a patient can tolerate and in which proportions.

Digestive enzyme supplements could potentially be useful after the elimination and reintroduction phase of the low FODMAP diet, but one should always take such supplements after consultation with a doctor and/or clinical dietitian. Possible useful digestive enzyme supplements are as follows:

Lactase enzyme (β-galactosidase). This enzyme helps in the digestion of lactose to form galactose and glucose so that they can be easily absorbed. These enzymes have been used for a while, and they have been shown to work in people with mild to medium lactose intolerance, even though recent reviews still question the existence of convincing evidence of their efficacy. The efficacy of the lactase supplement is short-lived, so it should be taken 5-30 minutes before eating the lactose-containing meal.

Recently, research has suggested the use of a combination of specific probiotic strains for lactose intolerance. Specifically, *Lactobacillus* and *Bifidobacterium* have been shown to help with lactose intolerance in both preclinical and clinical studies because these bacteria have β-galactosidase activity, which helps in the digestion of some of the lactose in the human gut. This evidence shows the potential for probiotics and probiotic-containing foods to decrease the symptoms of lactose intolerance in patients.

Alpha-galactosidase (also called Beano). This enzyme helps to breakdown GOS (oligosaccharides) because most of the us lack the enzymes in our bodies. The Monash FODMAP group recently published a study and recommends the use of alpha-galactosidase to help people with IBS tolerate GOS-containing foods. Evidence from their study showed that the enzymes should be consumed with food (half of a dose immediately before the meal and half during the meal) to ensure effectiveness. Enzyme supplementation helped with a significant decrease in abdominal symptoms such as pain, bloating and general IBS symptoms.

Xylose isomerase. This enzyme can help convert excess fructose to glucose for those people suffering from the excess fructose part of the FODMAPs, even though much more research and evidence are required to show it if it can help with a significant reduction in IBS symptoms related to excess fructose.

Pancrealipase. This enzyme will facilitate the breakdown of fat into smaller molecules. Fat is a common culprit of gastrointestinal symptoms such as bloating, gas, cramping and urgent diarrhea, and many people suffering from IBS have tummy troubles after they consume foods with high fat content. Fat is not a FODMAP; however, enzymes to break it down might help people with IBS-D.

It is important to look at the ingredients in the package in order to make sure that there are no hidden FODMAP ingredients in the supplement that would cause abdominal symptoms. There are many different forms of over-the-counter digestive enzymes that are available and mostly considered safe, but always choose well-known brands with a good history and reputation because supplements are not as strictly regulated by the Food and Drug Administration as other medicines are.

Always take the supplements with food. When using supplements for IBS, some studies have shown decreased IBS symptoms if the supplement is taken either shortly before or at mealtimes.

Exercise

Frequent and moderate exercise helps with IBS symptoms. Be active one way or another every day. One randomized controlled study showed improvements in symptoms with exercise, particularly among individuals who suffer from IBS-C. In general, moderate exercise is highly recommended for symptom management and overall health. Take a walk after lunch or dinner, or take a morning or afternoon stroll to unwind. Use your bike instead of car to get to short distances. Sign up for a yoga, dancing, or water aerobics class to get your heart pumping. Play group sports, get out and walk in a park or go for a hike with friends and family and forget about any stress or worries. However, be careful with intense exercise, which may have negative effects and make symptoms worse. For example, runners are often affected by increased gut motility and runner's diarrhea due to the intensity of their sport.

Yoga has recently received much attention for its positive effect on IBS symptom management. A recent randomized study used 59 IBS patients placed on either the low FODMAP diet or a yoga regimen twice a week for 12 weeks. The results showed that yoga alone (with no changes in diet) was equally as effective as the low FODMAP diet, with 82% of the patients in the yoga group saying that their symptoms had seriously improved.

Teas (Ginger and Turmeric)

Ginger can calm spasms in the gut as well as nausea. Ginger root extract in preliminary studies has been shown to be effective in reducing intestinal inflammation markers, which may contribute to a decreased risk of colon cancer and therefore may inhibit microscopic inflammation in IBS. However, more studies are needed to further investigate these initial findings and applications in IBS and IBD.

You can cut a small piece or a few thin slices of fresh ginger root and infuse it in boiling water to make a tea.

The same applies for **turmeric**, which has anti-inflammatory properties and can ease stomach pain and flatulence, even though research on the benefits of symptom management is still limited.

Peppermint oil

Peppermint oil is an essential oil and provides a natural way to help manage IBS symptoms. The findings show that enteric-coated peppermint oil capsules help to decrease pain and bloating, diarrhea and flatulence and manage flareups. Peppermint is an antispasmodic, so it helps the muscles of the gut to relax. It can also affect the microbiota in the gut and control the frequency of stools and immunity and inflammation in the gut, which is particularly important for IBS-D.

In a double-blind placebo-controlled study of 90 IBS patients who took enteric-coated peppermint, their pain and quality of life significantly improved. Furthermore, a literature search evaluating the efficacy of peppermint oil in IBS or abdominal pain in children revealed that in 8 out of 12 placebo-controlled studies, peppermint oil showed greater symptom improvement than did the placebo. Finally, in the most inclusive meta-analysis to date published in 2019, peppermint oil was shown to be a safe and effective therapy for pain and symptom relief in adults with IBS.

When taking the peppermint oil pill, take it at least 30 minutes before your meal. If you find that it causes a burning sensation when you go to the bathroom, then decrease the dose. Compared to those who take other spasmodics, people who supplement with peppermint oil tend to have fewer adverse effects.

Apply heat when bloated or in pain. Heat applied via microwave heating pads, hot water bottles or chemical pads can help with symptoms. When heat is applied, the heat receptors are switched on, which block the pain receptors so that pain is no longer perceived. The relief will probably be short-lived and occur only when the heat is applied, but it will definitely make you feel better.

Become a squatter when using the bathroom, as it helps with proper stool movement and reduces straining.

Address the mind-body connection

Stress affects the brain, which in turn borrows energy from the gut and initiates some distinct GI effects: reduced blood flow to the intestines, decreased mucus production, reduced movement of food through the GI tract and increased gastrointestinal sensitivity. All of these can trigger abdominal pain, bloating and stool changes.

There is no argument that behavioral therapies work for functional gastrointestinal disorders. Importantly, we see that gastroenterologists recommend such therapies without hesitation to their patients as adjunct therapy to manage IBS symptoms. Cognitive behavioral therapy is very person-specific and tailor-made to identify and work on the specific patient's needs. The purpose of cognitive behavioral therapy is to find ways to change the type of thinking and behavior of the patient, which may have a negative impact on the way the person feels. Cognitive behavioral therapy and gut-directed hypnosis aim to reduce stress in certain patients. This type of stress management helps reduce the psychological issues that impact our physical well-being. Relaxation techniques, meditation and the practice of mindfulness (i.e., training the mind to focus on the present moment) are also important.

Gut-directed hypnotherapy has been used in randomized controlled trials, which have shown its high effectiveness. Basically, with hypnosis, the therapist works with the subconscious mind, which is a normal state of mind, to determine where the emotional issue originates. That way, once the root cause is identified, the hypnotherapist and patient work to initiate mind changes that will produce the best and most long-lasting results.

A recent randomized clinical study compared the short- and long-term effectiveness of gut-directed hypnotherapy versus the low FODMAP diet. Seventy-four patients were randomly placed in one of three groups: hypnotherapy, low FODMAP diet or both. The scientists concluded that gut-directed hypnotherapy provided similar efficacy to the low FODMAP diet in the duration of relief from gastrointestinal symptoms. When hypnotherapy and the low FODMAP diet were combined, however, there was no additive effect.

Meditation can help address stress. Try a meditation session or a meditation app on your phone or computer. Dedicate a few minutes per day to this activity and other forms of self-care. Take some deep belly breaths. Place one hand on your chest and the other one on your belly and feel how each moves up and down when you inhale and exhale deeply.

The practice of mindfulness trains the mind to focus on the present moment, which is important because it forces us to forget about stressful situations and to dwell only on the present moment.

Chapter 9:
Action Plan

Putting the low FODMAP diet into Practice

The low FODMAP diet was designed to be administered by a registered clinical dietitian or nutritionist who is trained in the diet to ensure the success of the nutritional therapy.

The diet is very restrictive, especially during the elimination phase, and unless you eat a great variety of low FODMAP foods, your nutrition can become compromised very easily. This is especially important if you have limitations in your diet due to other medically prescribed therapies or if you follow a vegan or vegetarian diet. A clinical dietitian/nutritionist will help you develop a meal plan tailored to your needs to ensure that you consume all the nutrients that your body needs. A dietitian can also tailor your diet based on the severity of your symptoms and determine how strict you need to be.

Children and the low FODMAP diet

Although much research supports the use of a low FODMAP diet in adults with IBS, very little research has been conducted in children. A recent study is promising, suggesting that a low FODMAP diet may improve IBS symptom control in children, but more research is needed to confirm these results.

If children are subjected to a restricted diet, such as the low FODMAP diet, this process must be supervised by a specialized clinical pediatric dietitian, as restricted diets can have negative consequences in growing children, such as food fears, nutritional inadequacies and possible eating disorders.

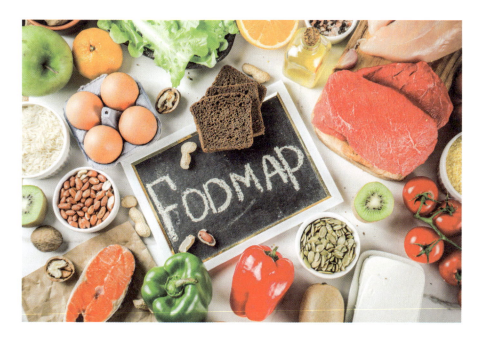

Vegans/Vegetarians

The low FODMAP diet can be challenging for most vegans and vegetarians because many vegan and vegetarian staples are also high FODMAP foods, such as beans and many soy products. Expert advice and guidance is very important to ensure a nutritionally adequate diet.

Prepare for your appointment with the registered dietitian/nutritionist

Keep a Food and Symptom Diary

Once all tests have been carried out and medical issues have been excluded, we advise keeping a food diary. Keeping a food diary for at least two weeks will help your dietitian or medical provider determine which foods and food combinations bother you, as well as how frequently you have symptoms.

Keeping a food diary is an effective way of identifying which foods trigger your gastrointestinal symptoms. It requires some discipline, but your belly will thank you at the end of the day. Remember that the more entries you add to your food diary, the easier it will be to determine the exact foods that bother you. You can use this insert as your guideline.

In your diary, record the following:

- What you eat and drink, as well as the amounts, in detail.
- What times you eat the food and where you are (e.g., home, office, restaurant, on the go).
- Your symptoms in detail; these can be bloating, gas, pain, headaches, diarrhea, constipation, urgency, and changes in energy levels.

DAY	MEAL DESCRIPTION	SYMPTOMS
Breakfast		
Snack		
Lunch		
Snack		
Dinner		
Snack		

You can print a template for a full week of the food and symptoms diary from our website:

http://www.digestivenc.com/en/resources/54-weekly food-symptoms-diary.html

Consider these first steps to help tame your digestive distress

When you are suffering from digestive issues, it is helpful to consider a number of simple steps you can take to help alleviate symptoms of bloating, gas, belly aches, diarrhea or constipation. Follow these dietary and lifestyle recommendations as your first line of change towards gut health and symptom relief.

- Eat your food slowly. Eating too fast and not chewing well can cause air swallowing, which can lead to **bloating** and discomfort.
- If spicy foods seem to bother you and cause symptoms, we propose that

you minimize their intake and see if that helps alleviate the symptoms.

- Caffeine is a gut stimulant affecting gut motility. If you find that caffeine consumption is associated with your symptoms, reduce caffeine intake.
- Avoid alcohol if it poses a gut trigger for you. Alcohol is known to affect gut motility and acid secretion in the gut.
- Avoid fried or very fatty foods, which can cause dyspepsia, abdominal pain, bloating, gas and diarrhea.
- Keep in mind that carbonated drinks and drinking with a straw can lead to bloating.
- Drink water to stay hydrated but also to facilitate digestion and help food move easily and readily through your gut. Aim for 1.5-3 L a day of fluid intake, preferably water.
- Add some fermented foods, such as lactose-free yogurt, lactose-free kefir, tempeh, pickles and olives in brine.
- If you find that milk and dairy products bother you, try following a low lactose diet to see if symptoms are reduced. Just make sure you compensate with other sources of calcium to avoid calcium deficiencies.
- Eat your food mindfully, avoiding distractions from the phone, computer or social media and making sure to devote sufficient time so you can enjoy your food and start the digestion process correctly.
- Avoid wearing tight clothing that can make you feel more uncomfortable when bloated.
- Avoid eating heavily processed foods that contain gut-irritating food chemicals, additives and emulsifiers. Instead, choose whole-grain, whole-food options and always aim to eat a variety of whole foods.
- Avoid snacking continuously throughout the day. Instead, allow for 3-4 hours between meals for cleansing to take place in the intestines. When we are not eating, the intestines undergo a repetitive cleaning wave called the migrating motor complex. This process ensures that the intestines are clean before the next load of food comes along. Without this cleaning wave, microbes, toxins and food would not move along and would accumulate in the area. Do not graze or eat throughout the day.

> **!** If symptoms still remain after these general dietary principles have been followed, then the low FODMAP diet can be implemented, but only for a short period of time.

The low FODMAP diet

It is so exciting to see a diet plan that works and brings relief to such a large proportion of patients whose lives are hindered by gut issues. The low FODMAP diet is science-based and scientifically backed and has been shown to work for 50-80% of people suffering from IBS. It was developed approximately 10 years ago by researchers at Monash University in Melbourne, Australia, where foods were analyzed and identified based on their FODMAP content.

We know that FODMAPs can cause bloating and other gut symptoms in patients. To comprehend the impact of FODMAPs, the University of Michigan team created the bucket concept, in which our guts are compared to a bucket into which FODMAPs are dumped while the body tries to digest and absorb them. If there are too many FODMAPs or if they fill the bucket too quickly, the body may not be able to digest and absorb them quickly enough, so they accumulate over time and cause symptoms. Some buckets are large, and some buckets are small, based on the amount of FODMAPs each person can handle at a time. The idea of the FODMAP diet is to first eliminate the FODMAPs and empty our buckets and then start reintroducing them slowly. This process is ideally performed under the supervision of a trained registered dietitian.

The diet consists of three distinct steps.

Step 1: The elimination phase
The first step involves strict adherence to the low FODMAP diet, usually for a period of 2 to 6 weeks, to improve symptoms and identify whether the diet works on the patient.

Step 2: The reintroduction phase
The elimination phase is followed by a 6- to 10-week reintroduction phase, in which FODMAP foods are rechallenged and then reintroduced into the diet on a sequential and patient-by-patient basis, depending on each patient's response.

Step 3: The personalization and maintenance phase
This phase considers the variation in the quantities and types of FODMAP-containing foods that each patient can eat.

With respect to the bucket analogy, the elimination phase cleans the bucket and allows our gut to calm down, while the reintroduction phase slowly introduces one type of FODMAP at time back into our system. This process allows us to determine which FODMAPs and what amount of the FODMAP our bodies can handle. The final phase then allows us to customize our bucket accordingly, given our knowledge of which foods we can and cannot eat, as well as the quantities that our body can tolerate. This is very personal and patient-specific.

This plan does, in fact, work. As you know, both of us suffer from GI symptoms and we have tried the diet and found immense symptom relief. You can actually start having relief immediately after cutting down on FODMAPs. Some people need more time, some people less time, and each person's body will respond to the diet differently. However, clinical and research evidence shows that results can be seen even within a week of being on the diet. So, go ahead and give it a try!

Remember, the low FODMAP diet is Not a forever diet

Of course, we all know that following this type of diet, especially in its elimination phase, requires tremendous effort and dedication, given all the temptations. However, the elimination phase is short in duration, and it is very important to move away from this phase after 2-6 weeks to include a variety of foods in the diet, increase one's chances of sticking with the diet, and decrease the effects of the diet on the gut microbiome. This process is very important, even for individuals who experience a significant reduction in their symptoms and who may be reluctant to give up the low FODMAP elimination diet. Studies have shown that the restrictive diet has an impact on gut microbiota, although its long-term impact on health has not yet been determined. Long-term FODMAP elimination is very restrictive, unnecessary and often difficult to maintain. Hence, the individual's diet during the personalization phase should be both healthy and varied and be as similar as possible to what would be considered a 'normal' diet. It should be rich in fiber and balanced so that it will promote gut health while minimizing unpleasant gut symptoms.

The low FODMAP diet is Not a No FODMAP diet

The low FODMAP diet does not mean no FODMAPs at all. This means that many of the FODMAP-containing foods are removed from the diet to minimize gut symptoms. You will remove high FODMAP foods from your diet during the elimination phase of the diet, but this removal will be temporary, and high FODMAP foods will then be reintroduced in small quantities in the second phase of the diet. Follow our lists of high and low FODMAP foods, as well as Monash University's app on your phone or tablet, to determine which foods are high and low in FODMAPs and the quantities that are acceptable in the low FODMAP diet. The low FODMAP thresholds assigned allow people to engage in food stacking, or having more than one serving of different low FODMAP foods in one meal. The lists will help you with your grocery shopping, cooking and navigation of restaurant menus when eating out.

Over time, you may notice that the lists of acceptable low FODMAP foods or their green serving portions change slightly, as the Monash app is updated quite regularly. Do not fret! After all, the diet is not a FODMAP-free diet but is instead a low FODMAP diet, and even with these small changes, the principal idea of reducing FODMAPS is still the basis of the diet, and the diet works!

High FODMAP Foods
Fruits
Apples, apricots, blackberries, boysenberries, pears, peaches, plums, prunes, currants, dates, figs, nectarines, cherries, mangos, tamarillos, watermelons, feijoas, unripe guavas, goji berries, lychees, persimmons, pomegranates, dried fruit
Vegetables
Artichoke (globe and Jerusalem), asparagus, beetroot, broccoli (stalks only), cabbage (savoy), cauliflower, chayote, chicory root, sugar snap peas, garlic, leeks, onions (red, white, Spanish, shallots), spring onions (white part), sweet corn, mushrooms, karelas, peas, taro, yucca root
Legumes, Tofu and Seeds
Black beans, red kidney beans, navy beans, lima beans, butter beans, chickpeas, fava beans, mung beans, split peas, soybeans (soy flour, soymilk and other products made with whole soybeans), silken tofu

Nuts
Pistachios, cashews

Grains
Rye, wheat (bulgur, couscous, semolina), barley, emmer (farro), freekeh, kamut, spelt, einkorn

Flours
Amaranth, barley, einkorn, emmer (farro), coconut, wheat, kamut, spelt, rye

Bread, cereals and pasta
Breads, cereal and pasta made with amaranth, barley, rye, wheat, emmer (farro), freekeh, kamut, spelt, einkorn
Naan or roti bread
Oatmeal bread
Gnocchi
Noodles (egg noodles, hokkein, udon pot noodles, supernoodles, ramen)
Granola, muesli, fine oatmeal
Flakes (of wheat, corn, rice, and oats) with dried fruits and nuts
Rice crisps

Dairy and Alternatives
Milk (cow's, goat's), A2 milk, yogurt, buttermilk, custard, kefir, coconut milk, oat milk, soymilk (soybeans)

Sweeteners
Agave, honey, high-fructose corn syrup, sorbitol, mannitol, maltitol, isomalt, xylitol

Other
Ketchup and pasta sauce (containing garlic and onion), onion and garlic (salt, dried, powders and extracts), stocks, stock cubes, ready meals, gravy, dressings, breaded fish and poultry, tempura batter, biscuits, crackers, cakes, pastry goods Sugar-free items: desserts, gum, supplements and medications

Ingredients to avoid

Fructose, fructose syrup, glucose-fructose syrup, fructose-glucose syrup, high-fructose corn syrup, high-fructose corn syrup solids, fruit juice concentrate, fructo-oligosaccharides (FOS), inulin, oligofructose, chicory root

 Note: Garlic and onion are often used in foods and are labeled as flavor and natural flavor.

Drinks

Teas (chai, oolong, fennel, dandelion, chamomile and strong black tea, strong herbal tea)

Alcohol

Rum, dessert wine

Reference: Monash University (booklet, low FODMAP App, website blog), Kings College (booklet, low FODMAP App), published studies, USDA nutrient database.

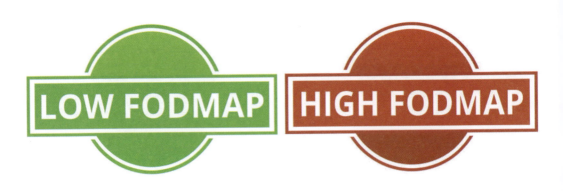

Low FODMAP Foods

 Use the Monash FODMAP app for serving recommendations that are low FODMAP (green-light servings).

Fruits

A maximum of 1 serving of fruit per meal

1 unripe banana, blueberries (<30 berries), breadfruit, clementine, dragon fruit, grapes, kiwifruit, kumquats, lemons, limes, oranges, mandarins, passion fruit, papayas, pineapples, raspberries (<30 berries), rhubarb, star fruit, strawberries

Vegetables

Arugula, alfalfa, bamboo shoots, bean sprouts, bok choy, broccoli (whole and heads only), celeriac, Chinese cabbage, carrot, choy sum, cucumber, collard greens, cabbage (common, red), eggplant, endive, green beans, ginger, kale, kohlrabi, lettuce (butter, iceberg, radicchio, red coral), plantain, canned pumpkin, Japanese pumpkin, parsnip, pepper (red), potato, radish, rutabaga, scallion (green part only), sweet potato, chicory leaves, snake beans, spinach, Swiss chard, squash, tomato, turnip, water chestnut, yam, olives (black, green), seaweed (nori), silverbeet, spaghetti squash, oyster mushrooms

Grains and Pasta

Rice, rice bran, buckwheat groats, millet, polenta, quinoa, teff, sorghum

Rice noodles, buckwheat noodles

Wheat-free or gluten-free pasta

Quinoa pasta

Cereals

Buckwheat groats (cooked)

Flakes of corn (gluten-free)

Quinoa flakes

Rice flakes

Oatmeal (coarse)

Whole-grain oat cereal biscuits

Oats (rolled)

Oats (UK)

Oat bran

Oat groats

Bread

Wheat-free and gluten-free bread (check the ingredients)

Wheat-free and gluten-free pizza base, pita bread, naan bread (check the ingredients)

100% sourdough spelt bread

Bread made from rice, corn, potato, millet, buckwheat, tapioca flours

Corn tortillas

Millet bread

Flour

Wheat-free or gluten-free flour

Arrowroot flour, buckwheat flour, corn flour, green banana flour, maize flour, millet flour, polenta, potato flour, pounded yam flour, rice flour, sorghum flour, teff flour

Baking

Baking powder, bicarbonate of soda, cream of tartar

Legumes and Tofu

Tofu (firm)

Tofu (plain)

Tempeh (plain)

Mung beans (sprouted)

Urid dal (boiled)

Edamame (frozen)

Nuts
Brazil nuts, chestnuts, peanuts, pecans, pine nuts, tigernuts, walnuts, macadamias Peanut butter
Seeds
Chia seeds, hemp seeds, poppy seeds, sesame seeds, sunflower seeds, pumpkin seeds
Protein
Chicken, fish, beef, egg, seafood, pork, turkey
Spices
Allspice, cardamom, chili powder, cinnamon, clove, coriander seeds, cumin, curry powder, fennel seeds, fenugreek seeds, five spice, mustard seeds, nutmeg, oregano, paprika, pepper (black), saffron, anise, thyme, turmeric
Herbs
Basil, bay leaves, cilantro, coriander, curry leaves, fenugreek leaves, kaffir lime leaves, lemongrass, mint, parsley, rosemary, sage, tarragon, thyme, watercress
Plant-based dairy alternatives
Almond milk, rice milk, soy milk (protein)
Dairy
Lactose-free ice cream, lactose-free milk, lactose-free yogurt
Cheese
Brie, Camembert, lactose-free cottage cheese, feta, Havarti, haloumi, mozzarella, pecorino, cheddar, colby, Swiss
Beverages
Coffee, diet soda, sucrose-sweetened soda Tea (except chai, oolong, fennel, dandelion, chamomile and strong black tea, strong herbal tea)

Sweeteners
Artificial sweeteners not ending in 'ol', aspartame, sugar, glucose, maple syrup (pure), Stevia

Other
Olive oil, baking powder, baking soda, vanilla essence, barbeque and tomato sauce without onion, garlic or other high FODMAP ingredients, Dijon mustard, tamarind paste, agar agar, egg replacer

Reference: Monash University (booklet, low FODMAP App, website blog), Kings College (booklet, low FODMAP App), published studies, USDA nutrient database.

Lactose is a FODMAP.
Are You Lactose Intolerant? Do You Have Any Symptoms Soon after Consuming Milk or Dairy Products?

Being lactose intolerant means your body is unable to digest lactose, a type of sugar primarily found in milk and dairy products. This means that your body has a shortage or a deficiency of an enzyme called lactase.

Lactase is needed for the breakdown of lactose into two simple forms of sugar—glucose and galactose—which can be easily absorbed into the bloodstream.

Following the consumption of lactose, individuals with lactose intolerance may experience flatulence, diarrhea, a bloated stomach, stomach cramps, pains and nausea. These symptoms typically start to develop 30 minutes to 2 hours after the lactose is consumed.

There are three types of lactose intolerance:

(a) Primary lactose intolerance

This is the most common type of lactose intolerance. As people age, their bodies produce lower quantities of lactase enzyme, and symptoms start to develop. Usually, this occurs after the age of two, although the symptoms are only noticeable in adulthood.

This type of lactose intolerance is caused by an inherited genetic mutation that runs in the family. It affects 65% of the human population, being most common in East Asia, where it affects more than 90% of the adult population, and in people of West African, Arab, Jewish, Greek, and Italian descent. Furthermore, lactose intolerance has the lowest prevalence in populations with a long history of dependence on milk products as an important food source.

(b) Secondary lactose intolerance

This type of lactose intolerance occurs when the small intestine decreases lactase production after an illness, injury or surgery involving the small intestine. It can occur at any age.

Possible causes are gastroenteritis, inflammatory bowel disease, celiac disease, chemotherapy or the long-term use of antibiotics. It can be only temporary but may become permanent if its cause is a long-term condition. This condition can also occur as people age and as the body's ability to produce lactase decreases.

(c) Congenital or developmental lactose intolerance

This condition is a rare genetic disorder in which little or no lactase is produced from birth.

Do not confuse a milk allergy with milk intolerance!

Milk allergy can potentially be life threatening because it involves the over-reaction of the immune system to a specific protein in the milk. When there is consumption of the specific food protein, the body can trigger an allergic reaction. Symptoms can vary from mild (rashes, hives, itching, swelling, etc.) to severe (trouble breathing, wheezing, loss of consciousness, etc.)

Ways to Manage Lactose Intolerance

The severity of symptoms depends on the individual, as people have different levels of tolerance. Some people may be able to tolerate small amounts of lactose without any symptoms, while others may not even be able to have a small amount. Finding the amount of lactose in milk products and how much can be tolerated requires some trial and error.

- Choose reduced-lactose milk and milk products
- Avoid consuming milk on an empty stomach
- Consume dairy options with less lactose
- Use over-the-counter pills or drops that contain the lactase enzyme

Common foods with lactose are milk, creams, ice creams, yogurt, soft cheeses and butter. Lactose may also be added to some canned, frozen, boxed and other prepared foods. Make sure to check the ingredient label. Look for these words that indicate that the product probably contains lactose: milk, cream, butter, milk solids, margarine, cheese, whey and curds. Additionally, watch out for 'nondairy' foods that contain sodium caseinate, which can be expressed as 'caseinate' or 'milk derivative' on the label and may contain low levels of lactose.

Note that the terms 'lactose-free' or 'lactose-reduced' are not the same and are not regulated by the US Food and Drug Administration (FDA). A lactose-reduced item may still contain lactose and could cause symptoms.

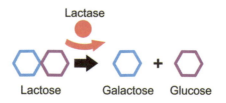

Lactose Content of Food

High Lactose

Food	Lactose Content
Evaporated milk (1 cup)	24 grams
Sweetened condensed milk (½ cup)	15 grams
Milk (3.3%, 2%, 1%, skim) (1 cup)	12-13 grams
Buttermilk (1 cup)	9 grams
Half-and-half (1 cup)	10 grams
Goat's milk (1 cup)	11 grams
Chocolate milk (1 cup)	10 grams
Coffee latte made with milk, 175 ml (¾ cup)	7 grams
Yogurt (Note: the cultures in yogurt help digest lactose), 180 grams (¾ cup)	8-14 grams
Pudding and custard made with milk (½ cup)	6 grams

Moderate Amount of Lactose

Food	Lactose Content
Frozen yogurt (½ cup)	4.5 grams
Ice cream (½ cup)	3-6 grams
Cottage cheese, 120 grams (½ cup)	3 grams
Greek yogurt, 180 grams (¾ cup)	5-6 grams

Low Lactose

Food	Lactose Content
Sour cream, 60 ml (¼ cup)	2 grams
Evaporated milk, 15 ml (1 tbsp)	1.5 grams
Cream cheese, 50 grams (1½ oz)	1.5 grams
Blue cheese, 50 grams (1½ oz)	1 gram
Butter, 5 ml (1 tsp)	Trace
Margarine, 5 ml (1 tsp)	Trace
Cheese slice (sharp cheddar, Parmesan, Swiss), 1 slice (1 oz)	Less than 1 gram
Mozzarella cheese, 30 grams	0.02 grams
Feta, 30 grams	1 gram
Haloumi, 30 grams	1 gram

Watch Your Calcium If You Are following a Dairy-Free low FODMAP diet

Calcium is important for strong bones and teeth, the dilation and contraction of the blood vessel wall and the proper function of our muscles and nerves. The daily requirements for men and women 19-50 years of age is 1,000 mg/day. Women over 50 years of age are advised to consume 1,200 mg/day.

Generally, we obtain much of our calcium from eating dairy foods. If you are following a dairy-free low FODMAP diet, then your calcium intake might be very low. However, by including lactose-free dairy, such as lactose-free yogurt and milk, as well as hard cheeses that are low in lactose, you can ensure that you consume adequate amounts of calcium. If you are removing dairy products from your diet, make sure you replace these foods with alternatives that are fortified with calcium or make sure that you include calcium-rich plant foods.

To meet calcium recommendations, consider not only the food content of calcium but also its bioavailability. Bioavailability is the degree to which a nutrient is absorbed and utilized by the body; it is the fraction of dietary calcium that is absorbed and incorporated into bone.

Dairy products (milk, cheese and yogurt) and tofu with calcium have good bioavailability of calcium (approximately 30 to 35%), but some plant foods have even better bioavailability (e.g., bok choy and kale, which have approximately 50-60% bioavailability; Chinese cabbage flower leaves, Chinese spinach and mustard greens, which have approximately 40% bioavailability).

Calcium bioavailability from plant foods can be affected by their oxalate and phytate content; these substances are inhibitors of calcium absorption. For example, cooked spinach contains 115 mg calcium per serving (125 mL or ½ cup), but only an estimated 5% of this calcium is actually absorbed in the body. Nuts and seeds also contain inhibitory phytic acid, which reduces calcium absorption.

Low FODMAP food choices and calcium bioavailability

Food Type	Serving size (g)	Calcium content (mg)	Fractional absorption (%)	Estimated absorbable calcium (mg)
Lactose-free dairy products	240 (1 cup)	300	32	96.3
Hard cheese	42	300	32	97.2
Firm tofu with calcium (check the label for the presence of calcium)	126	258	31	80
Broccoli	71	35	61	21.5
Bok choy	85	79	53.8	42.5
Kale	85	61	49.3	30

Calcium bioavailability in certain fish is also noteworthy. Calcium in fish comes from the bones. Fish with soft bones, such as sardines, anchovies and salmon (canned with bones) will have the most calcium. Shellfish are also a fair source of calcium.

The FODMAP Reintroduction Phase

Once you have followed the elimination phase for 2-6 weeks and have seen an improvement in your symptoms, it is time to test which FODMAP foods are problematic for you and which foods you can tolerate. The objective is to obtain an understanding of your individual tolerance levels to each of the FODMAP groups to ensure a nutritionally adequate diet. This is particularly important for prebiotic fructans (FOS) and galactans (GOS), which act as a fertilizer for the good bacteria in your gut and are linked to gut and overall health. Therefore, this phase involves rechallenging and reintroducing FODMAPs.

Determining your Trigger Foods

The rechallenge phase will help you find which foods you can tolerate without any symptoms and which high FODMAP foods trigger your symptoms. The FODMAP rechallenge phase is a series of food challenges that help identify tolerance levels for high FODMAP groups. You should test one FODMAP subtype per week.

The FODMAP rechallenge rules

- Test only one food per week.
- Choose foods that contain only one type of FODMAP.
- Stick to the same food as day 1 for challenge days 2 and 3.
- Test a normal-sized portion of food as part of a meal than by itself.
- Stick to a strict low FODMAP diet while completing the rechallenge phase.
- Avoid trigger foods/drinks (alcohol, caffeine) or keep them as consistent as possible.
- Test the challenge food, but remember that if you pass a challenge, you will still need to avoid those foods while undergoing the remaining FODMAP challenges. Reintroduce only once you have finished with all the FODMAP challenges.
- You need to be symptom free for at least 3 consecutive days before you start testing the next FODMAP group.
- Avoid eating out during the challenge days.

- Consult with your dietitian if you develop moderate to severe symptoms.
- Test again the trigger foods at a later time, as FODMAP tolerance can change over time.
- After you have finished all the challenges that contain one type of FODMAP, you can test foods containing more than one FODMAP type. However, test these foods in smaller amounts initially, beginning with a 40-gram portion and increasing it to a 120-to-150-gram portion.

There are two ways to test FODMAPS in the reintroduction phase:

Option 1
Rechallenge plan: 3 days in a row

Day 1
Eat a small portion of a high FODMAP challenge food and monitor your symptoms.

If symptoms appear, stop the challenge. Continue with your low FODMAP diet until symptoms resolve and you are symptom-free for 3 days.

Day 2
If you have no symptoms, test a medium-sized portion of the high FODMAP challenge food and monitor symptoms.

If symptoms appear, stop the challenge. Continue with your low FODMAP diet until symptoms resolve and you are symptom-free for 3 days.

Day 3
If you have no symptoms, test a large portion of the high FODMAP challenge food and monitor symptoms.

If symptoms appear, stop the challenge. Continue with your low FODMAP diet until symptoms resolve and you are symptom-free for 3 days.

Day 4/Day 5/Day 6
Washout period.

Follow a low FODMAP diet during these days.

Day 7
If you do not have any symptoms, start the next challenge.

Option 2
Alternative testing schedule

Day 1

Rechallenge day: Eat a small portion of the high FODMAP challenge food and monitor symptoms.

If symptoms appear, stop the challenge. Continue with your low FODMAP diet until symptoms resolve and you are symptom-free for 3 days.

Day 2

Rest day: Monitor symptoms.

Day 3

Rechallenge day: Eat a medium-sized portion of the high FODMAP challenge food and monitor symptoms.

If symptoms appear, stop the challenge. Continue with your low FODMAP diet until symptoms resolve and you are symptom-free for 3 days.

Day 4

Rest day: Monitor symptoms.

Day 5

Rechallenge day: Eat a large portion of the high FODMAP challenge food and monitor symptoms.

If symptoms appear, stop the challenge. Continue with your low FODMAP diet until symptoms resolve and you are symptom-free for 3 days.

Day 6

Rest day: Monitor symptoms

Day 7

Rest day: Monitor symptoms

Day 8

Rest day: Monitor symptoms

Day 9

If you do not have any symptoms, start the next challenge.

There are up to 10 main rechallenges to be completed

One rechallenge is required for each of the following FODMAPs: fructose, lactose, galactans (galacto-oligosaccharides, GOS), sorbitol, and mannitol. Additionally, 5 more rechallenges are required to test various fructans (fructo-oligosaccharides, FOS). This is due to the presence of various different food categories that contain fructans in variable amounts.

Example of a rechallenge program

Rechallenge FODMAP categories	QUANTITY
Rechallenge 1: Fructose Test one food from this group.	1 teaspoon of honey, increasing to 2 tablespoons. ½ medium fresh fig, increasing to 2 medium figs.
Rechallenge 2: Sorbitol (polyols) Test one food from this group.	3 blackberries, increasing to 10 blackberries. ¼ of an avocado, increasing to a whole avocado. 100 grams fresh coconut, increasing to 200 grams. ¼ peach, increasing to 1 whole peach.
Rechallenge 3: Mannitol (polyols) Test one food from this group.	¼ stick celery, increasing to 2 sticks. 100 grams of sweet potato, increasing to a 200-grams serving. 30 grams cauliflower, increasing to a 90-grams serving.
Rechallenge 4: Lactose (disaccharides) Test one food from this group.	½ cup (120 ml) milk, increasing to 1½ cup (360 ml) of milk. ½ cup (120 grams) of plain yogurt, increasing to 1 ½ cup (360 grams) yogurt

Rechallenge 5 and 6: Fructans (FOS-oligosaccharides) Bread, cereals, grains: Test two foods from this group (bread and pasta).	1 slice of white wheat bread, increasing to 3 slices of wheat bread. 100 grams wheat pasta, increasing to 200 grams (use the cooked weight of the pasta). 50 grams couscous, increasing to 150 grams (use the cooked weight). 20 grams of cereal, increasing to 60 grams.
Rechallenge 7 and 8: Fructans (FOS-oligosaccharides) Vegetables. Test two foods from this group (garlic and onion).	¼ of a clove of garlic, increasing to 1 clove of garlic. ¼ of a medium leek, increasing to ½ leek (white and green sections). 1 tablespoon chopped onion, increasing to 6 tablespoons. ½ spring onion, increasing to 2 spring onions.
Rechallenge 9: Fructans (FOS -oligosaccharides) Fruit. Test one food from this group.	½ medium grapefruit, increasing to 1 large grapefruit. ¼ cup pomegranate seeds, increasing to 1 cup. 1 tablespoon raisins or currants, increasing to 4 tablespoons. 2 tablespoons dried cranberries, increasing to 6 tablespoons. 1 dried date or fig, increasing to 4 pieces.
Rechallenge 10: Galactans (GOS – oligosaccharides) Test one food from this group.	2 tablespoons of chickpeas, black beans or peas, increasing to 6-table-spoon servings. 15 almonds, increasing to 25 almonds.

While the rechallenging process helps you identify trigger foods, reintroducing FODMAPs into the diet allows you to determine what combination and amount of FODMAPs you can have without experiencing symptoms. This reintroduction occurs via a trial-and-error process that will help you obtain a clear picture of your tolerance levels during a meal and throughout the day.

Following the completion of these steps, you will know whether or not you can eat high FODMAP foods with every meal, every day or every other day. Figuring out how many FODMAPs you can combine before reaching the tipping point and experiencing symptoms will help you develop a longer-lasting, more personalized FODMAP diet plan. This personalization will offer you greater flexibility when planning your meals, as you will be able to consume a greater variety of foods while managing your symptoms.

High FODMAP foods with more than one type of FODMAP

High FODMAP foods usually contain more than one type of FODMAP. Thus, after the rechallenge task, it is important to check the FODMAP content of foods to help reintroduce and combine foods so you can identify your tolerance level.

You can use the following tools to help you find high FODMAP foods that contain more than one type of FODMAP:

- The Monash FODMAP app
- http: //myginutrition.com/downloads/High_FODMAP_foods.pdf

Fiber in the low FODMAP diet

I really want to eat more fiber while on a low FODMAP diet. How do I do it?

Optimal fiber intake is important for all. However, the emphasis on fiber (e.g., the different types of fiber, how much you should consume and how to eat more of it) can be daunting. With this book, we aim to provide all the tools you need to increase your fiber intake gradually, even during the elimination phase of the diet, and to maximize gut health while minimizing gut symptoms.

All of these efforts will ultimately be worthwhile. While the diet may appear to be difficult at first, the results you will see and feel will be almost immediate. Studies show that it only takes 3 days for gut bacteria diversity to be affected by an increase or a decrease in the amount of fiber we consume. Therefore, we need to help our gut bacteria by providing them with enough fiber to thrive and maintain their diversity, and in return, they will work hard to keep us healthy.

Assess your current fiber intake

Step 1: Assess your current fiber intake from your food diary.

You can use this quick assessment to determine an approximate value for your daily fiber consumption.

Look at your food diary and assess how many servings of the following foods you consume on a daily basis. Then, add it all up and obtain the total daily amount.

Food type	Serving size	Servings per day	Grams of fiber per serving	Total amount of fiber intake per serving
FRUITS				
Raspberries	1 cup		x 8	=
Apple with skin	1 medium		x	=
Banana	1 medium		x 3	=
Blueberries	1 cup		x 4	=
Cantaloupe	1 cup		x 1	=
Cherries	10 cherries		x 1.5	=
Clementine	1 fruit		x 1.5	=
Grapes	1 cup		x 1	=
Honeydew melon	1 cup		x 1	=
Nectarine	1 medium		x 2	=
Orange	1 medium		x 3	=
Peach	1 medium		x 2	=
Pear	1 medium		x 4	=

Pineapple	1 cup	x 2	=
Plum	1 medium	x 1	=
Prunes, dried	5 prunes	x 3	=
Strawberries	1 cup	x 3	=
Watermelon	1 cup	x 1	=
Consider your other fruit intake			=
VEGETABLES			
Avocado	⅓ medium (50 grams)	x 3	=
Artichoke, boiled	1 medium	x 6	=
Asparagus	6 spears	x 1.5	=
Broccoli, boiled	½ cup	X 2.5	=
Brussels sprouts, boiled	½ cup	x 2	=
Carrot	1 medium	x 2	=
Celery	1 stalk	x 1	=
Cauliflower, boiled	½ cup	x 2	=
Cucumber	½ cup, sliced	x 0.5	=
Corn, on the cob	1 ear	x 2	=
Eggplant, boiled	½ cup	x 1	=
Green beans, boiled	½ cup	x 2	=
Mushroom	½ cup	x 0.5	=
Peas	½ cup	x 4	=
Potato, baked with skin	1 medium (240 grams)	x 5	=
Potato, boiled	1 medium (240 grams)	x 2	=
Pumpkin, canned	½ cup	x 5	=
Tomato	1 medium	x 1	=
Spinach, raw	1 cup	x 1.5	=

Mixed green salad	1 cup		x 1	=
Consider your intake of other vegetables			x	=
NUTS/SEEDS (i.e., peanuts, almonds, sunflower seeds)	28 grams/1 oz/about ¼ cup		x 3	=
Chia seeds	2 tablespoons		x 10	=
Nut butters	2 tablespoons		x 2	=
BEANS/LEGUMES/ LENTILS	½ cup		x 6-9	=
GRAINS				
BREAD				
Whole-grain bread	1 slice		x 2	=
White bread	1 slice		x 1	=
CEREAL				
Breakfast cereal	1 cup		x 0-1	=
Whole-grain breakfast cereal	1 cup, cooked		x 3	=
Bran cereal	½ cup		x 6-14	=
Oats, rolled	½ cup		x 5	=
Oatmeal	½ cup		x 2	=
WHOLE GRAINS/PSEUDOGRAINS				
Pasta (whole-grain)	1 cup		x 4-6	=
Rice, brown	1 cup		x 3	=
Quinoa	1 cup		x 5	=
Buckwheat	1 cup		x 5	=
REFINED GRAINS				
Pasta	1 cup		x 2	=
Rice, white	1 cup		x 1	=
TOTAL AMOUNT OF FIBER per DAY			=	

Fiber values were rounded to the nearest 0.5 gram.

Step 2: Tips for increasing your fiber consumption

Of course, the whole point of counting fibers is to have an indication of how much fiber you consume so you can aim to reach the recommended amounts. We do not want you to obsess over counting fibers or count each and every one precisely. The objective is to enjoy a healthy, balanced diet that also includes the recommended proportion of fiber.

> Now that you have calculated the total amount of your daily fiber intake, here are our tips for increasing your fiber consumption while still following the low FODMAP diet. Remember to choose low FODMAP serving sizes, as recommended in the Monash Low FODMAP app.

Abrupt additions or changes in fiber can have undesirable GI consequences. Increase fiber intake gradually if you do not want to experience intestinal issues.

1. Make a small change in your eating habits every day. Do not eat all your fiber in one meal. Spread your fiber intake throughout the day. This helps your gut bacteria handle the fiber and reduce the chances of suffering from bloating or other intestinal issues.
2. Increase your fiber intake up 5 grams per week. It may take a month or two until you adjust your fiber intake. Remember that fibers affect everyone differently, so try another type if you cannot tolerate a specific one.
3. Choose some foods high in soluble fiber that will help you consume 6-8 grams of soluble fiber per day (about ¼ of your daily fiber intake). We created a table of low FODMAP foods high in soluble fiber to help you with this.
4. Cut back on fiber intake if you have symptoms.
5. Aim to drink at least eight glasses of water or other fluids throughout the day. Fibers that are both soluble and insoluble need water to function properly. Fiber can take up to 30 to 40 hours to pass throughout the gut, and water is needed throughout the process.
6. Aim to have at least five servings of low FODMAP vegetables and two servings of low FODMAP fruit per day.
7. Focus on whole, unprocessed foods. Aim to have four to six servings of whole-grain products throughout the day. These products could include quinoa, oats, buckwheat and millet.

8. Eat nuts and seeds. Add one tablespoon of chia seeds, which provides five grams of fiber.
9. Add low FODMAP servings of beans.

Be careful with the type of fiber!

In the past, increasing fiber intake was the first line of therapy for IBS patients. However, we now know that different types of fiber have different effects and that fiber tolerance in IBS is variable, with certain fibers actually making IBS symptoms worse.

For example, a placebo-controlled trial that compared psyllium fiber, which is soluble, to bran fiber, which is insoluble, showed that IBS patients handled the psyllium much better than the insoluble fiber from bran.

Maximizing fiber intake without ingesting a great quantity of rapidly fermentable fibers is the best way to go with IBS. Insoluble fiber appears to be less well tolerated in IBS. Include FODMAP-friendly whole grains, such as oats, oat bran, quinoa, quinoa flakes, and low FODMAP fruit and vegetables. Inulin and FOS are frequently found in cereal and granola bars, breads, other cereals and even yogurts, so be careful.

Specific recommendations for fiber in IBS

As we have said, the effect of fiber on IBS is variable and specific to the type of fiber consumed. We generally opt to decrease the intake of highly fermentable fibers (such as fructo-oligosaccharides and galacto-oligosaccharides, inulin and wheat bran) when following a low FODMAP diet because these fibers can produce a large amount of gas in a short amount of time and exacerbate symptoms such as bloating, gas and overall discomfort in IBS patients. Conversely, clinical studies show that soluble fiber supplements such as linseed, methylcellulose, partially hydrolyzed guar gum, and psyllium have a positive therapeutic effect, particularly in patients with IBS-C. In cases of IBS-D, the recommendation is to increase fiber that is soluble with good water holding and gel forming properties, while psyllium, oats, oat bran, methylcellulose or calcium polycarbophil can be added to the diet, as studies have shown symptom improvement.

Low FODMAP foods high in soluble fibers.

Choose low FODMAP serving sizes recommended in the Monash Low FODMAP app.

	Serving Size	Total Fiber (grams)	Insoluble Fiber (grams)	Soluble Fiber (grams)
VEGETABLES				
Broccoli	½ cup	2.5	1.2	1.2
Brussels sprouts	⅓ cup	2	0.8	1.2
Carrots, cooked	1 cup	5.2	3	2.2
Collard greens, cooked	1 cup	5.3	2.1	3.1
Eggplant, cooked	1 cup	2.5	1.8	0.7
Kale, cooked	1 cup	2.6	1.2	1.4
Parsnip, cooked	1 cup	6.2	2.6	3.6
Potato, baked with skin	1 medium	5	2.9	2.1
Turnip, cooked	½ cup	3	1.3	1.7
Sweet potato, cooked	½ cup	2	1.3	0.7
Spinach, cooked	½ cup	2.2	1.5	0.7
FRUITS				
Orange	1 medium	3.1	1.3	1.8
Passion fruit	1 medium	1.9	0.5	1.4
Strawberries	½ cup	1.7	1.3	0.4
Banana	1 medium	3	2.3	0.7
CEREALS and GRAINS				
Oat bran	1 tablespoon	1.5	0.8	0.7
Oatmeal	½ cup	4.3	2.3	2
Flaxseeds	1 tablespoon	4	2.8-3.4	0.6-1.2
Sunflower seeds	¼ cup	3	2	1

LEGUMES/PULSES				
Edamame (frozen soybeans only)	½ cup	5	3.5	1.5
Lentils	¼ cup	4	3.8	0.2

Recommendations regarding fiber supplements in IBS

- Soluble fibers (such as psyllium) may be especially effective in IBS. Psyllium may be useful in reducing constipation in IBS-C. However, psyllium may not be universally tolerated, as it is highly fermented, so care should be taken in consumption.
- Oats/oat bran may help with constipation, abdominal bloating and pain in IBS; however, more studies are required to confirm this finding.
- Linseeds/flaxseeds (up to 2 tablespoons/day) may improve constipation, abdominal pain and bloating in IBS.
- Insoluble fibers (such as wheat bran) are ineffective and may make abdominal pain and bloating worse.
- Sterculia and methylcellulose have helpful properties, since they are non-fermentable and form a gel-like consistency in the intestines, thus making the stool softer. This would help in IBS-C; however, few well-designed studies have been performed to show their benefits.
- The efficacy of wheat dextrin as a fiber supplement in IBS has not been formally examined.
- Partially hydrolyzed guar gum (PHGG) seems to have prebiotic properties and help in the growth of probiotic bacteria, such as lactobacilli and bifidobacteria, in the large intestine. It may be well tolerated and might help people with either IBS-C or IBS-D; however, more studies are required to confirm this benefit.
- Fiber supplements that contain wheat bran, fructo-oligosaccharides (FOS) and galacto-oligosaccharides (GOS) and that can produce a large amount of gas in a short amount of time in the large intestine appear to make IBS symptoms worse.
- Inulin is highly fermentable and can make gas symptoms worse in IBS patients. Avoid fiber supplements that have inulin from chicory root (which is high in the FODMAP fructan).
- Other fiber supplements to be aware of are those that contain sugar alcohols, such as sorbitol.

Prebiotic Foods in the low FODMAP diet

Many prebiotic foods fall in the category of high FODMAPs; and, in many people with functional gastrointestinal disorders, they result in symptoms such as bloating, flatulence and abdominal discomfort and pain upon their consumption. For this reason, a low FODMAP elimination diet tends to restrict many of these offenders, for example, garlic and onion. It is therefore extremely important to gradually reintroduce high FODMAP prebiotic foods into our diet during the reintroduction phase to ensure that we promote the growth of good bacteria in our gut.

Even during the elimination phase of the diet, however, it is fundamental to consume a variety of prebiotic foods in their small, safe low FODMAP serving size. It is also important to remember that the elimination phase lasts only for a short period of time of 2-6 weeks.

Here is a list of foods that have prebiotic properties and that can be included in the low FODMAP diet in their low FODMAP serving size based on the Monash FODMAP app:

> **Fruit:** Banana, pomegranate, rambutan, dried paw paw, raisins, currants, rhubarb, kiwifruit
>
> **Vegetables:** Potato, beetroot, butternut pumpkin, savoy cabbage, corn, snow peas, cassava, taro, common or red cabbage (not cooked)
>
> **Bread:** Gluten-free multigrain, whole meal
>
> **Pulses (check the Monash FODMAP app for low FODMAP serving recommendations):** Red/green lentils, boiled; canned lentils; canned chickpeas and butter beans; lima beans, boiled; mung beans, boiled
>
> **Grains:** Oats, oat bran, rice bran, corn, puffed amaranth, buckwheat kernels
>
> **Seeds:** Flaxseeds
>
> **Nuts:** Almonds, hazelnuts

What are some good food sources of resistant starch that are also low in FODMAPs?

At this point, there are no official intake recommendations for resistant starch. The literature has suggested that 20 g of resistant starch per day is needed for optimal gut health.

Note that the whole-grain versions of foods contain more resistant starch than do the refined versions.

Low FODMAP serving size	Resistant starch content (grams)
Underripe banana, 1 medium	4.7
Rolled oats, ¼ cup, uncooked	4.4
Hi-maize resistant starch, 1 tablespoon	4.5
Lentils, ½ cup, cooked	3.4
Millet, 1 cup, cooked	3.0
Chickpeas, ½ cup, cooked, canned	2.3
Buckwheat groats, ¾ cup cooked	2.2
Oats, 1 cup, cooked	0.5
White rice (100 grams)	1.2
Brown rice (100 grams)	1.7
Potato, boiled, mashed or baked (100 grams)	0.6
Corn polenta (½ cup)	1.0

How to Get your Fiber While on the low FODMAP diet

The tables give the amount of fiber for food items allowed on the low FODMAP diet. Check the Monash FODMAP app for the low FODMAP serving sizes for each of the food items in the table.

Fruits	Serving size	Fibers (grams)
Banana	1 medium	3
Plantain	1 medium	3.5
Blueberry	20 berries	0.5
Breadfruit	¼ fruit (100 grams)	5
Cantaloupe	½ cup	0.5

Fruits	Serving size	Fibers (grams)
Clementine	1 medium	1.5
Kumquats, unpeeled	1 fruit	1.5
Dragon fruit	1 medium	5
Durian	1 cup, cubed	5.5
Grapes	1 cup	2
Guava ripe	1 medium	6
Honeydew melon	½ cup	1
Kiwifruit, gold and green	1 small	2.5
Mandarin	1 small	1
Orange	1 medium	3
Passion fruit	1 fruit	2
Papaya (paw paw)	1 cup	2.5
Pear, prickly	1 medium	6.5
Pineapple	1 cup, cubed	2
Raspberry	10 berries	1.5
Rhubarb	1 cup	2.5
Strawberry	10 medium	3
Star fruit	1 medium	3.5

Vegetables	Serving size	Fibers (grams)
Alfalfa	1 cup	1
Arugula	1 cup	1.5
Bok choy	1 cup	1
Broccoli	½ cup	2.5
Cabbage, common or red	½ cup	1
Carrot, raw	1 medium	2
Choy sum	1 cup, chopped	2

Vegetables	Serving size	Fibers (grams)
Eggplant	1 cup	2.5
Green Bean	10 beans	1.5
Lettuce (butter, iceberg, red coral, romaine, rocket, radicchio)	1 cup	1
Olives (green, black)	10 small olives, pitted	1
Parsnip	1 medium	3.5
Bell Pepper	1 medium	1.5
Potato, baked with skin	1 medium (120 grams)	2.5
Potato	1 medium (120 grams)	1
Japanese pumpkin, raw	½ cup	0.5
Pumpkin, boiled	½ cup	1.5
Spinach (baby)	1 cup	1
Spinach, boiled	1 cup	4.5
Swiss chard	1 cup	1
Swiss chard, boiled	1 cup	4
Tomato	1 small	1.5
Tomato, cherry	4 tomatoes	1
Cucumber	½ cup	0.5
Water chestnuts	½ cup	2
Turnip	½ turnip	3
Yam	1 cup	3
Kale, raw	1 cup	2
Kale, boiled	1 cup	3
Chili red	1 small	0.5
Chili green	1 small	0.5

Vegetables	Serving size	Fibers (grams)
Collard greens, cooked	1 cup	5.5
Seaweed (nori)	1 piece	1
Mushrooms, oyster	1 cup	2
Corn	4 tbsps	2
Sweet potato	½ medium	2

Legumes, Tofu, Nuts and Seeds	Serving size	Fibers (grams)
Chestnuts, boiled	10 nuts	2,5
Brazil nuts	10 nuts	3
Peanuts	30 nuts	2.5
Macadamias	15 nuts	2.5
Pecans	15 halves	3
Walnuts	10 halves	2
Chia seeds, black and white	1 tbsp	5
Flaxseeds	1 tbsp	4
Pine nuts	1 tbsp	0.5
Sunflower seeds	1 tbsp	0.75
Sesame Seeds	1 tbsp	1.5
Pumpkin seeds	1 tbsp	0.5
Tahini	1 tbsp	2
Tofu, firm	½ cup (100 grams)	0.5
Tofu, plain	½ cup (100 grams)	0.5
Tempeh, plain	100 grams	5
Edamame (frozen soybeans only)	½ cup	5

Legumes, Tofu, Nuts and Seeds	Serving size	Fibers (grams)
Low FODMAP pulses Check Monash FODMAP app for suitable serving sizes	¼ cup-½ cup	3-7

Bread, Cereals, Grains and Pseudograins	Serving size	Fibers (grams)
Gluten-free bread (white)	1 slice	1-2
Sourdough bread (white)	1 slice	1-2
Sourdough bread (spelt, whole-grain)	1 slice	2-3
Corn tortillas	1 tortilla	1
Gluten-free bread (brown)	1 slice	2-3
Flakes of corn, gluten-free	½ cup	0.5
Flakes of quinoa	½ cup	0.5
Oats, rolled	½ cup (40 grams)	4

Flours	Serving Size	Fibers (grams)
Arrowroot	½ cup, 67 grams	2
Buckwheat	½ cup, 67 grams	4-5
Corn	½ cup, 67 grams	4
Millet	½ cup, 67 grams	4
Quinoa	½ cup, 67 grams	4-5
Rice	½ cup, 67 grams	1
Brown rice	½ cup, 67 grams	3.5
Sorghum	½ cup, 67 grams	4
Teff	½ cup, 67 grams	8
Starch (maize, potato, tapioca)	½ cup, 67 grams	0

Grains/Pasta	Serving Size	Fibers (grams)
Oat bran, unprocessed	1 tbsp	1.5
Rice bran, unprocessed	1 tbsp	1.5
Buckwheat groats, cooked	½ cup	2.5
Noodles, rice	1 cup, cooked	2
Pasta, gluten-free	1 cup, cooked	2
Pasta, quinoa	1 cup, cooked	5
Polenta	½ cup, cooked	2
Quinoa (black, red, white)	1 cup, cooked	5
Rice, brown	1 cup, cooked	3.5
Rice, white	1 cup, cooked	1

Fiber values are rounded to nearest 0.5 grams.

Chapter 10:
Our Clean low FODMAP diet

Our Take on the low FODMAP det.
The Mediterranean Twist!

We love the Mediterranean diet and lifestyle, specifically, the idea of how our grandparents used to live so close to nature, consuming mostly plant-based foods (lots of legumes, vegetables, olives, whole grains), lots of olive oil and, every now and then, animals that were grass-fed out in the pasture. We are also passionate about gut health, aiming to reduce gut symptoms without compromising a healthy, balanced diet. The low FODMAP diet is the first dietary plan that actually works to relieve symptoms in so many people suffering from IBS, and we wanted to marry that with the Mediterranean diet, which is scientifically famous for its health benefits.

Many epidemiological studies and clinical trials have shown that following a Mediterranean diet decreases the risk of all-cause mortality and several chronic diseases. Although few such studies have investigated the effect of diet on gut microbiota, current results show that the Mediterranean diet induces favorable microbiota profiles and the production of favorable metabolites. Additionally, this research shows that the more one adheres to the diet, the greater the positive effect on gut microbiota diversity, more specifically, a lower ratio of Firmicutes: Bacteroidetes. Furthermore, there is a vast amount of evidence that it is more beneficial to include a greater variety and quantity of plant-based foods instead of excluding animal-based foods.

Therefore, with the Mediterranean diet having so many benefits and the low FODMAP diet working for so many people, we could not help but envision a low FODMAP diet that is healthy, balanced and Mediterranean-influenced.

Our Clean low FODMAP diet

We love healthy, unprocessed food made with fresh ingredients and prepared in a pure manner. We also like to use ingredients with the greatest nutritional value and aim to eat a balanced diet, heavy on plant-based foods. Finally, we try as much as possible to source locally and use ingredients that are in season.

With this in mind, we have developed our unique Clean low FODMAP diet (with a Mediterranean twist), which includes a great variety of foods in our everyday diet and aims to maximize fiber intake.

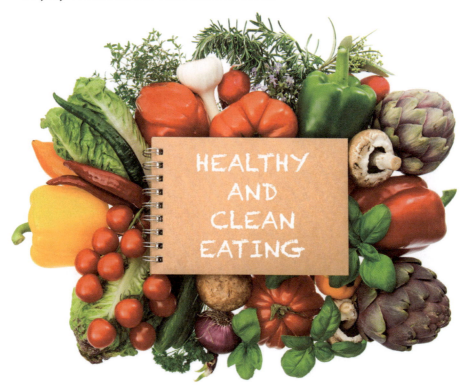

We choose whole grains and natural sugars and minimize overprocessed foods that contain preservatives and additives. Our recipes use plenty of olive oil, vegetables, legumes (as much as is allowed by Monash FODMAPs), olives, fruits, whole grains and lean protein sources. We also try to minimize salt intake and choose foods that are free of chemical flavorings, artificial colors, antibiotics, pesticides.

Our Clean low FODMAP approach makes the following recommendations based on Our Clean low FODMAP Plate.

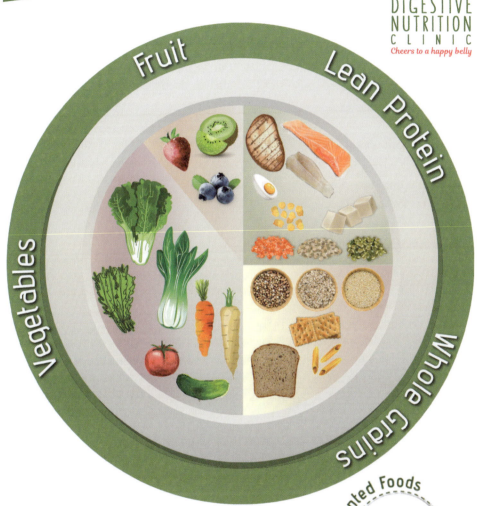

Fruit

Lean Protein

Vegetables

Whole Grains

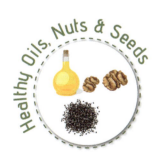

Healthy Oils, Nuts & Seeds

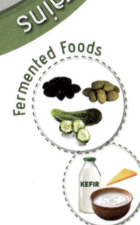

Fermented Foods

KEFIR

Vegetables
- Eat more vegetables and aim for a variety of low FODMAP vegetables during the day.

Fruit
- Limit one portion of low FODMAP fruit per meal.
- Aim for a variety of low FODMAP fruit during the day.
- Limit concentrated sources of fruit, such as dried fruit and fruit juices.

Grains
- Choose unprocessed whole grains/pseudograin products. Whole grains do not cause a spike effect in blood sugar and insulin after consumption and are therefore a better option than white refined grains. Choose quinoa, buckwheat, teff, sorghum, and oats.

Proteins from animal sources
- Choose sustainable fish, eggs and poultry, and limit red meat (beef, pork and lamb).
- Avoid processed meats (deli, bacon, sausages and hot dogs).
- Choose to eat pastured eggs.
- Aim to consume meat that is derived from 100% grass-fed animals and not from animals raised in animal feeding operations in which they are often fed antibiotics at low doses to promote growth.
- Choose low-fat dairy options (lactose-free if you cannot tolerate lactose).
- Choose sustainable fish that live in nonpolluted waters. Avoid fish bred in aquaculture environments where they are also exposed to low levels of antibiotics for growth.
- As a general rule of thumb, bear in mind that the bigger the fish is, the longer it has lived and the longer time it has had to accumulate toxins from the sea or ocean. Small wild-caught fish, such as sardines, anchovies and herring, are good examples of fish with a lower contamination risk and are great choices for seafood.

Proteins from plant sources
- Consume seeds and nuts low in FODMAPs and free of sulfites as a preservative.
- Choose organic firm tofu and tempeh.

- Go for these tested low FODMAP legumes in their recommended low FODMAP servings:
- o   Chana dal, boiled
- o   Urid dal, boiled
- o   Lentils, canned/preferably in carton
- o   Lentils (green or red), boiled
- o   Mung beans, sprouted
- o   Edamame, frozen
- o   Chickpeas, canned/preferably in carton

Oils

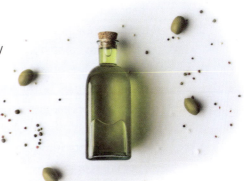

- Use cold-pressed healthy oils instead of animal fats.
- We recommend the use of a good-quality extra-virgin olive oil.
- Due to its high saturated fat content, use virgin coconut oil only occasionally and not as an everyday staple.
- Limit butter to occasional use.
- Avoid partially hydrogenated oils.

We also encourage the consumption of foods containing probiotics (good bacteria for the gut). Such low FODMAP foods are lactose-free yogurt, lactose-free kefir, tempeh, olives, pickles and sauerkraut (low FODMAP portion is 1 tablespoon).

Choosing the Healthiest Eggs

Eggs are not a source of FODMAPs, and we enjoy both eating them and using them in our recipes. A large egg provides 6 grams of high-quality protein and 50% of our daily needs of B12. Eggs provide 13 important nutrients, such as folate, iron, zinc, choline, lutein and zeaxanthin (antioxidants), and vitamins A, D, and E.

However, all the terminology surrounding eggs today can be very confusing. Brown eggs, pasture-raised, organic, hormone-free, free-range, cage-free: what does this mean and why are the distinctions important? We would like to help you decipher some of these labels and allow you to make the best choice for your needs.

For example, this is how eggs are regulated and labeled in the United States.

Where Are the Hens Raised?

1. **Eggs from Pasture-Raised versus Caged/Conventional Hens**

   We prefer eggs from pasture-raised hens because the hens are allowed to move about and graze in the pasture all day, eating lots of grass, worms and bugs. Their food may be supplemented with a little bit of feed but only if required. The hens can roam around in plenty of space during the day, specifically, at least 108 square feet (10 square meters), and they are moved into the barn at night.

   It should be noted, however, that the term pasture-raised is not regulated by the US Department of Agriculture (USDA), as standards for this terminology have not been officially disclaimed. A third-party certification called the "Certified Humane®" pasture seal certifies that these hens are allowed to roam freely in the pasture during the daylight hours.

   On the other hand, most eggs in supermarkets come from hens that are caged. Caged/conventional hens are confined to a small space, generally a 67-square-inch (0.04-square-meter) area where movement is very limited. They are kept in those cages for their whole lifespan and are given corn or a soy feed with added vitamins and minerals.

   Some studies have shown increased omega-3 fatty acid content in eggs from pastured hens versus those from caged hens.

2. **Eggs from Cage-Free Hens**

   This label is regulated by the USDA, but it only means that the hens are not in a cage and that they have slightly more room than caged hens to move. However, the space is still small; each is given up to 1.5 square feet, and the hens remain inside and are fed the same diet of corn or soy.

3. **Eggs from Free-Range Hens**

   According to the USDA, free-range eggs come from hens that are "allowed access to the outside." This is not the same as pasture-raised because it does not guarantee that the hens are roaming free outside. The term is loosely regulated, which means that the barn may have small doors that could allow the hens to go outside during their egg-laying cycle. However, the outside could just be a cemented yard and not a pasture that would allow free roaming and feeding by the hens. These hens may still eat a corn- or soy-based diet like the caged/conventional hens.

What Are the Hens Fed?

1. **Eggs from Vegetarian-Fed Hens**

   This is an interesting category and a major source of confusion. We tend to think that vegetarians are healthier, but chickens are not supposed to be vegetarians; they are in fact omnivorous, meaning that they eat both plants and animals. Therefore, vegetarian-fed hens should not be considered healthier.

2. **Eggs High in Omega-3s**

   These eggs are enriched with fatty acids. Specifically, they may contain 400 mg EPA and DHA omega-3 fatty acids. This is because the hens are fed a diet supplemented with extra omega-3 fatty acids. Other than that, however, the hens that produce these eggs are kept under the same conditions as caged/conventional ones. A study has shown that omega-3-enriched eggs have five times as much omega-3 fatty acids as conventional eggs and 39% less arachidonic acid, an inflammatory omega-6 fatty acid. If you cannot get enough omega-3 fatty acids from other sources, choose omega-3-enriched eggs.

3. **Organic Eggs**

   Hens producing organic eggs are kept in the same way as conventional hens or are allowed some movement. However, it is important to note that they are not treated with antibiotics, and their food is organic without exposure to any pesticides or fertilizers.

4. **Hormone-Free Eggs**

   No chickens in the US, Europe or other parts of the world are given added hormones, so essentially, all eggs are hormone-free.

A Couple of Whimsical Points to Bear in Mind

A hen will start producing eggs at 19 weeks of age and will lay, on average, 259 eggs a year. Additionally, brown eggs are not any healthier than white eggs. They are just different in color because they come from a different breed of hens.

> **Our Choice: Pastured Eggs**
>
> Studies have shown that pastured eggs are probably the healthiest type of eggs. They are higher in vitamin A, vitamin E and omega-3 fatty acids, as well as lower in cholesterol and saturated fat, and contain three to four times the amount of vitamin D than do eggs from hens raised in a cage.

Choosing Sustainable Seafood

As defined by the Monterey Bay Aquarium Seafood Watch, sustainable seafood is "shellfish and fish caught or farmed in environmentally responsible ways."

Furthermore, aquaculture –which is described as fish farming– is often promoted as an efficient way to boost fish and shellfish production while protecting wild fisheries. Keep in mind, however, that aquaculture practices vary from region to region, as well as their specific ecological impact.

For more information on these ratings, check out the Monterey Bay Aquarium's Seafood Watch® website (https: //www.seafoodwatch.org/).

Additionally, you can check country-based seafood guidelines on fish farming and seafood sustainability on the Monterey Bay Aquarium website under the Resources section. (https: //www.seafoodwatch.org/resources)

 Is there a catch to eating fish?

Some types of fish may contain high levels of mercury, PCBs (polychlorinated biphenyls), dioxins and other environmental contaminants. Older, larger predatory fish and marine mammals tend to have higher levels of such substances.

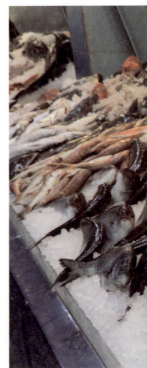

The benefits and risks of eating fish vary greatly depending on a person's age. For instance, the US Environmental Protection Agency (EPA) and the US Food and Drug Administration (FDA) released their latest advice on eating fish and shellfish in 2017.

Based on this report, adults should consume two to three servings of a variety of cooked fish, with a typical serving of 4 ounces (113 grams) of fish, which is measured prior to cooking. Thus, 8 to 12 ounces (226 to 340 grams) of fish should be consumed on a weekly basis. Furthermore, women who weigh less than the average weight (165 pounds or 75 kilos) may wish to eat smaller portions or eat only two servings per week.

Children should consume a variety of fish once or twice a week. Children's serving sizes should be as follows:

- 1 ounce (28 grams) for children aged 2 to 3 years;

- 2 ounces (56 grams) for children ages 4 to 7 years old;
- 3 ounces (85 grams) for children ages 8 to 10 years old; and
- 4 ounces (113 grams) for children 11 years and older.

These US agencies have concluded that the following population groups should eat more fish that is lower in mercury to help with important developmental and health benefits:

- Women of childbearing age (16 to 49 years old);
- Pregnant and breastfeeding women; and
- Young children.

Fish choices high in omega-3 fatty acids and low in mercury	
Anchovies	Sardines
Herring	Shad
Mussels	Trout
Salmon (wild)	

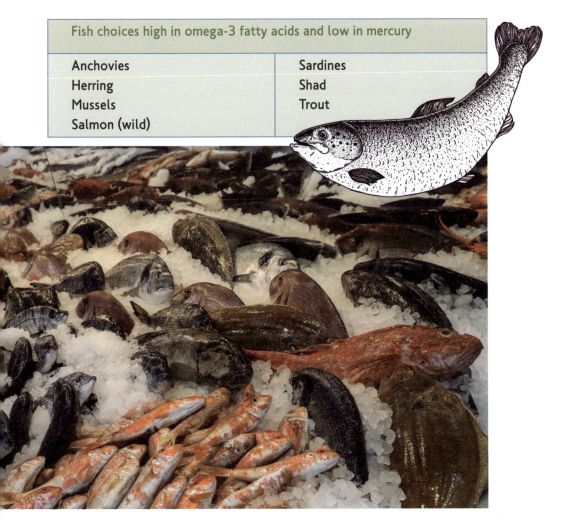

Best fish choices with low levels of mercury

Eat 2-3 servings a week
Atlantic croaker
Atlantic mackerel
Black sea bass
Butterfish
Catfish
Clam
Cod
Crab
Crawfish
Flounder
Haddock
Hake
Lobster (American and spiny)
Mullet
Oyster
Pacific chub mackerel
Perch
Pickerel
Plaice
Pollock
Scallop
Shrimp
Skate
Smelt
Sole
Squid
Tilapia
Tuna, canned light (includes skipjack)
Whitefish
Whiting

Fish choices to avoid due to high mercury levels
Swordfish
Shark
King mackerel
Gulf tilefish
Marlin
Orange roughy
Tilefish (Gulf of Mexico)
Tuna (bigeye, ahi)

Limit the consumption of the following fish:
Grouper
Chilean sea bass
Bluefish
Buffalo fish
Carp
Chilean sea bass/Patagonian toothfish
Halibut
Mahi mahi/dolphinfish
Monkfish
Sheepshead
Snapper
Striped bass (ocean)
Tilefish (Atlantic Ocean)
Sablefish (black cod)
Spanish mackerel (Gulf)
Fresh tuna (except skipjack)
Weakfish/seatrout
White croaker/Pacific croaker

Watch Out for Emulsifiers and Other Additives in Food

Food additives are detergent-like chemicals that are added to many processed foods. Emulsifiers are added for the following reasons: to improve food appearance, texture and mouthfeel; to enhance flavor or to add flavor to low-fat foods; and to keep the quality and stability of food or to preserve it. Examples of food additives are preservatives, coloring agents, flavor enhancers, humectants, anti-foaming agents, bulking agents, sweeteners and more. Foods that commonly contain emulsifiers are gluten-free and low-fat products, ice cream wine and pickles. These chemicals are approved as safe, but strict regulations exist to control the amount found in foods.

Animal studies show increased inflammation in the gut and a change in gut microbiota composition due to the consumption of emulsifiers and additives in our food. Our intestine is protected from gut bacteria by the thick layer of mucus that lines it. The mucus stops the bacteria from reaching the inner lining of the intestine and causing inflammation. Unfortunately, emulsifiers can destroy this intestinal mucus layer, leaving the wall unprotected from the microbiota that reside there. Thus, bacteria can start causing inflammation in the gut wall. In fact, epidemiological, cellular and animal studies have shown links between emulsifier consumption and inflammatory bowel disease, especially Crohn's disease.

More specifically, when two dietary emulsifiers, namely, polysorbate-80 and carboxymethyl cellulose, were given to mice (along with their regular diet) in doses that were well within the limits that humans consume, they brought about obesity, intestinal inflammation, and problems with metabolism. What was even more interesting was that the addition of these emulsifiers to mice that had no microbiota (germ-free mice) did not bring about any of the consequences, while when microbiota was transferred from the emulsifier-treated mice to the germ-free mice, they induced the observed effects of obesity, inflammation and metabolic issues.

There is limited evidence to directly link emulsifiers and thickeners to human disease, but multiple potential pathogenic mechanisms exist. Knowledge of actual dietary intake and high-quality interventional studies are needed to clarify the risks associated with their intake.

It should also be noted that excess fat, refined grains, sugar and artificial sweeteners also negatively influence our gut microbiota. High fructose corn syrup (HFCS) has been associated with fatty liver and the presence of inflammatory bacterial toxins.

All of these findings highlight the importance of the consumption of whole instead of processed foods.

What is the Bt Toxin? Is it Safe in Genetically Modified Foods?

Bt toxins are a group of proteins that are naturally produced by the bacterium Bacillus thuringiensis. This bacterium is a gut pathogen for many organisms. The bacterium produces these toxins, which, through a sequence of events, become activated and kill the organism by forming holes in the membranes of the organism's gut lining.

Bt is used in agricultural sprays to destroy pests. This has been shown to pose no health risk because it degrades very quickly in daylight and thus does not end up being eaten by people.

Genetically modified (GM) organisms that express Bt toxin, such as cotton, corn and soybeans, are also commercially made. Through genetic modification, these organisms contain the genes that allow them to produce Bt toxin, which makes them resistant to pests. The problem is that evidence shows that the Bt toxins produced in these genetically modified crops are vastly different from the naturally occurring ones. Naturally occurring Bt proteins are large, insoluble and nontoxic molecules that require specific chemical conditions to become active toxins. In the case of GMOs, however, the Bt proteins are very similar in structure to the toxic active molecules and do not require many steps and conditions to become actively toxic.

When these crops are ingested by animals and people, the Bt protein is also ingested, and studies have shown the Bt protein from GM foods to be present in human blood. It has also been detected in fetal blood, suggesting that it probably can be passed from the mother to the next generation.

Currently, the impact of the toxicity of Bt toxins and the impact on the gut microbiome upon consumption of such toxins from genetically modified crops is not known, and more research is necessary to clarify this phenomenon.

Sprouting and Activating Foods

Legumes, including all types of beans and peas, can be problematic for people with a sensitive gut. On the other hand, the health benefits of legumes are well documented. Legumes are low in fat, have a low GI index, are high in fiber and contain a variety of phytochemicals. Phytochemicals may decrease the risk of various diseases, including certain cancers, diabetes, hypertension and heart disease, by acting as antioxidants and nutrient protectors or by preventing cancer-causing agents from forming. Therefore, it is very important to try to incorporate legumes into our diets in various quantities and via different cooking and processing methods.

We address a few of the common questions regarding legumes, seeds, grains and nuts.

 Should I soak my dried legumes (pulses)?

Only very small amounts of dried pulses are allowed during the elimination diet, but they do not need to be strictly avoided by people following a low FODMAP diet.

Soaking dried legumes is absolutely necessary, as the processes of soaking and draining (or cooking and draining) reduce the FODMAP content. Legumes are naturally high in oligosaccharides, including galacto-oligosaccharides (GOS) and fructans, which need to be reduced in people following the low FODMAP diet. Oligosaccharides dissolve in water and leach out of the legumes into the water, so cooking, canning and processing methods can decrease the amount of these FODMAPs in legumes.

 Should I sprout my foods? Are sprouted foods healthier than nonsprouted foods?

Sprouting involves periodically soaking, draining and then rinsing the seeds, legumes or grains until they germinate or sprout.

Very little research has been performed on whether sprouted foods are more beneficial than nonsprouted foods. It is complicated to compare different products when one must take into account varying ingredient contents and both processing and production methods, which may ultimately change the food's nutritional value.

While we cannot truly say whether sprouted foods are healthier than nonsprouted foods, there are few studies that show an enhancement in the nutritional value of grains and legumes through sprouting by increasing the protein concentration, digestibility and amounts of disease-fighting antioxidants. Sprouting can also cause a reduction in antinutrients such as phytic acid, lectins and protease inhibitors that are especially concentrated in grains and legumes and that can be problematic in people with a sensitive gut. The reduction in antinutrients can make important minerals, such as iron, zinc, calcium, magnesium and manganese, more bioavailable.

 ## Can sprouting affect the FODMAP content of foods?

This answer comes straight from Monash University, where the following foods have been tested: wheat grain, barley grain, rye grain, chickpeas, red kidney beans and mung beans.

The researchers found that sprouting decreases the FODMAP content in these foods, with the exception of chickpeas, in which the FODMAP content was slightly increased.

The reduction in the FODMAP content of mung beans and barley was sufficient to change their rating from red to green on the Monash app (and thus obtain a safe serving rating for somebody following the low FODMAP diet). Sprouting can thus affect the FODMAP content of foods, and we advise checking the Monash app to choose the right amount for each food. Furthermore, our advice is to test your tolerance by trying a small amount of each of these foods and monitoring your symptoms.

Safe sprouting

Sprouting may carry the risk of contamination with salmonella, *E. coli*, listeria, or other bacteria due to the warm, humid conditions.

Bacteria can enter the seeds prior to sprouting, and they are practically impossible to eliminate. Homegrown sprouts can also be dangerous if they are consumed without being cooked. Regardless of your level of cleanliness, these harmful bacteria can develop during the sprouting process.

To reduce this risk, the FDA offers the following advice:
- *Avoid eating raw sprouts of any kind (including alfalfa, clover, radish, and mung bean).*
- *Cook sprouts thoroughly, as it significantly reduces the risk of illness.*
- *Check sandwiches and salads purchased at restaurants and delicatessens. They may often contain raw sprouts. Request that raw sprouts not be added to your food.*
- *Refrigerate sprouts that you buy.*

❓ Should I activate nuts before consuming them?

Eating large amounts of raw nuts may place an extra strain on your digestive system. Hence, it may be worthwhile to activate nuts. *Activated nuts* have been soaked in water and salt for a certain amount of time, thus initiating germination or sprouting, and are then dehydrated at a low temperature (approximately 65°C/149°F) for 12-24 hours before consumption.

Activation may improve nutrient absorption and digestion by reducing antinutrients and enzyme inhibitors. By binding minerals such as calcium and iron, antinutrients may make it more difficult for your gut to absorb them. However, antinutrients are not necessarily bad, as they play an important role as antioxidants and anti-inflammatories. Keep in mind that with regard to the way our body absorbs nutrients, we must consider the food combination rather than a single food.

We advise that if you have a sensitive gut, you can try activated nuts, as antinutrients and enzyme inhibitors can make the food harder to digest. Try activated nuts in small quantities and test your tolerance and symptoms.

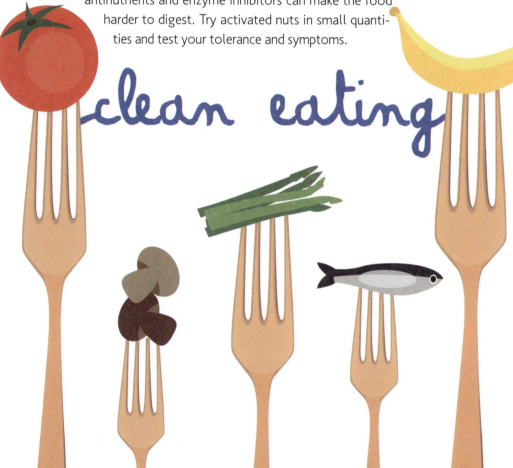

Section 3

Chapter 11:
Tips for Following a low FODMAP diet

Is the low FODMAP diet a Gluten-Free diet?

The low FODMAP diet is not a gluten-free diet. However, it is understandable that a gluten-free diet may be confused for a low FODMAP diet because many of the gluten-containing grains are also high in FODMAPs (particularly oligo-fructans) and are therefore removed from the diet during the elimination phase.

We recommend that while on the low FODMAP diet, one aims for whole-grain gluten-free options over refined gluten-free options as much as possible. Over-consumption of refined gluten-free options leads to a higher intake of rice, which is a source of trace amounts of arsenic, a known carcinogen. Lately, evidence has shown increased arsenic levels in people following a gluten-free diet, and even though this finding has not been linked directly to rice, we try to minimize our consumption of rice and increase consumption of other grains and seeds instead.

Moreover, studies associate whole-grain intake with improved health and protection against heart disease. In other studies, long-term dietary intake of gluten was not associated with the risk of coronary heart disease. However, subsequent concern is that the avoidance of gluten may result in a decrease in the consumption of beneficial whole grains, which can increase one's cardiovascular risk. For example, compared to groups with the lowest intake (less than 2 servings per day) of whole grains, groups with a high consumption of whole grains (2-3 servings a day) showed significantly lower rates of heart disease, stroke, type 2 diabetes and deaths from all causes. Thus, the consumption of processed gluten-free products could result in a decrease in the intake of whole grains, which could have a negative impact on cardiovascular health.

Moreover, research on patients with celiac disease who followed a gluten-free diet showed an increased risk of obesity and metabolic syndrome. This could be justified partly by the fact that these patients have improved absorption now due to the healing of their gut lining but also due to the increased consumption of processed gluten-free foods that are high in calories, sugar, saturated fats, sodium and low in nutrients. A gluten-free diet changes certain cardiovascular risk factors and should therefore be evaluated further, as its overall effect on cardiovascular risk is not clear. We therefore encourage the consumption of whole grains even during the low FODMAP diet and the limitation of processed gluten-free products. If you do not have problems with gluten, add whole grains such as wheat, rye and barley back into your diet according to your rechallenge results of the low FODMAP reintroduction phase.

Want to Make your Cooking low FODMAP?

Here are 10 Easy Ways to Do That

1. Use citrus fruits to add flavor. Add orange, mandarin, lemon and lime zest as well as small amounts of freshly squeezed citrus juice. Keep in mind that grapefruit is high in FODMAPs.
2. Substitute honey or agave syrup with maple syrup.
3. Prepare garlic- or onion-infused oils. Sauté garlic or onions in oil to infuse it with those flavors. Discard the garlic and onion and only use the oil.
4. Use chives and the green stems of spring onions, scallions and leeks to add oniony flavors to foods. Do not use the white parts.
5. Vinegars are great for taste, and most are FODMAP friendly. Restrict balsamic vinegar to 1 tablespoon per serving and do not consume unfiltered apple cider vinegar.
6. Use mustards that contain no garlic, onion or other ingredients high in FODMAPs.
7. Spices add flavor and are low in FODMAPs. Use allspice, freshly ground black pepper, cardamom, cloves, cinnamon, cumin, nutmeg, paprika, saffron, star anise and turmeric.
8. If you can tolerate spice, choose curry and chili powders that do not contain FODMAP ingredients.
9. Fresh herbs are your best friends! Basil, parsley, cilantro, oregano, mint, lemongrass, coriander, tarragon, rosemary, curry leaves, sage, watercress and thyme add deliciousness to your cooking.

10. Replace milk with lactose-free milk or plant-derived milk, such as almond, coconut (long life) and quinoa (unsweetened) milk.

Tips for Enjoying a Meal at a Restaurant While on a low FODMAP diet

- Prior to the outing, check the restaurant's menu online or call the restaurant ahead of time to determine if there are low FODMAP options.
- Ask the people you are going out with to let you choose the restaurant and go with a place you have visited before or a restaurant that you know will provide gut-friendly choices.
- Choose a FODMAP-friendly and healthy appetizer option right away so you avoid overindulging on bread until the main course arrives.
- Good options for meals at a restaurant are grilled fish or shellfish, poultry and red meat served with vegetables or salad, quinoa, and potatoes. Avoid fried or very fatty foods, as they can cause dyspepsia, abdominal pain, bloating, gas and diarrhea.
- Ask for gluten-free, quinoa or buckwheat pasta as an alternative to wheat-based pasta.
- Ask if your food can be prepared without onion or garlic (including onion and garlic powders).
- Ask for the dressing or sauces to be served on the side. Additionally, you can replace the salad dressing with extra-virgin olive oil and vinegar.
- Know your worst triggers, let the waiter know what your worst triggers are, and ask if the cook could accommodate these requests so that you are not stressed during your outing about the outcome of the evening.
- Stay away from pasta sauces or creamy, heavy dishes that tend to contain onion and garlic and that may be high in dairy products (lactose) and other high FODMAP ingredients.
- Avoid eating heavily processed foods that contain gut-irritating food chemicals, additives and emulsifiers.
- Avoid spicy foods if they tend to cause abdominal pain and/or diarrhea.
- You may consider a gluten-free meal, but bear in mind that those are not necessarily low in FODMAPs. Many times, gluten-free items are packed with high FODMAP onion, garlic, dried fruits and fruit juices, among other high FODMAP ingredients.
- Avoid alcohol if it poses a gut trigger for you. If your tummy can handle

alcohol, avoid drinking rum, which is high in FODMAPs. Drink one or two drinks only, and make sure you eat first before consuming the alcohol.

- Avoid the consumption of very cold beverages, juices, and fizzy drinks, and avoid drinking with a straw.
- Be careful when choosing desserts. As tempting as they are, they are usually high in FODMAPs. Go for one serving of low FODMAP fruit (or fruit salad), dark chocolate or another dessert that you have previously had without any negative results.
- If going out for breakfast or brunch, choose an egg-based dish (for example, omelets, frittatas, or scrambled eggs) with a salad or some fruit instead of bagels, muffins, pancakes or other very doughy foods that may cause bloating and other tummy issues.

Do you not have enough time for low FODMAP cooking?

Use our clean low FODMAP plate and our simple recommendations to create super easy, mix-and-match yummy dishes. Note that the portion sizes given are only applicable for those with FODMAP restrictions.

Fill ½ the plate with low FODMAP vegetable options
- 2 cups boiled kale = 6 grams of fiber
- 1 cup boiled carrots + 1 cup boiled spinach (English) = 7 grams of fiber
- 1 cup grated carrot + ¾ cup red cabbage = 5 grams of fiber
- 2 cups lettuce + 5 cherry tomatoes + ½ cup sliced cucumber + 1 medium red bell pepper = 5.5 grams of fiber
- 1 cup grated carrot + 1 ½ cup baby spinach + 1 cup cucumber + 5 cherry tomatoes = 7 grams of fiber
- 1 cup boiled mustard greens + 1 cup boiled carrots = 6 grams of fiber
- 2 cups grated carrot = 6 grams of fiber

Fill ¼ of the plate with whole grains
- 1 cup (180 grams) cooked red or white quinoa (see recipe page 364)
- 1 cup (184 grams) cooked millet (see recipe page 364)
- ¾ cup cooked (135 grams) buckwheat groats (see recipe page 364)
- 1 cup 100% quinoa pasta

Fill ¼ of the plate with protein
- Rotisserie/roasted chicken

- Any fish or chicken
- Pan-fried chicken (see recipe page 242)
- Pan-fried fish or salmon (see recipe page 240)
- Firm tofu (see recipe page 233)
- Pastured eggs

Add

- ½ cup (90 grams) boiled edamame
- ½ cup (46 grams) canned lentils
- ½ cup (42 grams) canned chickpeas (recipe for roasted chickpeas page 231)
- ½ cup (46 grams) urid dahl (boiled)
- Pan-fried haloumi cheese (see recipe page 362)
- Feta cheese

Garnish with herbs

- Mint
- Basil
- Parsley
- Cilantro

Add dressing (see recipes)

- Raspberry vinaigrette (page 240)
- Classic French vinaigrette (page 237)
- Balsamic vinaigrette (page 357)
- Passion fruit dressing (page 242)
- Thai orange dressing (page 231)
- Yoghurt dressing (page 299)
- Peanut orange sauce (page 233)
- Tahini orange sauce (page 361)
- Or use extra-virgin olive oil and vinegar or lemon juice

Add a low FODMAP fruit (see page 109)

Top with nuts, olives, seeds, fermented vegetables.

Add chia seeds if you want to boost your fiber intake.

Meal prep strategies:

- Decide on your meal plan.
- Write the ingredients that you are going to need.
- Create a shopping list.
- Go shopping.
- Start meal prepping and enjoy!

Small steps you can take to make things easier:

- Wash and chop your veggies ahead of time.
- Portion out your ingredients.
- Prepare 2 dressings ahead of time and have them ready to use during the week.
- Batch cooking: cook a large batch of quinoa or buckwheat and enjoy it throughout the week.
- Cook a whole chicken to use through the week.
- Prepare veggie burgers and quinoa muffins and freeze them.
- Make a suitable bread to have for the week.
- Make oat crackers to have for a week.
- Portion some roasted chickpeas to add to a salad and have them on the go.
- Portion some nuts and seeds to have on the go.
- Choose a suitable vegetable option to fill your plate.
- Add any suitable whole grain that has been prepared without any high FODMAP ingredients such as onion and garlic (choose boiled plain quinoa, millet, or any gluten-free pasta).
- Add protein that you are certain has been prepared without any high FODMAP ingredients, like onion and garlic. Check labels or ask. (Choose plain rotisserie chicken, grilled chicken, grilled plain fish/shrimp/salmon or boiled eggs.)
- Use olive oil and wine vinegar or lemon juice as dressings.

Chapter 12:
Meal plan and Recipes

Our Proposed 7 Day low FODMAP Menu Plan

Here is our proposed meal plan, which you can follow during the low FODMAP elimination phase. It is designed to be balanced and varied and to help you maximize your fiber intake, even during the elimination phase of the diet. You can find all the delicious recipes in the recipe section of this book.

For vegan/vegetarian menu ideas, check our recipes for vegans/vegetarians.

Bear in mind that a rapid increase in fiber consumption can result in excess gas being produced by the gut microbes that will ferment it, which can cause you tummy aches, bloating and flatulence. Therefore, be careful with how you introduce extra fiber in the diet. If your daily fiber intake is less than the recommended amount, increase the fiber in your diet slowly. Do not go for this meal plan in its entirety right away. Omit some foods, such as extra fruit and seeds, from this meal plan and work by adding them gradually (5 grams of fiber at a time) into your diet until you reach your fiber goal. This approach should help you avoid unpleasant intestinal issues caused by a sudden and sharp increase in fiber intake.

7 DAY LOW FODMAP MENU PLAN

Day 1	Day 2	Day 3
Breakfast	**Breakfast**	**Breakfast**
2 kiwifruits	2 poached eggs	½ cup rolled old fashioned oats
(150 grams)	smoked salmon	fiber 4 grams
fiber 3 grams	5 cherry tomatoes	lactose-free yogurt
¼ cup walnuts	(75 grams)	¼ cup (40 grams) heaped
fiber 2 grams	fiber 1 gram	blueberries
lactose-free yogurt	1 slice buckwheat bread	fiber 1 gram
maple syrup	(page 207)	2 teaspoons chia seeds
Lunch	fiber 3grams	fiber 3 grams
1 cup grated carrot	**Lunch**	**Lunch**
1 ½ cup baby spinach	Polenta- crusted chicken	1 cup grated carrot
1 cup cucumber	tenders	¾ cup red cabbage
5 cherry tomatoes	(page 319)	fiber 5 grams
fiber 7 grams	fiber 4 grams	1 cup (180 grams) cooked
¾ cup (135 grams) cooked	Coleslaw	white quinoa
buckwheat groats	(page 344)	fiber 5 grams
(page 364)	fiber 3 grams	Pan-fried chicken or rotisserie chicken
fiber 4 grams	Roasted vegetables	(page 242)
½ cup (90 grams) boiled	(page 340)	½ cup (42 grams) canned
edamame	fiber 4 grams	chickpeas
fiber 4 grams	10 medium strawberries,	fiber 2 grams
Peanut orange sauce	chopped	cilantro leaves
(page 233)	(150 grams)	vinaigrette
Dinner	fiber 3 grams	(page 237)
Fennel chickpea stew	**Dinner**	**Dinner**
(page 267)	Sweet potato burger	Grilled sardines or any
fiber 7 grams	(page 276)	other fish
Carrot ribbons salad	fiber 6 grams	Oven-roasted baby
(page 246)	¾ cup (75 grams) broccoli	potatoes
fiber 5 grams	fiber 2 grams	(page 339)
1 star fruit	Oven-roasted baby	fiber 2 grams
(95 grams)	potatoes	Carrot ribbons salad
fiber 3 grams	(page 339)	(page 246)
Snack	fiber 2 grams	fiber 3 grams
Green kiwi smoothie	Tahini orange sauce	1 orange
(page 174)	(page 361)	(140 grams)
fiber 4 grams	fiber 1 gram	fiber 3 grams
	Snack	**Snack**
	Macadamia milk	Strawberry smoothie bowl
	(page 171)	(page 178)
	fiber 3 grams	fiber 3 grams
	Oat crackers	2 teaspoons chia seeds
	(page 214)	fiber 3 grams
	fiber 1 gram	
	1 orange	
	fiber 3 grams	
TOTAL	**TOTAL**	**TOTAL**
39 GRAMS FIBER	**36 GRAMS FIBER**	**34 GRAMS FIBER**

Day 4	Day 5	Day 6	Day 7
Breakfast	**Breakfast**	**Breakfast**	**Breakfast**
slice buckwheat bread (page 207) fiber 3 grams	Frittata (page 197) fiber 2 grams	30 raspberries (60 grams) fiber 2 grams	Quinoa muffins with spinach and cheese (page 187) fiber 4 grams
teaspoons peanut utter fiber 1 gram	¼ cup (40 grams) heaped blueberries fiber 1 gram	¼ cup (30grams) Quinoa granola (page 199)	1 orange (140 grams) fiber 3 grams
medium banana 00 grams) fiber 3 grams	**Lunch** 2 cups grated carrot fiber 6 grams	fiber 3 grams 1 cup low-fat lactose-free yogurt	**Lunch** Whole roasted fish (page 293)
aple syrup	tofu, plain (page 233)	**Lunch**	Roasted root vegetables (page 342)
unch neapple chicken salad age 242) fiber 6 grams	Peanut orange sauce (page 233) 1 cup pineapple	Kale quinoa pasta (page 257) fiber 10 grams	fiber 4 grams Oven-roasted baby potatoes (2 servings)
orange 40 grams) er 3 grams	fiber 2 grams ¼ cup (28 grams) roasted peanuts	10 medium strawber-ries, chopped (150 grams)	(page 339) fiber 4 grams
inner cups boiled kale er 6 grams	fiber 2 grams **Dinner** Oyster mushroom	fiber 3 grams ⅔ cup whole baby carrots	¾ cup (75 grams) broc-coli fiber 2 grams
n-fried salmon/fish or icken ages 240, 242)	buckwheat risotto (page 258) fiber 8 grams	(100 grams) fiber 3 grams **Dinner**	1 orange (140 grams) fiber 3 grams
ive oil cup (180 grams) cooked d quinoa	3 cups green salad fiber 3 grams 2 kiwifruits	Lean lamb chops with orange sauce (page 325)	**Dinner** Thai chicken soup (page 227)
age 364) er 5 grams	(150 grams) fiber 3 grams	Quinoa tabbouleh salad (page 250)	fiber 4 grams 1 cup chopped
ack uinoa bar age 203) er 3 grams	**Snack** Chocolate cardamom smoothie (page 173)	fiber 5 grams Roasted root vegetables (page 342) fiber 4 grams	(75 grams) Chinese broccoli fiber 2 grams
ack cup grapes er 1 gram	fiber 4 grams **Snack** Macadamia milk	**Snack** 2 servings oat crackers (page 214)	1 star fruit (95 grams) fiber 3 grams
cup lactose-free yogurt tablespoon chia seeds er 5 grams	(page 171) fiber 2 grams Chocolate pumpkin	fiber 2 grams 2 tablespoons peanut butter	**Snack** 1 cup pineapple fiber 2 grams
	muffin (page 183) fiber 3 grams	fiber 2 grams 1 orange fiber 3 grams	¼ cup (28 grams) pecans fiber 5 grams
	¼ cup (28 grams) walnuts fiber 2 grams		
OTAL **5 GRAMS FIBER**	**TOTAL** **38 GRAMS FIBER**	**TOTAL** **37 GRAMS FIBER**	**TOTAL** **36 GRAMS FIBER**

Additional Menu Ideas Using Our Recipes

Breakfast

½ cup rolled oats 30 raspberries (60 grams) 1 teaspoon 100% pure maple syrup 2 teaspoons (7 grams) chia seeds Almond milk	9 grams of fiber
Overnight quinoa 1 tablespoon peanut butter (16 grams) 10 medium strawberries, chopped (150 grams)	8 grams of fiber
2 kiwifruits (150 grams) 5 halves walnuts Low-fat lactose-free yogurt 1 teaspoon 100% pure maple syrup 2 teaspoons (7 grams) chia seeds	7 grams of fiber
Poached eggs Smoked wild salmon 5 cherry tomatoes (75 grams) ⅔ cup baby carrots 1 slice buckwheat bread (1 serving)	7 grams of fiber
1 slice buckwheat bread (1 serving) 2 teaspoons peanut butter 1 medium unripe banana (100 grams) 1 teaspoon 100% pure maple syrup	7 grams of fiber
Quinoa crepes (1 serving) 9 halves pecans Chia raspberry jam	7 grams of fiber
Buckwheat pancakes 30 raspberries (60 grams) 1 tablespoon 100% pure maple syrup	6 grams of fiber
Chocolate cardamom smoothie 7 halves walnuts 2 teaspoons (7 grams) chia seeds	8 grams of fiber

2 slices buckwheat bread (2 servings) 2 teaspoons peanut butter Chia blueberry jam (1 serving)	7 grams of fiber
30 raspberries (60 grams) ¼ cup (30 grams) quinoa granola Low-fat lactose-free yogurt 2 teaspoons (7 grams) chia seeds	8 grams of fiber
Quinoa crepes 2 teaspoons 100% pure maple syrup 10 medium strawberries, chopped (150 grams) 2 teaspoons (10 grams) chia seeds	8 grams of fiber
Buckwheat pancakes 100% pure maple syrup 1 tablespoon peanut butter (16 grams) 10 medium strawberries, chopped (150 grams)	7 grams of fiber
Chia pudding 30 raspberries (60 grams) ¼ cup (30 grams) grain-free quinoa granola	8 grams of fiber

Lunch/Dinner

Kale quinoa pasta (1 serving) 10 medium strawberries, chopped (150 grams) ⅔ cup whole baby carrots (100 grams)	16 grams of fiber
Thai chicken soup (1 serving) 1 cup kale 2 passion fruits (46 grams)	11 grams of fiber
Lamb and potato stew (1 serving) 2 teaspoons (7 grams) chia seeds ¾ cup (75 grams) broccoli 1 orange (140 grams)	11 grams of fiber
Polenta-crusted chicken tenders (1 serving) Coleslaw (1 serving) 10 medium strawberries, chopped (150 grams)	9 grams of fiber

Sweet potato burger (1 serving) Roasted root vegetables (1 serving) Tahini orange sauce (1 serving) 2 kiwifruits (150 grams)	13 grams of fiber
Chicken curry 1 cup quinoa 1 star fruit (95 grams)	14 grams of fiber

Snacks

10 medium strawberries, chopped (150 grams) 1 oz/28 grams walnuts	5 grams of fiber
1 medium (100 grams) unripe banana 5 Brazil nuts (20 grams)	5 grams of fiber
Macadamia milk 1 medium (100 grams) banana unripe	5 grams of fiber
1 cup cubed (150 grams) durian 1 oz/28 grams walnuts	5 grams of fiber
Chocolate cardamom smoothie	4 grams of fiber
1 cup chopped (140 grams) papaya (paw paw) 1 oz/28 grams walnuts	4 grams of fiber
2 passion fruits (46 grams) Lactose-free yogurt	4 grams of fiber
Green kiwi smoothie	4 grams of fiber
1 cup grapes 1 oz/28 grams walnuts 2 teaspoons (7 grams) chia seeds	5 grams of fiber

Our 101 Clean low FODMAP Recipes

All of the recipes in our book follow our clean FODMAP approach and are all suitable for when you are following the low FODMAP elimination phase.

The low FODMAP diet is by no means a gluten-free diet. You will notice that our recipes are gluten-free, as they were designed to also help people who have issues with gluten.

If you are following a **gluten-free diet**, please ensure that the following ingredients are gluten-free when making our recipes:

Chocolate, baking powder, sauces, mustard, herbs, blended seasonings, peanut butter, yeast extracts, dry roasted nuts, tamari, buckwheat noodles, quinoa pasta, polenta, quinoa, buckwheat, tofu and oats.

No special equipment is necessary to create our recipes; they are easy to make in any kitchen. A food processor is recommended.

Special Notes

 Vegetarian Recipes marked lacto-ovo Vegetarian include eggs, butter and milk.

 Vegan Recipes marked Vegan contain no animal ingredients.

 Gluten free

 Dairy free

 See page 166

 See page 166

Our Phase 1 diet

If you take a look at the recipes in this book, you will see that they are labeled with a sticker for either Phase 1 or Phase 2 diet.

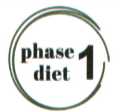 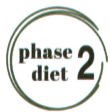

Our low FODMAP recipes for the Phase 1 diet are designed for patients with active gastrointestinal (GI) distress, such as diarrhea, gas, bloating and multiple bowel movements. Once your active GI distress is over, you can include recipes labeled Phase 2.

Our Phase 1 diet takes into consideration the following recommendations:

- Try to avoid raw vegetables.
- Include more cooked low FODMAP vegetables.
- Avoid gut stimulants, such as coffee, spices and alcohol.
- Avoid foods that stimulate gas production, such as these sulfur-rich vegetables: cabbage, broccoli, cauliflower, brussels sprouts, bok choy, and related vegetables, onions, shallots, garlic and leeks.
- Avoid lactose, sugar alcohols and whole grains.

Coconut

Desiccated coconut is dried and shredded coconut that is made from the flesh of a mature coconut. According to Monash University, a ¼-cup serving of desiccated coconut is low FODMAP. Large servings contain moderate to high levels of polyols.

Coconut flour is a byproduct of coconut milk production and is high in FODMAPS. A ¾ cup (100 grams) contains high levels of GOS, fructans and excess fructose content, as well as sorbitol.

We use organic citrus when zesting. Why?

Fruit waxing is the process of covering fruits with either natural or petroleum-based artificial waxing material to prevent water loss and spoilage and to improve appearance. None of these chemicals are approved for use in organic produce, so we recommend buying organic citrus, zesting the peel and freezing the zest. In this way, you do not have to worry about chemicals on your citrus zest.

Recipes

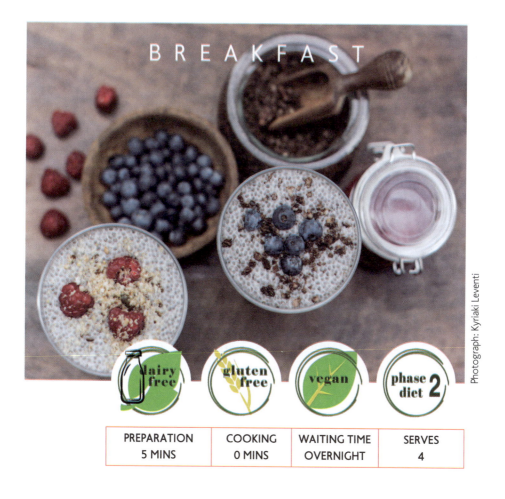

Photograph: Kyriaki Leventi

dairy free · gluten free · vegan · phase diet 2

PREPARATION	COOKING	WAITING TIME	SERVES
5 MINS	0 MINS	OVERNIGHT	4

Nondairy Milks
(almond and macadamia)

Almonds are high FODMAP in large servings, but because almonds comprise only a small proportion of almond milk, almond milk is safe to consume.

INGREDIENTS

- 1 cup (120 grams) raw almonds or 1 cup (125 grams) raw macadamias, preferably organic
- 2-4 cups (480-960 ml) water, plus more for soaking (and possibly more water to thin out the milk)
- 1 teaspoon (5 ml) pure vanilla extract
- 1-2 teaspoons (5-10 ml) 100% pure maple syrup, to taste, optional

INSTRUCTIONS

Soak nuts in water overnight or soak for 2-3 hours in hot water.

Drain and rinse well.

Peel the skins off if the nuts have skin.

Combine the nuts with 2 cups of fresh water, vanilla extract and maple syrup (if using).

Blend at a high speed until smooth.

Line a sieve with a piece of cheese cloth.

Place the lined sieve over a large bowl.

Gather the cheese cloth together and **squeeze** to drain as much liquid as possible.

You can dry out the solids and make almond or macadamia flour if you want.

Add water accordingly if you need to thin out the milk consistency.

Store milk in the refrigerator for up to 3 days.

For chocolate nondairy milks, add the following to the mix:

1 teaspoon (2.3 grams) Ceylon cinnamon

1 teaspoon (5 ml) 100% pure maple syrup

1 teaspoon (2 grams) raw cacao

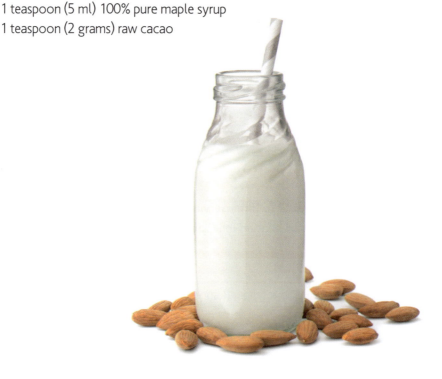

SMOOTHIES AND SMOOTHIE BOWLS
Chocolate Cardamom Smoothie

PREPARATION	COOKING	SERVES 1
5 MINS	0 MINS	(SERVING SIZE: 300 ML)

INGREDIENTS

- 1 frozen medium (100 grams) unripe banana, peeled
- 1 teaspoon (4.6 grams) cocoa nibs
- 1 teaspoon (5 ml) 100% pure maple syrup
- 1 teaspoon (2 grams) fresh peeled chopped ginger
- Seeds from 2 cardamom pods
- ½ cup (120 ml) ice
- ½ cup (120 ml) almond milk (**see recipe for nondairy milks page 171** or use unsweetened almond milk)

INSTRUCTIONS

Blend all ingredients together until smooth.

Nutrition Facts	
Per serving: 170 kcal	38 grams carbohydrates
2 grams protein	4 grams fiber
2 grams total fat	High in riboflavin
0 grams saturated fat	B6, manganese

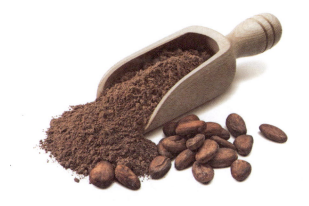

Green Kiwi Smoothie

PREPARATION 5 MINS	COOKING 0 MINS	SERVES 1 (SERVING SIZE: 190 ML)

INGREDIENTS

- 2 small kiwis (140 grams) (2 slices saved for decoration)
- ½ cup (15 grams) baby fresh or frozen spinach leaves
- ¼ cup (60 ml) ice cubes
- 2 tablespoons (30 ml) fresh lime juice
- 2-3 cm (0.8-1.2 inches) fresh knob of peeled chopped ginger
- ¼ teaspoon turmeric powder or 2-3 cm (0.8-1.2 inches) fresh knob of peeled chopped turmeric
- ⅛ cup (6 grams) mint leaves, plus 4 sprigs for garnish
- Add a pinch of salt

INTRUCTIONS

Blend everything until smooth.

Nutrition Facts	
Per serving: 110 kcal	27 grams carbohydrates
3 grams protein	4 grams fiber
1 gram total fat	High in potassium, folate, manganese, and vitamins A, C, and K
0 grams saturated fat	

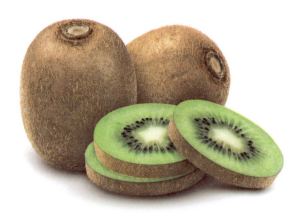

Orange Banana Smoothie

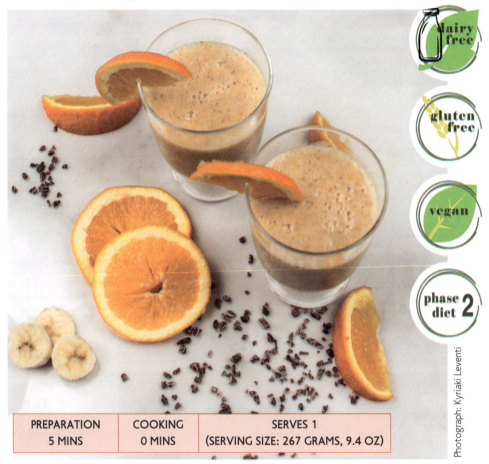

Photograph: Kyriaki Leventi

PREPARATION 5 MINS	COOKING 0 MINS	SERVES 1 (SERVING SIZE: 267 GRAMS, 9.4 OZ)

INGREDIENTS

- ½ orange (43 grams), peeled segments separated and frozen
- ⅓ cup (33 grams) unripe frozen banana, peeled, sliced
- ½ cup (120 ml) almond milk (**see recipe for nondairy milks page 171** or use unsweetened almond milk)
- ¼ cup (60 ml) ice cubes
- 1 teaspoon (5 ml) 100% pure maple syrup
- 1 teaspoon (4.6 grams) cocoa nibs
- ¼ teaspoon (0.5 grams) organic orange zest

INSTRUCTIONS

Blend all ingredients together until smooth.

Nutrition Facts

Per serving: 120 kcal	26 grams carbohydrates
2 grams protein	2 grams fiber
1.5 grams total fat	High in vitamin C
0 grams saturated fat	

Pineapple Green Smoothie Bowl

PREPARATION 5 MINS	COOKING 0 MINS	SERVES 1

INGREDIENTS

- ½ cup (70 grams) frozen pineapple cubes
- ½ cup (15 grams) fresh baby spinach
- 1 small kiwi (70 grams), peeled and cut into chunks
- ½ cup (140 grams) **lactose-free** yogurt

INSTRUCTIONS

Blend until smooth.

Nutrition Facts

Per serving: 140 kcal	23 grams carbohydrates
7 grams protein	2 grams fiber
2 grams total fat	High in calcium, phosphorous, riboflavin and vitamins C, and K
1.5 grams saturated fat	

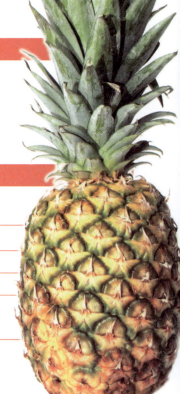

Banana Green Smoothie Bowl

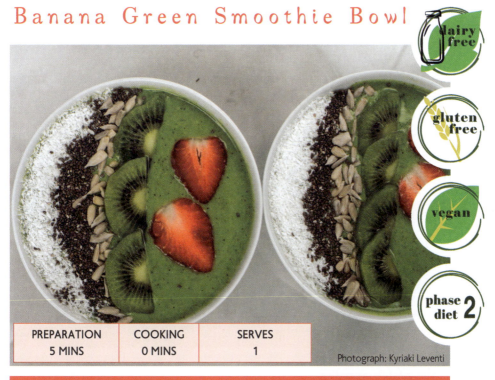

dairy free

gluten free

vegan

phase diet 2

PREPARATION	COOKING	SERVES
5 MINS	0 MINS	1

Photograph: Kyriaki Leventi

INGREDIENTS

- ½ medium (50 grams) unripe banana, peeled, sliced and frozen
- ½ cup (15 grams) fresh baby spinach leaves
- 1 cup (30 grams) fresh baby kale leaves
- ⅛ cup (20 grams) blueberries
- ½ cup (120 ml) almond milk (**see recipe for nondairy milks page 171** or use unsweetened almond milk)
- ½ tablespoon (5.5 grams) flaxseed meal

INSTRUCTIONS

Blend until smooth.

Nutrition Facts	
Per serving: 140 kcal	23 grams carbohydrates
7 grams protein	2 grams fiber
2 grams total fat	High in calcium, riboflavin, folate, copper, manganese, and vitamins A, C, and K
1.5 grams saturated fat	

Strawberry Smoothie Bowl

PREPARATION	COOKING	SERVES
5 MINS	0 MINS	1

INGREDIENTS

- 10 medium (140 grams) frozen strawberries
- ½ cup (140 grams) **lactose-free** yogurt
- 1 tablespoon (11 grams) chia seeds
- 2 teaspoons (10 ml) 100% pure maple syrup

INSTRUCTIONS

Blend until smooth.

Nutrition Facts	
Per serving: 200 kcal	35 grams carbohydrates
8 grams protein	5 grams fiber
4 grams total fat	High in vitamin C and manganese
1.5 grams saturated fat	

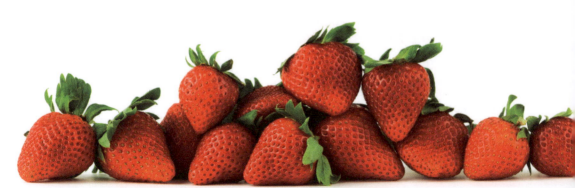

PANCAKES, CREPES, MUFFINS AND MORE
Buckwheat Banana Pancakes

PREPARATION 5 MINS	COOKING 20 MINS	SERVES 6 (SERVING SIZE: 2 SMALL PANCAKES, 100 GRAMS, 3.5 OZ)

INGREDIENTS

- 1 cup (135 grams) buckwheat flour
- 1 tablespoon (15 ml) 100% pure maple syrup
- 1 tablespoon (15 ml) cold-pressed vegetable oil
- 1 cup (240 ml) low-fat **lactose-free** milk or almond milk **(page 172)**
- 1 medium (100 grams) ripe banana, mashed
- 1 pastured egg
- 2 teaspoons (9.6 grams) **gluten-free** baking powder
- ¼ teaspoon (1.5 grams) salt
- Vegetable oil for cooking

INSTRUCTIONS

Mix the buckwheat flour, baking powder and salt in a large bowl.

Whisk together milk, egg, maple syrup, oil and mashed banana.

Add dry ingredients to the milk mixture and whisk until moistened.

Heat a nonstick skillet over medium heat.

Moisten a paper towel with the vegetable oil.

Rub skillet with oiled paper towel.

Scoop 2 tablespoons of batter onto the skillet.

Spread batter into a round shape.

Cook for a few minutes until brown.

Flip the pancake with a spatula and brown the other side.

Rub the skillet with oil and continue with the rest of the batter.

Nutrition Facts

Per serving: 150 kcal	24 grams carbohydrates
5 grams protein	3 grams fiber
4.5 grams total fat	High in calcium, phosphorous, and manganese
3 grams saturated fat	

Quinoa Crepes

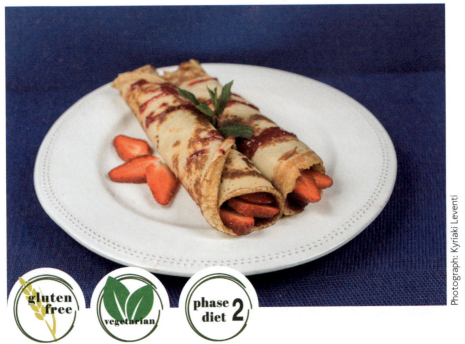

Photograph: Kyriaki Leventi

PREPARATION 5 MINS	COOKING 20 MINS	SERVES 9 (SERVING SIZE: 50 GRAMS EACH, 1.8 OZ)

INGREDIENTS

2 flax eggs

Omit this step if using eggs

- 2 tablespoons (21 grams) ground flaxseed meal
- 6 tablespoons (90 ml) of warm water

Crepes

- 1 cup (112 grams) quinoa flour
- 1 cup (240 ml) low-fat **lactose-free** milk or almond milk **(see recipe page 171)**
- 1 tablespoon (15 ml) 100% pure maple syrup
- 2 tablespoons (30 ml) cold-pressed vegetable oil
- 2 flax eggs or 2 pastured eggs
- Vegetable oil for cooking

INSTRUCTIONS

Step 1: Make flax eggs, if using

Stir two tablespoons ground **flaxseed** meal with six tablespoons of warm water.

Let it sit for 10 minutes to thicken.

Step 2

Whisk together milk, eggs, maple syrup and oil.

Add quinoa flour to milk mixture and whisk until smooth.

Heat a nonstick skillet over medium heat.

Moisten a paper towel with oil.

Rub skillet with oiled paper towel.

Scoop ¼ cup batter onto the skillet.

Tilt the pan with a circular motion so that the batter coats the surface evenly.

Cook for approximately 2 minutes until the bottom is light brown. Loosen with a spatula, turn and cook the other side.

Rub the skillet with oil and continue with the rest of the batter.

Served with fresh fruits and chia jam.

Nutrition Facts	
Per serving: 100 kcal	1 gram saturated fat
4 grams protein	12 grams carbohydrates
4.5 grams total fat	2 grams fiber

Quinoa Pancakes

PREPARATION	COOKING	SERVES 6
5 MINS	20 MINS	(SERVING SIZE: 2 PANCAKES, 102 GRAMS, 3.6 OZ)

INGREDIENTS

2 Flax eggs

- 2 tablespoons (21 grams) ground flaxseed meal

- 6 tablespoons (90 ml) of warm water

Pancakes

- 1 cup (112 grams) quinoa flour
- 1 cup (240 ml) almond milk **(see recipe page 171)**
- 1 medium (100 grams) ripe banana, mashed
- 1 teaspoon (5 ml) pure vanilla extract
- 1 tablespoon (15 ml) 100% pure maple syrup
- 1 tablespoon (15 ml) cold-pressed coconut oil, melted
- 2 flax eggs
- 2 teaspoons (9.6 grams) gluten-free baking powder
- ¼ teaspoon (1.5 grams) salt
- Coconut oil for cooking

INSTRUCTIONS

Step 1: Make flax eggs

Stir one tablespoon ground flaxseed meal with three tablespoons of warm water.
Let it sit for 10 minutes to thicken.

Step 2

Mix together the quinoa flour, baking powder and salt in a large bowl.
Whisk together almond milk, flax eggs, maple syrup, vanilla, coconut oil and the
   mashed banana.
Add dry ingredients to milk mixture and whisk until moistened.
Heat a nonstick skillet over medium heat.
Melt the coconut oil and moisten a paper towel with it.
Rub skillet with oiled paper towel.
Scoop 2 tablespoons of batter onto the skillet.
Spread batter into a round shape.
Flip the pancake with a spatula and allow to brown on both sides.
Rub the skillet with oil and continue with the rest of the batter.

Nutrition Facts	
Per serving: 160 kcal	2 grams saturated fat
4 grams protein	25 grams carbohydrates
6 grams total fat	4 grams fiber

Chocolate Pumpkin Muffins

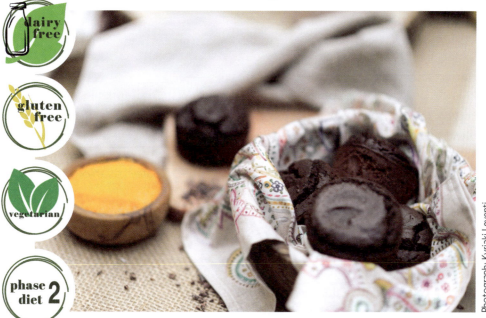

Photograph: Kyriaki Leventi

dairy free

gluten free

vegetarian

phase diet 2

PREPARATION 10-15 MINS	COOKING 35 MINS	TO PREPARE PUMPKIN PUREE: 50 MINS	SERVES 12 (SERVING SIZE: 50 GRAMS EACH, 1.8 OZ)

INGREDIENTS

- 1 cup plus 1 tablespoon (120 grams) almond meal
- 4 tablespoons (24 grams) raw cacao
- 70 grams (2.5 oz) melted dark chocolate 70-85% cocoa solids
- ½ teaspoon (3 grams) salt
- ½ teaspoon (2.3 grams) baking soda
- 1 teaspoon (4.6 grams) **gluten-free** baking powder
- ½ cup (120 ml) 100% pure maple syrup
- 2 pastured eggs
- 1 teaspoon (5 ml) pure vanilla extract
- ¾ cup (183 grams) Japanese pumpkin puree, readymade or make your own **(see recipe below)**
- ¼ cup (22.5 grams) coconut, shredded, dried

Desiccated coconut (dried and shredded coconut that is made from the flesh of a mature coconut, see page 166)

INSTRUCTIONS

Step 1: Pumpkin puree

Cut the pumpkin in large pieces.

Scrape out the seeds and pulp from the center.

Place pumpkin pieces on a baking sheet face up.

Roast in a 177°C/350°F oven for 45 minutes or until pumpkin is fork-tender.

Peel off the skin from the pumpkin pieces.

Blend the pumpkin in a food processor or with a potato masher.

> If it is watery, transfer the puree to a saucepan and simmer over medium-low heat, stirring frequently. Continue to simmer until the puree has thickened to the right consistency.

Refrigerate for up to four days or freeze in an airtight container.

Step 2

Preheat oven to 177°C/350°F.

Line a muffin tin with 12 muffins liners.

Grind coconut into flour using a food processor.

Mix coconut, almond meal, baking soda, baking powder, raw cacao and salt.

Beat the eggs, vanilla, and maple syrup in a food processor until well combined.

Add the pumpkin and beat for a few seconds.

Add the dry ingredients to the wet and pulse to combine.

Allow the mixture to sit for 5 minutes, until the coconut flour absorbs the liquids.

Melt the chocolate (bring about an inch of water to a simmer in a small saucepan; set a heatproof bowl in the mouth of the pot and stir chocolate until it softens).

Add the chocolate.

Divide batter evenly among 12 muffin cups.

Bake for 25-35 minutes or until a toothpick comes out clean and the tops of the muffins are just slightly golden brown.

Nutrition Facts	
Per serving: 160 kcal	17 grams carbohydrates
4 grams protein	3 grams fiber
10 grams total fat	High in manganese
3 grams saturated fat	

> ❗ *Use dried and shredded coconut (desiccated coconut) that is made from the flesh of a mature coconut. According to Monash University, a ¼-cup serving of desiccated coconut is low in FODMAPs. Large servings contain moderate to high levels of polyols.*
>
> *Coconut flour is a byproduct of coconut milk production and is high in FODMAPS. A ¾-cup (100 grams) serving contains high levels of GOS, fructans, excess fructose and sorbitol.*

Zucchini Chocolate Muffins

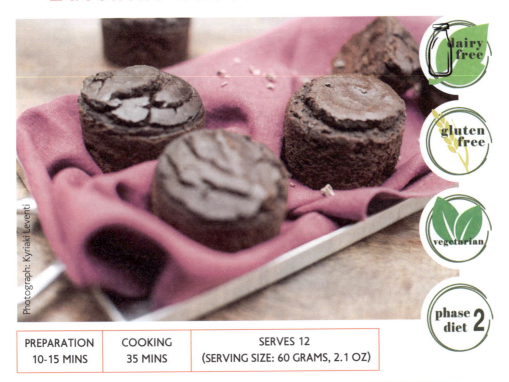

Photograph: Kyriaki Leventi

dairy free

gluten free

vegetarian

phase 2 diet

PREPARATION 10-15 MINS	COOKING 35 MINS	SERVES 12 (SERVING SIZE: 60 GRAMS, 2.1 OZ)

INGREDIENTS

- 1 cup (95 grams) shredded unpeeled zucchini (after excess moisture has been squeezed out)
- 40 grams/1.4 oz almonds
- ½ cup (45 grams/1.6 oz) desiccated coconut (dried and shredded coconut that is made from the flesh of a mature coconut, see page 166)

- 150 grams/5.3 oz banana
- 4 pastured eggs
- ⅓ cup (80 ml) 100% pure maple syrup
- 2 tablespoons (30 ml) of extra-virgin olive oil
- 2 teaspoons (9.2 grams) gluten-free baking powder
- ¼ teaspoon (1.5 grams) salt
- 60 grams/2.1 oz melted dark chocolate (70-85% cocoa solids)
- 2 tablespoons (12 grams) raw cacao

INSTRUCTIONS

Preheat oven to 180°C/356°F.

Line a muffin tin with 12 muffins liners.

Grind the almonds and the coconut into flour.

Shred the unpeeled zucchini.

Gather shredded zucchini in a clean kitchen towel and squeeze to remove as much moisture as possible.

Combine coconut and almond flour with the baking soda and salt.

Beat the eggs, vanilla, maple syrup and oil until well combined.

Melt the chocolate (bring about an inch of water to a simmer in a small saucepan; set a heatproof bowl in the mouth of the pot and stir *chocolate* until it softens).

Add the dry ingredients to the wet ingredients and stir to combine.

Allow the mixture to sit for 5 minutes, until the coconut absorbs the liquids.

Add the zucchini, banana, vinegar and melted chocolate.

Mix until smooth and well combined.

Divide batter evenly among 12 muffin cups.

Bake for 25-35 minutes or until toothpick comes out clean and the tops of the muffins are just slightly golden brown.

Nutrition Facts	
Per serving: 150 kcal	14 grams carbohydrates
4 grams protein	3 grams fiber
11 grams total fat	High in manganese
4.5 grams saturated fat	

Quinoa Muffins

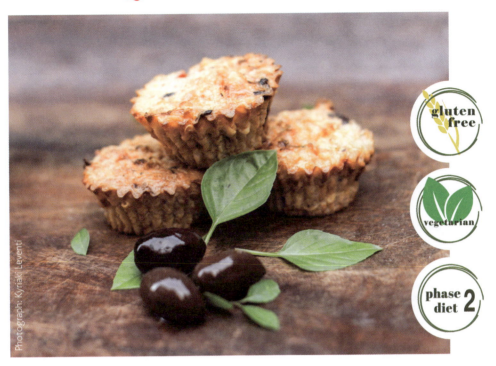

Photograph: Kyriaki Leventi

gluten free

vegetarian

phase diet 2

PREPARATION 15 MINS	COOKING 30 MINS FOR THE MUFFINS	COOKING QUINOA 15 MINS	ROASTED RED PEPPERS 25 MINS	SERVES 10 (SERVING SIZE: 2 MUFFINS, 55 GRAMS EACH, 1.9 OZ)

INGREDIENTS

Roasted red pepper
- 1 medium red bell pepper (119 grams)

Muffins
- 2 pastured eggs
- 2 egg whites (66 grams)
- 2 cups (360 grams) cooked quinoa (¾ cup (130 grams) dry quinoa; **page 364**)
- 2 cups (190 grams) shredded unpeeled zucchini (after excess moisture has been squeezed out)
- 3 cups (90 grams) spinach
- ½ cup (50 grams) grated Parmesan

- ½ cup (70 grams) feta, crumbled
- 1 medium oven roasted red pepper (119 grams/4.2 oz) cut into small pieces (you can use readymade red peppers in a jar)
- Salt and pepper

INSTRUCTIONS

Step 1: : Roasting bell peppers

Roast bell peppers (you can skip this step and use roasted red peppers in a jar).

Preheat your oven to 230°C/450°F.

Cut the peppers in half lengthwise.

Remove the stem and seeds.

Cover baking sheet with parchment paper.

Roast for approximately 25 minutes or until the skin is wrinkled.

Cover and let them cool.

Remove the skin and cut the peppers into small pieces.

Step 2: Prepare the muffins

Preheat oven to 180°C/356°F.

Whisk together eggs and egg whites in a large bowl.

Gather shredded zucchini in a clean kitchen towel and squeeze to remove as much moisture as possible.

Stir in the remaining ingredients.

Add salt and pepper (adjust salt according to your cheese).

Spoon into **silicone muffin liners** (muffins stick to paper liners and greased muffins trays).

Bake for 30 minutes or until a toothpick comes out clean when poked into a muffin.

Nutrition Facts	
Per serving: 100 kcal	10 grams carbohydrates
6 grams protein	2 grams fiber
4 grams total fat	High in vitamins A and C
2 grams saturated fat	

Quinoa Muffins with Olives and Feta Cheese

PREPARATION 15 MINS	COOKING 30 MINS FOR THE MUFFINS	COOKING QUINOA 15 MINS	SERVES 7 (SERVING SIZE: 2 MUFFINS, 55 GRAMS EACH, 1.9 OZ)

INGREDIENTS

- 2 pastured eggs
- 2 egg whites (66 grams)
- 2 cups (360 grams) cooked quinoa (¾ cup (130 grams) dry quinoa; **see recipe page 364**)
- 2 cups (190 grams) shredded unpeeled zucchini (after excess moisture has been squeezed out)
- ¼ cup (35 grams) feta, crumbled
- 20 black Kalamata olives, cut in small pieces
- 1 small (119 grams) fresh tomato, cut into small pieces

INSTRUCTIONS

Preheat oven to 180°C/356°F.

Whisk together eggs and egg whites.

Gather shredded zucchini in a clean kitchen towel and squeeze to remove as much moisture as possible.

Stir in the remaining ingredients.

Add salt and pepper (adjust salt according to your cheese).

Spoon into **silicone muffin liners** (muffins stick to paper liners and greased muffins trays).

Bake for 30 minutes or until a toothpick comes out clean when poked into a muffin.

Nutrition Facts	
Per serving: 130 kcal	7 grams carbohydrates
8 grams protein	<1 gram fiber
8 grams total fat	High in calcium and phosphorus
3.5 grams saturated fat	

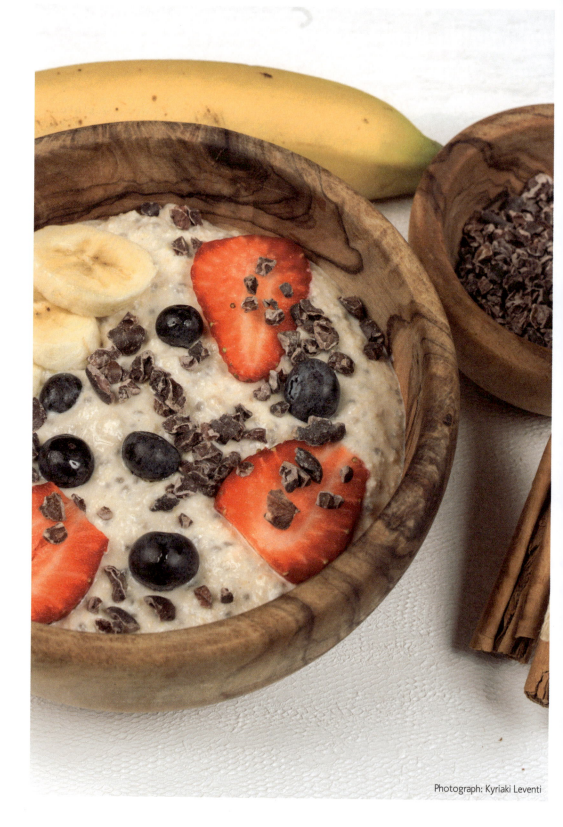

Photograph: Kyriaki Leventi

Overnight Quinoa

PREPARATION 2 MINS	COOKING 0 MINS	SERVES 3 (SERVING SIZE 125 GRAMS, 4.4 OZ)

INGREDIENTS

- ⅓ cup (80 grams) plain **lactose-free** Greek yogurt
- ¾ cup (75 grams) quinoa flakes
- ⅔ cup (180 ml) almond milk (**see recipe for nondairy milks page 171** or use unsweetened almond milk)
- 1 tablespoon (11 grams) chia seeds
- ½ teaspoon (2.5 ml) pure vanilla extract
- 2 tablespoons (30 ml) 100% pure maple syrup
- Pinch of salt

INSTRUCTIONS

Whisk all the ingredients together and place the mixture into a jar with a tight lid.
Store overnight (or at least for 4-6 hours).

Nutrition Facts
Per serving: 190 kcal
6 grams protein
4 grams total fat
0.5 grams saturated fat
33 grams carbohydrates
4 grams fiber
High in calcium, riboflavin, manganese, phosphorous, and magnesium

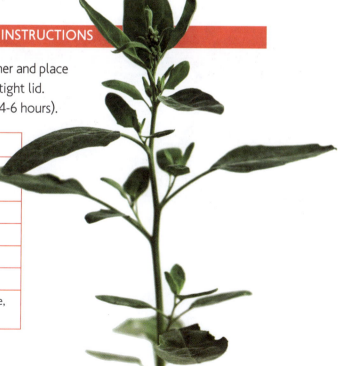

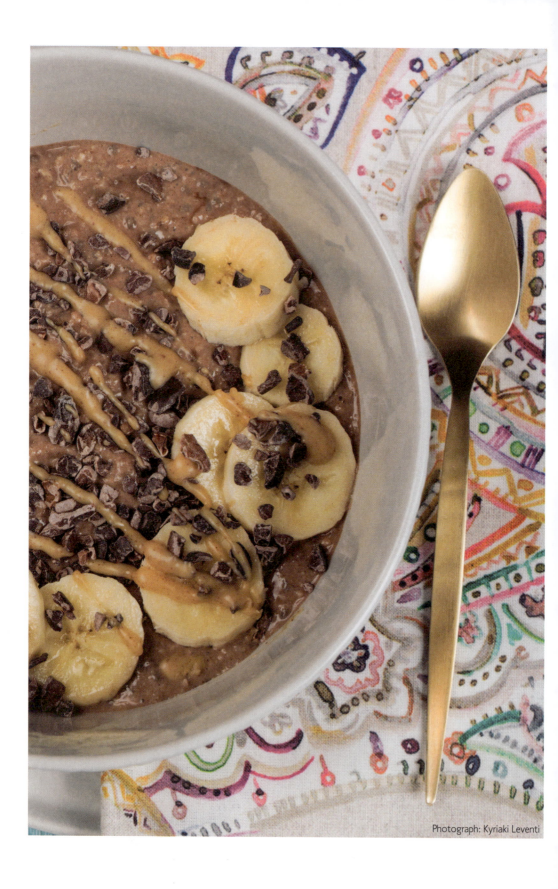

Photograph: Kyriaki Leventi

Overnight Buckwheat with Cocoa

PREPARATION 2 MINS	COOKING 0 MINS	SERVES 2 (SERVING SIZE 162 GRAMS, 5.7 OZ)

INGREDIENTS

- ⅓ cup (80 grams) plain **lactose-free** Greek yogurt
- ½ cup (45 grams) buckwheat flakes
- ⅔ cup (180 ml) almond milk (**see recipe for nondairy milks page 171** or use unsweetened almond milk)
- 1 tablespoon (11 grams) chia seeds
- 2 teaspoons (4 grams) raw cacao
- ½ teaspoon (2.5 ml) pure vanilla extract
- 1 tablespoon (15 ml) 100% pure maple syrup
- Pinch of salt

INSTRUCTIONS

Whisk all the ingredients together and place the mixture into a jar with a tight lid. **Store** overnight (or at least for 4-6 hours).

Nutrition Facts	
Per serving: 220 kcal	39 grams carbohydrates
7 grams protein	4 grams fiber
4.5 grams total fat	High in calcium, riboflavin, and manganese

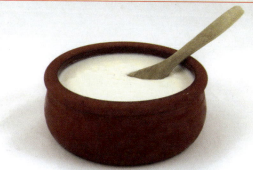

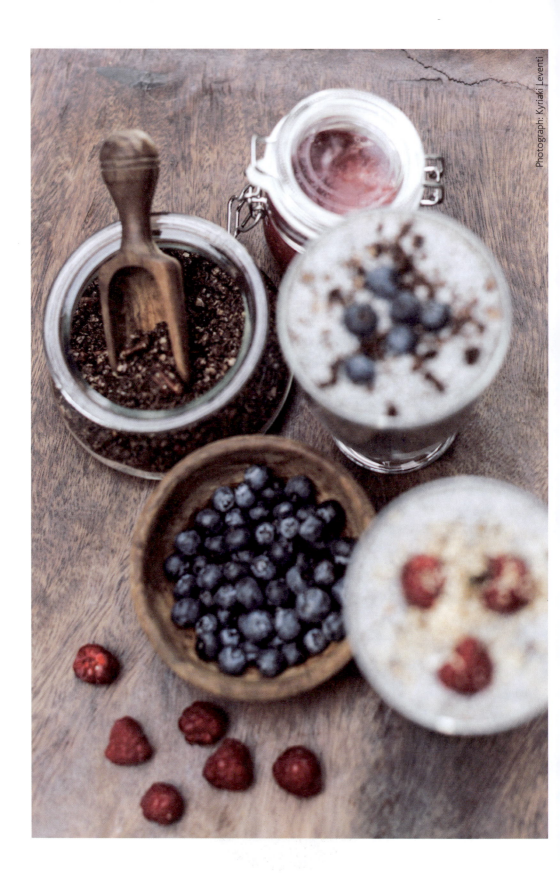

Photograph: Kyriaki Leventi

Chia Pudding

PREPARATION 2 MINS	COOKING 0 MINS	WAITING TIME OVERNIGHT	SERVES 6 (SERVING SIZE 90 GRAMS, 3.3OZ)

INGREDIENTS

- 2 cups (480 ml) of almond milk (**see recipe for nondairy milks page 171** or use unsweetened almond milk)
- 8 tablespoons (88 grams) chia seeds
- 1 tablespoon (15 ml) 100% pure maple syrup
- 1 teaspoon (5 ml) pure vanilla extract

INSTRUCTIONS

Whisk all the ingredients together and place the mixture into a jar with a tight lid.

Let sit for a few minutes and then whisk again.

Cover and refrigerate for 4-5 hours or overnight.

Add more chia seeds and stir if it is too runny.

Keep in the refrigerator for up to 5 days.

Nutrition Facts
Per serving: 90 kcal
2 grams protein
4 grams total fat
0 grams saturated fat
12 grams carbohydrates
4 grams fiber
High in calcium and magnesium

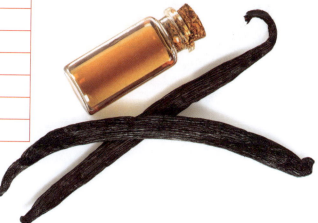

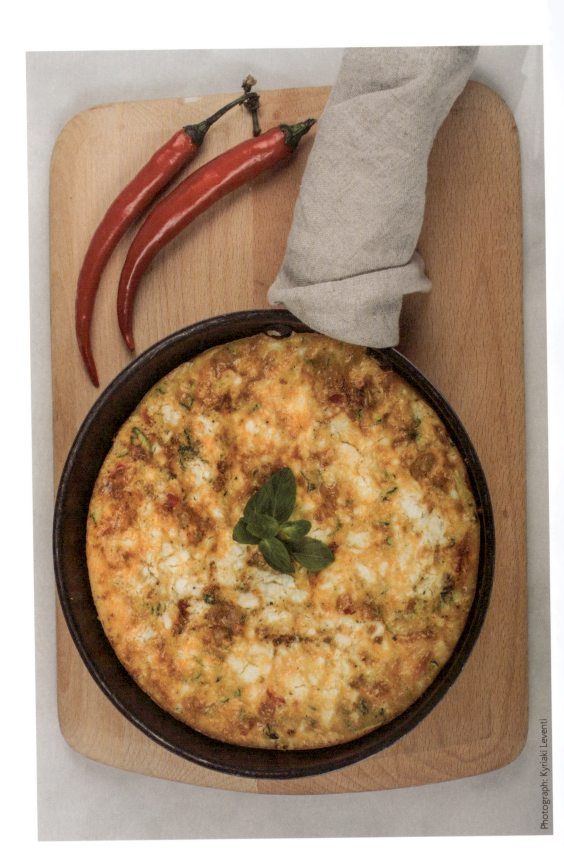

Photograph: Kyriaki Leventi

Zucchini and Red Pepper Frittata

PREPARATION 5-10 MINS	COOKING 12 MINS	SERVES 2 (SERVING SIZE 245 GRAMS, 8.6 OZ)

INGREDIENTS

- 1 medium (130 grams) zucchini, grated
- 1 small (74 grams) red pepper, cut into small pieces
- 4 medium pastured eggs
- ¼ cup (35 grams) feta, crumbled
- 1 spring onion (green parts only)
- ½ tablespoon (7.5 ml) olive oil
- Fresh chili (optional), to serve
- Fresh mint leaves, to serve
- salt and pepper

INSTRUCTIONS

Grate the zucchini.

Finely chop the green parts of the spring onion.

Heat a medium frying pan with the olive oil.

Sauté the pepper and zucchini over medium heat for a few minutes until softened.

Heat the grill to high.

Beat the eggs in a bowl with the salt and pepper.

Crumble the feta and stir about half into the egg mixture.

Add the finely chopped green parts of the spring onion.

Pour into the pan, letting the egg flow evenly through the vegetable mixture.

Cook for 4-5 minutes until the egg begins to just set on the base.

Add the rest of the feta.

Place under the hot grill and cook until just cooked through and golden.

Serve with mint leaves and fresh chili.

Nutrition Facts	
Per serving: 240 kcal	7 grams carbohydrates
15 grams protein	2 grams fiber
17 grams total fat	High in folate, selenium, phosphorus, riboflavin and vitamins C, A, D, B6, and B12
6 grams saturated fat	

Chocolate Buckwheat Granola

PREPARATION 5 MINS	COOKING 35-40 MINS	SERVES 27 (SERVING SIZE 30 GRAMS, ¼ CUP)

INGREDIENTS

- 2 cups (200 grams) buckwheat flakes
- 1 cup (109 grams) pecans (chopped)
- 1 cup (80 grams) unsweetened **desiccated coconut (dried and shredded coconut that is made from the flesh of a mature coconut, see page 166)**
- ½ cup (84 grams) golden flaxseed
- ¼ cup (48 grams) chia seeds
- ½ cup (120 ml) maple syrup
- ½ cup (48 grams) unsweetened raw cocoa
- 3 tablespoons (45 ml) cold-pressed virgin coconut oil
- 2 teaspoons (10 ml) pure vanilla extract
- ½ teaspoon (3 grams) salt

INSTRUCTIONS

Preheat oven to 180°C/356°F.

Toss buckwheat flakes, pecans, coconut, flaxseed and chia seeds on a rimmed baking tray.

Toast in the oven for 10-15 minutes, stirring once or twice until the coconut is golden brown.

Decrease the oven temperature to 150°C/302°F.

Place the buckwheat mixture into a large mixing bowl.

Add the raw cocoa and mix.

Mix the maple syrup, coconut oil, vanilla and salt and pour over the buckwheat mixture until it is uniformly coated.

Spread the mixture onto a rimmed baking tray and bake for 20-25 minutes, until it turns golden brown.

Remove from the oven and allow to cool.

The granola can keep in an airtight container for up to three weeks.

Nutrition Facts	
Per serving: 110 kcal	2.5 grams saturated fat
2 grams protein	9 grams carbohydrates
8 grams total fat	3 grams fiber

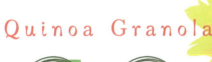

Quinoa Granola

PREPARATION 5 MINS	COOKING 35-40 MINS	SERVES 15 (SERVING SIZE 30 GRAMS, ¼ CUP)

INGREDIENTS

- 1 cup quinoa flakes (100 grams)
- ½ cup (60 grams) walnuts, chopped
- ½ cup (70 grams) sunflower seeds
- ½ cup (40 grams) unsweetened **desiccated coconut (dried and shredded coconut that is made from the flesh of a mature coconut, see page 166)**
- ¼ cup (42 grams) crushed golden flaxseeds
- ¼ cup (35 grams) macadamia nuts
- ¼ cup (60 ml) 100% pure maple syrup
- 3 tablespoons (45 ml) virgin coconut oil
- 1 teaspoon (5 ml) pure vanilla extract
- ¼ teaspoon (1.5 grams) sea salt

INSTRUCTIONS

Preheat oven to 180°C/356°F.

Toss quinoa flakes, walnuts, sunflower seeds, coconut, flaxseeds and macadamia nuts on a rimmed baking tray.

Toast in the oven for 10-15 minutes, stirring once or twice, until the coconut is golden brown.

Decrease oven temperature to 150°C/302°F.

Place the quinoa mixture into a large mixing bowl.

Mix the maple syrup, coconut oil, vanilla and salt and pour over the quinoa mixture until it is uniformly coated.

Spread the mixture onto a rimmed baking tray.

Bake for 20-25 minutes, until it turns golden brown.

Remove from the oven and allow to cool.

The granola can keep in an airtight container for up to three weeks.

Nutrition Facts	
Per serving: 160 kcal	4 grams saturated fat
3 grams protein	11 grams carbohydrates
11 grams total fat	2 grams fiber

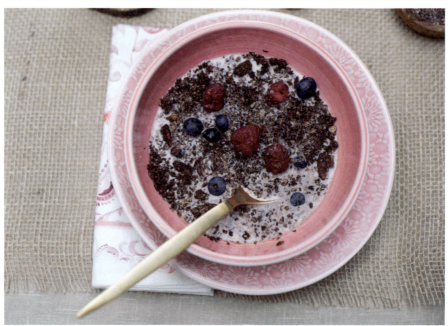

Photograph: Kyriaki Leventi

Buckwheat Bars

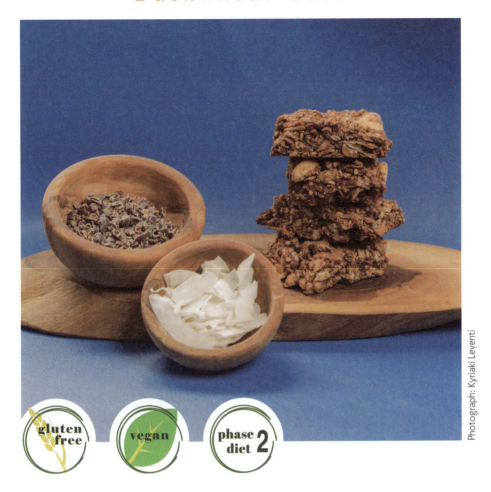

Photograph: Kyriaki Leventi

PREPARATION 5 MINS	COOKING 35 MINS	SERVES 17 (40 GRAMS, 1.4 OZ)

INGREDIENTS

- 1 cup (120 grams) sliced almonds
- 1 cup (140 grams) sunflower seeds
- ½ cup (84 grams) crushed golden flaxseeds
- 1 cup (120 grams) walnuts, chopped
- ½ cup (50 grams) buckwheat flakes

- 2 tablespoons (21 grams) chia seeds
- 4 tablespoons (30 grams) dried cranberries, chopped
- ½ cup (120 ml) 100% pure maple syrup
- 2 tablespoons (32 grams) peanut butter

INSTRUCTIONS

Preheat oven to 170°C/338°F.

Toss buckwheat flakes, walnuts, sunflower seeds, and almonds on a rimmed baking tray.

Toast in the oven for 10-15 minutes, stirring once or twice.

Place the buckwheat flake mixture into a large mixing bowl; add chia seeds, flaxseeds and cranberries.

Mix the maple syrup and peanut butter in a pan and stir over heat until the peanut butter is melted.

Pour the maple syrup and peanut butter over the buckwheat mixture until it is uniformly coated.

Line a baking sheet with parchment paper.

Spread the mixture onto the baking tray and press firmly.

Bake for 20 minutes, until it turns golden brown.

Remove from the oven and allow to cool; then **cut** to desired size.

The bars can keep in an airtight container for up to three weeks.

Nutrition Facts	
Per serving: 200 kcal	1.5 grams saturated fat
6 grams protein	15 grams carbohydrates
14 grams total fat	3 grams fiber

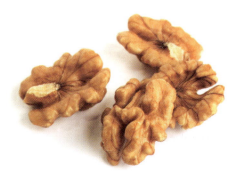

Quinoa Bars

PREPARATION 5 MINS	COOKING 35 MINS	SERVES 20 (40 GRAMS, 1.4 OZ)

INGREDIENTS

- 1 cup (120 grams) sliced almonds
- 1 cup (120 grams) peanuts, chopped
- ½ cup (87 grams) dark chocolate chips (70-85% cacao solids)
- 1cup (80 grams) unsweetened **desiccated coconut (dried and shredded coconut that is made from the flesh of a mature coconut see page 166)**
- ½ cup (50 grams) quinoa flakes
- ½ cup (70 grams) sunflower seeds
- ¼ cup (42 grams) crushed golden flaxseed
- ½ cup (60 grams) walnuts, chopped
- ½ cup (120 ml) 100% pure maple syrup
- 2 tablespoons (32 grams) peanut butter

INSTRUCTIONS

Preheat oven to 170°C/338°F.

Toss quinoa flakes, walnuts, sunflower seeds, coconut, almonds and peanuts on a rimmed baking tray.

Toast in the oven for 10-15 minutes, stirring once or twice until the coconut is golden brown.

Place the quinoa flake mixture into a large mixing bowl; add flaxseeds and chocolate chips.

Mix the maple syrup and peanut butter in a pan and stir over heat until the peanut butter is melted.

Pour the maple syrup and peanut butter over the quinoa mixture until it is uniformly coated.

Line a baking sheet with parchment paper.

Spread the mixture onto the baking tray and press firmly.

Bake for 20 minutes, until it turns golden brown.

Remove from the oven, allow to cool, and then **cut** to desired size.
The bars can remain in an airtight container for up to three weeks.

Nutrition Facts	
Per serving: 210 kcal	4.5 grams saturated fat
5 grams protein	14 grams carbohydrates
16 grams total fat	3 grams fiber

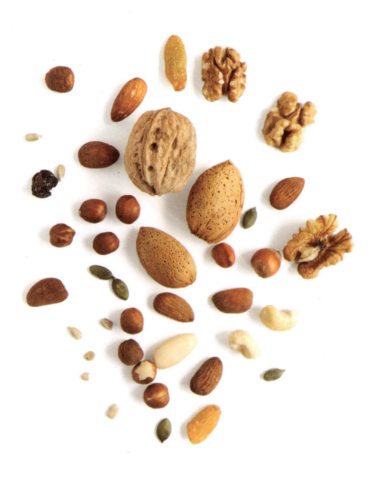

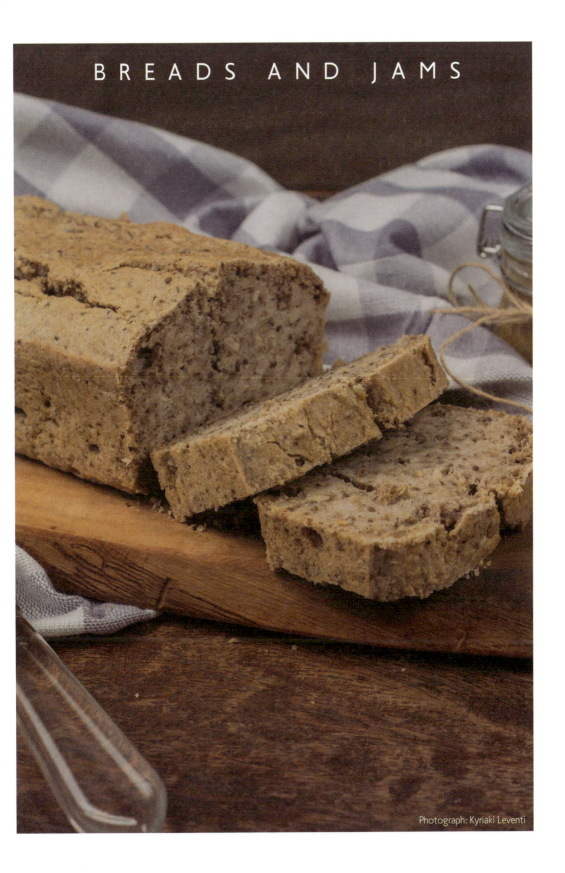

Photograph: Kyriaki Leventi

Buckwheat Quinoa Bread

PREPARATION 10 MINS	COOKING 40 MINS	COOKING TIME FOR CHIA JAM 20-30 MINS	SERVES 26 (30 GRAMS EACH, 1 OZ)

INGREDIENTS

Chia pineapple jam

(Use only ½ cup from this recipe; you can freeze the remaining jam)
- 3 ½ cups (500 grams) fresh or frozen pineapple, with heart of pineapple removed and pineapple chopped into small pieces
- 4 tablespoons (44 grams) chia seeds

Bread
- 2 cups (270 grams) buckwheat flour (100% whole-grain stone-ground)
- 1 ½ teaspoon (6.9 grams) baking soda
- ½ teaspoon (2.4 grams) **gluten-free** baking powder
- ½ teaspoon (3 grams) salt
- ½ cup (50 grams) quinoa flakes
- 1 ½ cup (360 ml) **lactose-free** kefir
- ½ cup (112 grams) pineapple chia jam

INSTRUCTIONS

Step 1: Make the jam

Place the pineapple pieces into a medium-sized pot and allow to boil.

Reduce the heat to medium and boil for approximately 10 minutes, stirring frequently, until the pineapple is soft.

Place the pineapple in a blender and blend until smooth.

Add the pineapple back into the pot and stir in the chia seeds.

Cook the jam on low until it thickens approximately 7-10 minutes, continuing to stir frequently.

Remove from heat and let it cool down.

Pour the jam in a glass jar and store in the refrigerator.

It can remain in the refrigerator for up to 2 weeks.

Step 2: Make the bread

Preheat oven to 180°C/356°F.

Generously grease an 8 x 4 x 2.5 inch (20 x 10 x 6 cm) loaf pan with olive oil.

Mix buckwheat flour, baking soda, baking powder, salt and quinoa flakes.

Mix kefir with pineapple jam (**let the jam cool first**).

Mix wet and dry ingredients until well combined.

Pour the batter in the greased loaf pan.

Bake for 30-40 minutes until golden and a toothpick or knife inserted into the center comes out clean.

Nutrition Facts	
Per serving: 60 kcal	0 grams saturated fat
2 grams protein	11 grams carbohydrates
1 gram total fat	1 gram fiber

Buckwheat Bread

PREPARATION 10 MINS	COOKING 90 MINS	WAITING TIME 2 HRS	SERVES 30 (33 GRAMS, 1.2 OZ)

INGREDIENTS

1 ¾ cups (310 grams) buckwheat groats

½ cup (70 grams) sunflower seeds

½ cup (64 grams) pumpkin seeds

½ cup (76 grams) sesame seeds

4 tablespoons (44 grams) chia seeds

1 cup (240 ml) water

3 tablespoons (45 ml) olive oil

2 teaspoons (9.6 grams) **gluten-free** baking powder

½ teaspoon (3 grams) salt

1 teaspoon (2 grams) mahleb (optional)

2 tablespoons mixed seeds (chia, sesame, and pumpkin) for topping

INSTRUCTIONS

Soak the buckwheat in enough water for 2 hours until it is soft enough.

Preheat oven to 160°C/320°F.

Grease a 8 x 4 x 2.5 inch (20 x 10 x 6 cm) loaf pan generously with olive oil.

Remove the excess water, but keep the slimy liquid. You need about **one cup of water** for this liquid.

Place the water-soaked buckwheat groats with 1 cup of the slimy liquid in a food processor and pulse until a dough is made. The mixture will be sticky.

Remove the dough from the processor and combine it with the chia seeds, stirring to mix. Let sit for approximately 10 minutes until thickened.

Combine the dough with the remaining ingredients, stirring to combine.

Scoop the mixture into the greased loaf pan.

Top with mixed seeds if desired.

Bake for 90 minutes or until a toothpick or knife inserted into the center comes out clean.

Nutrition Facts	
Per serving: 100 kcal	0.5 grams saturated fat
4 grams protein	11 grams carbohydrates
5 grams total fat	3 grams fiber

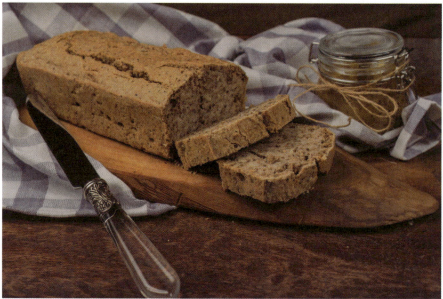

Photograph: Kyriaki Leventi

Buckwheat Pita Bread

PREPARATION 15 MINS	COOKING 80 MINS	WAITING TIME 1 HOUR 50 MINS	SERVES 12 (30 GRAMS)

INGREDIENTS

- ¾ cup (180 ml) warm **lactose-free** milk
- 1 envelope **gluten-free** active dry yeast (8 grams)
- 2 cups (270 grams) or more buckwheat flour
- 1 teaspoon (4 grams) raw sugar
- ¾ teaspoon (4.5 grams) salt
- 3 tablespoons (45 ml) extra-virgin olive oil

INSTRUCTIONS

Mix the yeast, raw sugar, and warm milk in a large bowl. (Do not boil the milk; maintain at 40-46°C/105-115°F)

Allow the mixture to activate approximately 15 minutes.

Foam will form along the surface.

Mix the buckwheat flour, salt and olive oil.

Add the yeast mixture.

Work slowly to make fairly firm dough.

Flour a work surface and knead the dough for 5 minutes until it no longer sticks.

Cover and allow the dough to rise in a warm spot for 1 hour.

Remove dough from bowl and place onto a floured work surface.

Cut dough into 12 pieces.

Cover dough pieces with lightly oiled plastic wrap and let rest for 30 minutes.

Sprinkle a small amount of flour on a work surface.

Take one piece at a time and roll out the dough into a round pita shape (approximately ¼ inch thick).

Place round pitas between two sheets of baking paper.

Let rest for 5 minutes.

Repeat with the remaining dough pieces.

Brush a cast-iron skillet with 1 teaspoon olive oil and place over medium-high heat.

Cook pita bread until it begins to puff up and the bottom has brown spots and blisters (approximately 3 minutes) (see photo on page 273).

Repeat on the other side.

Wrap them in a kitchen cloth towel and place them in a plastic bag (very important step to ensure that they will remain soft).

Reheat before use.

Nutrition Facts	
Per serving: 90 kcal	0 grams saturated fat
3 grams protein	13 grams carbohydrates
3 grams total fat	1 gram fiber

Chia Fruit Jams

PREPARATION 2 MINS	COOKING 12 MINS	SERVES 40 (1 TABLESPOON, 14 GRAMS)

INGREDIENTS

- 3 ½ cups (500 grams) blueberries/raspberries/strawberries (fresh or frozen)
- 1 teaspoon (5 ml) pure vanilla extract
- 3 tablespoons (45 ml) 100% pure maple syrup
- 4 tablespoons (44 grams) chia seeds

INSTRUCTIONS

Boil the fruit in a medium-sized pot.

Reduce the heat to low and boil for approximately 5 minutes, stirring frequently.

Mash the fruit with a potato masher or a fork.

Stir in the maple syrup and chia seeds.

Cook the jam on low until it thickens (approximately 5-7 minutes); continue to stir frequently.

gluten free

vegan

phase **2** diet

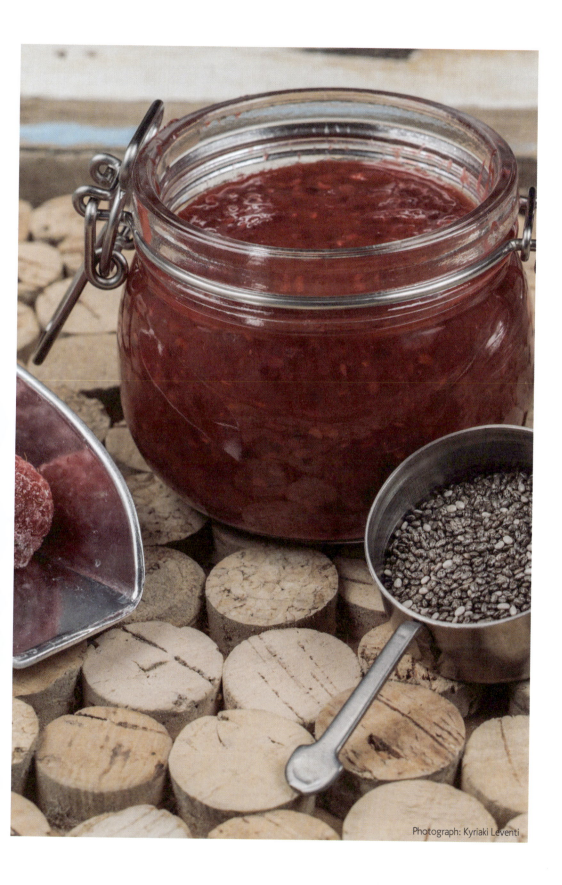

Photograph: Kyriaki Leventi

Remove from heat.

Stir in the vanilla extract.

Let the jam cool.

Pour the jam into a glass jar and store in the refrigerator.

It can be refrigerated for up to 2 weeks.

Nutrition Facts	
Per serving: 15 kcal	0 grams saturated fat
0 grams protein	3 grams carbohydrates
0 grams total fat	‹1 gram fiber

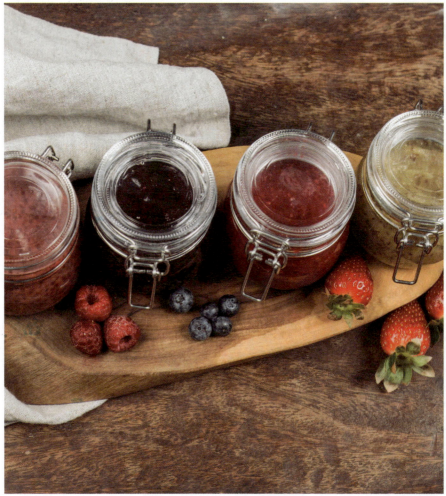

Photograph: Kyriaki Leventi

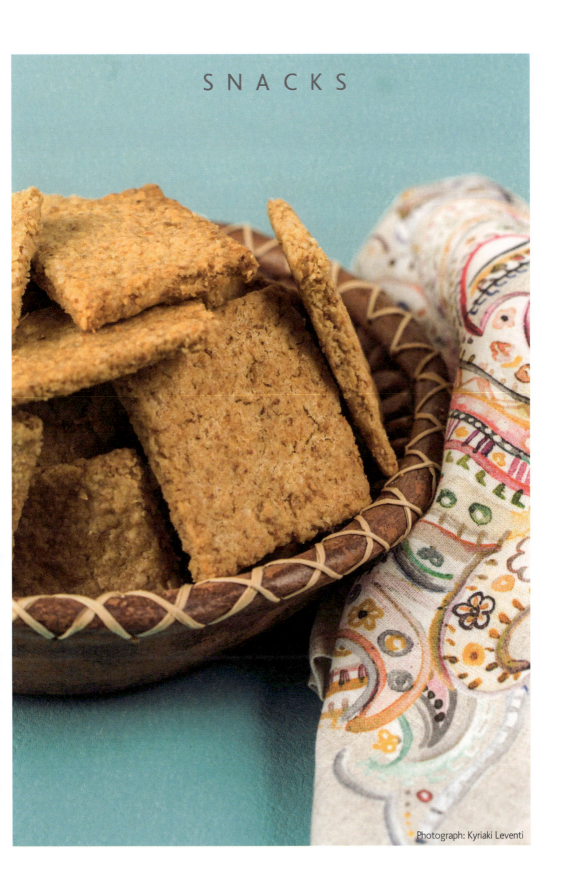

SNACKS

Photograph: Kyriaki Leventi

Oat Crackers

PREPARATION 10 MINS	COOKING 20 MINS	WAITING TIME 20 MINS	SERVES 12 (14 GRAMS, 0.5 OZ)

INGREDIENTS

- 1 cup (80 grams) **gluten-free** rolled oats
- ¾ teaspoon (3 grams) **gluten-free** baking powder
- 3 tablespoons (45 ml) of extra-virgin olive oil
- 3 tablespoons (45 ml) water
- Pinch of salt

INSTRUCTIONS

Preheat oven to 204°C/400°F.

Line a cookie sheet with parchment paper.

Grind oats in a food processor or blender until they become flour.

Pour and **mix** in a bowl the oat flour, baking powder and salt.

Add oil and water to the dry ingredients.

Knead the dough with your hands and add more water, a tablespoon at a time if needed, to form a soft (but not sticky) dough.

Let the dough rest for 20 minutes.

Roll the dough by using a rolling pin to form a thin layer approximately ⅛ inch thick.

Cut the dough in different shapes by using a cookie cutter.

Bake for 15-20 minutes or until golden brown.

Rotate the sheet once while baking.

Allow crackers to cool on a wire rack.

Store the crackers in an airtight container.

Nutrition Facts	
Per serving: 50 kcal	0.5 grams saturated fat
‹1 gram protein	5 grams carbohydrates
4 grams total fat	‹1 gram fiber

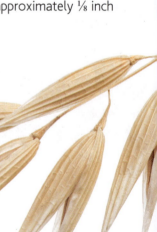

Plantain Chips

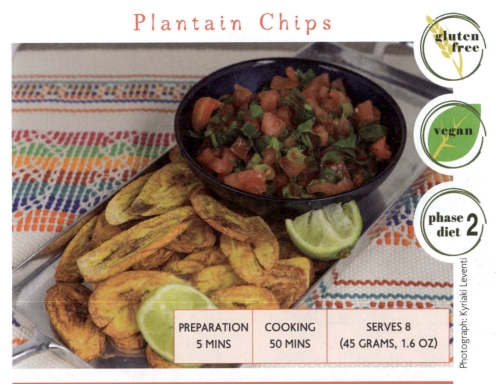

gluten free

vegan

phase diet 2

Photograph: Kyriaki Leventi

PREPARATION 5 MINS	COOKING 50 MINS	SERVES 8 (45 GRAMS, 1.6 OZ)

INGREDIENTS

- 2 unripe (green) plantains (360 grams/12.7 oz)
- 1 tablespoon (15 ml) olive oil
- Salt

INSTRUCTIONS

Peel the plantains and slice diagonally into thin pieces.

Brush both sides with olive oil.

Bake at 180°C/356°F until crispy (40-50 minutes), turning once halfway through.

Nutrition Facts	
Per serving: 70 kcal	0 grams saturated fat
‹1 gram protein	14 grams carbohydrates
2 grams total fat	1 gram fiber

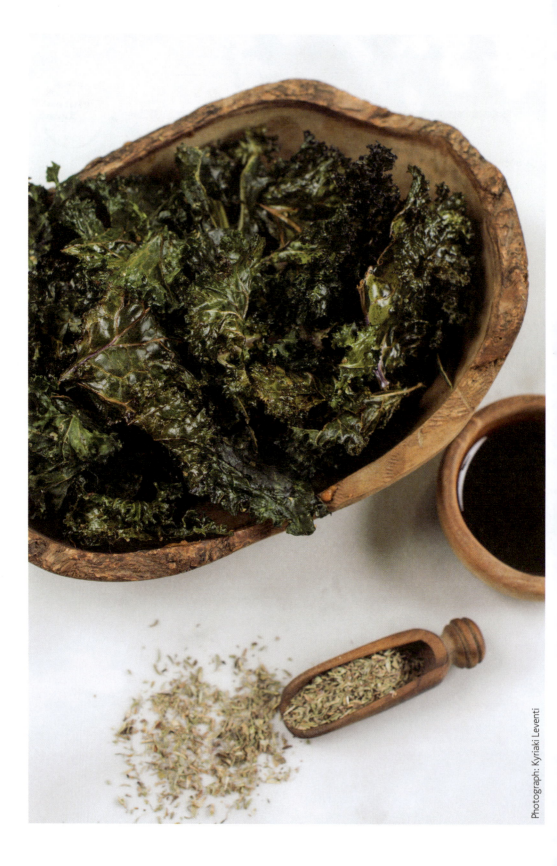

Kale Chips

PREPARATION 2 MINS	COOKING 25 MINS	SERVES 4 (52 GRAMS, 1.8 OZ)

INGREDIENTS

- 1 bunch (190 grams/7 oz) of kale (roughly chopped into large pieces, remove the stems)
- 1 tablespoon (15 ml) extra-virgin olive oil
- 2 teaspoons (4.6 grams) paprika
- ¼ teaspoon (1.5 grams) salt
- Freshly ground black pepper

INSTRUCTIONS

Preheat oven to 150°C/300°F.

Wash and spin until completely dry.

Line a baking tray with parchment paper.

Add the kale in a large bowl.

Massage kale leaves well with olive oil, salt, pepper and paprika until well coated.

Spread the pieces of kale on the tray and bake for 15 minutes.

Rotate the tray and bake for 10 more minutes.

Make sure to check on the kale, as it could burn easily.

Remove from oven when the kale is crispy but has not become dark in color.

Nutrition Facts	
Per serving: 60 kcal	5 grams carbohydrates
2 grams protein	2 grams fiber
4 grams total fat	High in copper and vitamins A, C, and K
0.5 grams saturated fat	

Oven Baked Plantains with Haloumi

PREPARATION 5 MINS	COOKING 45 MINS	SERVES 8 (77 GRAMS, 2.7 OZ)

INGREDIENTS

- 2 ripe (green) plantains (360 grams/12.7 oz)
- 8 slices (240 grams) of haloumi
- 1 tablespoon (15 ml) olive oil
- Salt to taste
- Chili pepper flakes (optional)

INSTRUCTIONS

Preheat the oven at 180°C/356°F.

Peel the plantains and slice down the middle lengthwise.

Brush both sides with olive oil and sprinkle with salt.

Bake the plantains for 30 minutes.

Add two slices of haloumi to each of the plantain slices. If you would like, sprinkle the haloumi with some chili pepper flakes.

Bake the plantains for 15 minutes or until the haloumi is lightly brown.

Nutrition Facts	
Per serving: 180 kcal	14 grams carbohydrates
7 grams protein	1 gram fiber
11 grams total fat	High in vitamin A
6 grams saturated fat	

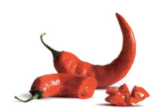

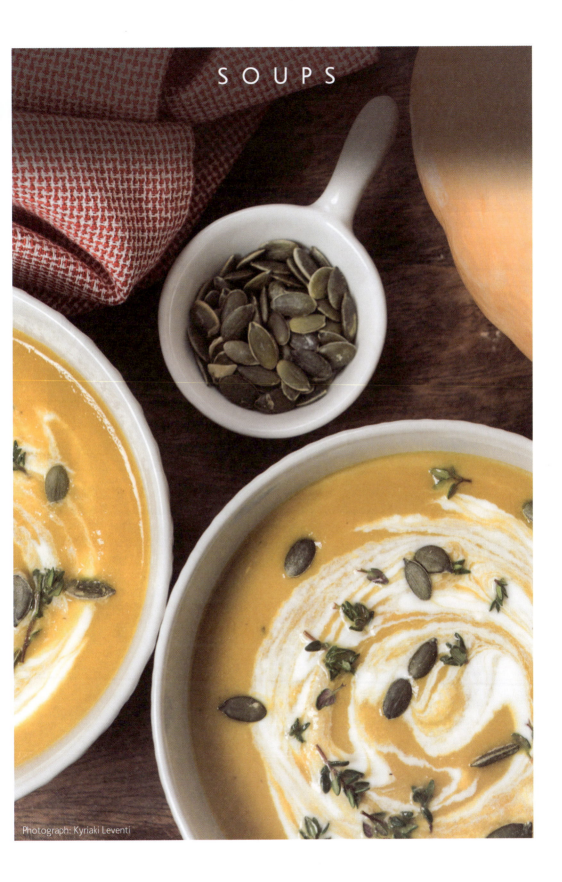

SOUPS

Photograph: Kyriaki Leventi

Pumpkin Soup

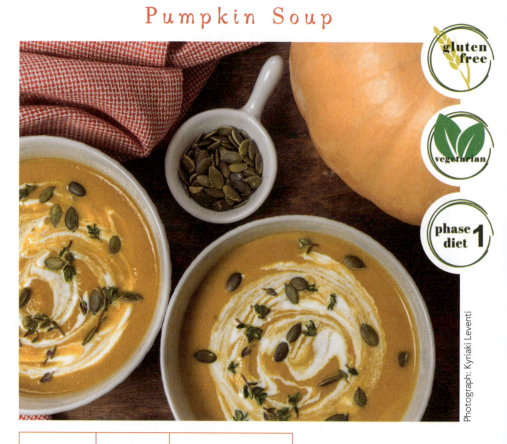

gluten free

vegetarian

phase diet 1

Photograph: Kyriaki Leventi

PREPARATION 15 MINS	COOKING 60 MINS	SERVES 7 (360 GRAMS, 12.7 OZ)

INGREDIENTS

- 1 kilo/2.2 pounds fresh Japanese pumpkin
- 2 medium (300 grams) potatoes, peeled
- 1 medium (119 grams) orange or red bell pepper
- 2 medium (220 grams) sized tomatoes
- 5 spring onions (green parts only)
- 2 leeks (green parts only)
- 2 (220 grams) carrots, peeled
- 1 tablespoon (6 grams) of fresh ginger
- 2 bay leaves

- ⅓ cup (80 ml) olive oil
- ½ teaspoon (1 gram) freshly ground black pepper
- 1 teaspoon (1.6 grams) dried thyme
- Salt to taste
- 2 cups (480 ml) water

INSTRUCTIONS

Chop the pumpkin, potatoes, pepper, tomatoes, spring onions, leeks and carrots into large pieces.

Mix all vegetables with chopped ginger, bay leaves, salt, pepper, dry thyme and olive oil and slow-cook for approximately half an hour, stirring occasionally. The vegetables will release a large amount of water.

Add water after the half hour to cover the vegetables and cook until the vegetables are soft.

Remove the bay leaves and blend in a blender until smooth.

Serve hot with a tablespoon of lactose-free yogurt.

Garnish with fresh thyme.

Nutrition Facts	
Per serving: 200 kcal	26 grams carbohydrates
4 grams protein	3 grams fiber
11 grams total fat	High levels of potassium, manganese, and vitamins A, C, E, K and B6
1.5 grams saturated fat	

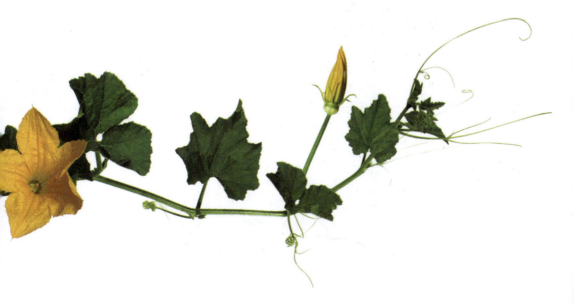

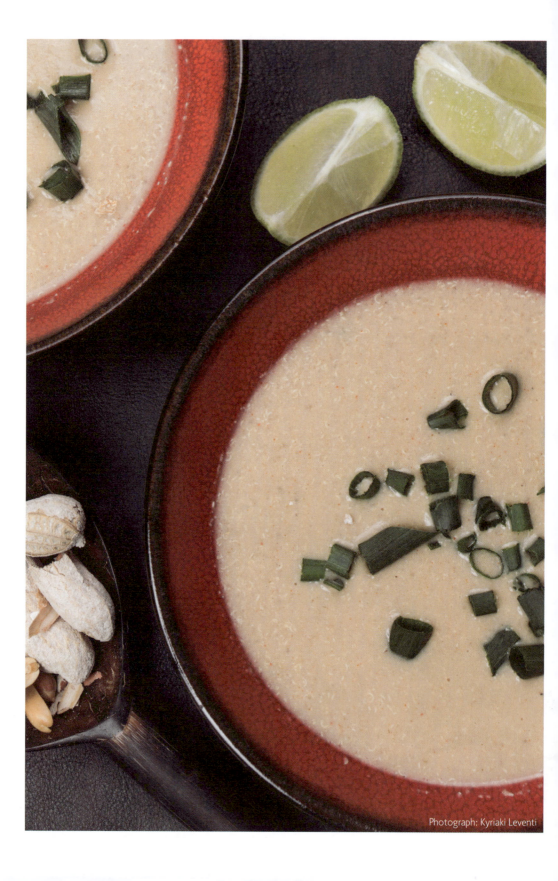

Quinoa Soup

PREPARATION 15 MINS	COOKING 60 MINS	SERVES 6 (305 GRAMS, 10.8 OZ EACH)

INGREDIENTS

- 1 ⅓ cups (240 grams) uncooked quinoa
- 3 cups (750 ml) of quinoa milk or almond milk **(see recipe page 171)**
- ¼ cup (65 grams) smooth peanut butter
- 1 teaspoon (2.3 grams) paprika
- 2 tablespoons (30 ml) olive oil
- Salt and pepper (to taste)
- Spring onion (the green parts only) for garnish

INSTRUCTIONS

Cook the quinoa **(see recipe page 364)**

Blend ⅓ of the cooked quinoa with quinoa milk, peanut butter, paprika, salt and pepper in a blender.

Add 2 tablespoons of olive oil in a large pot and sauté the remaining ⅔ of the cooked quinoa for a few minutes.

Add the blended quinoa to the pot with the sautéed quinoa and warm for 5 minutes. If the soup is too thick for your taste, you may need to add 500ml-750 ml of water to dilute it.

Garnish with the chopped green parts of a spring onion.

Nutrition Facts	
Per serving: 290 kcal	35 grams carbohydrates
8 grams protein	4 grams fiber
13 grams total fat	High in calcium, riboflavin, vitamin E, phosphorous, manganese, and folate
2 grams saturated fat	

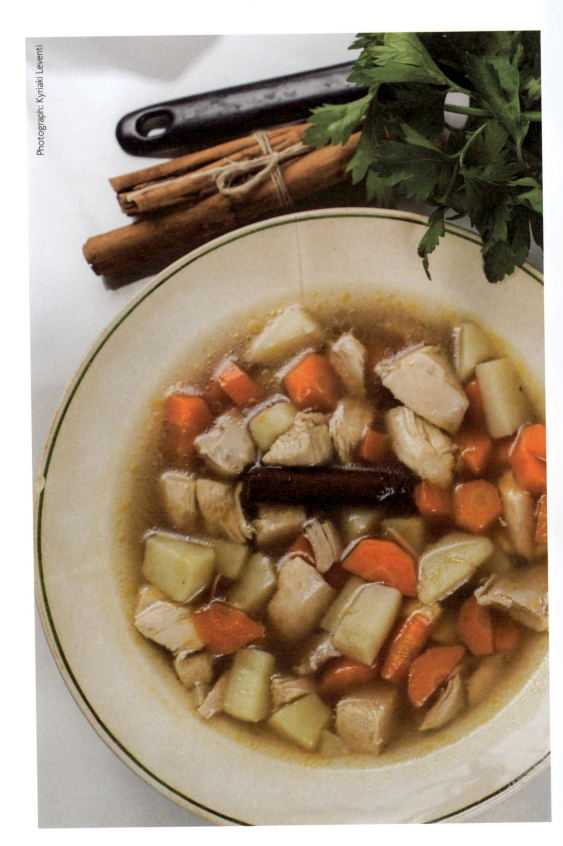

Photograph: Kyriaki Leventi

Grandma's Chicken Soup

PREPARATION 10 MINS	COOKING 70 MINS	SERVES 7 (352 GRAMS, 12.4 OZ)

INGREDIENTS

- 600 grams/1.3 pounds chicken (one bone-in skinless leg and one bone-less skinless breast)
- 5 cups (1.2 liters) water
- ¾ teaspoon (1.6 grams) freshly ground black pepper
- 8 cloves
- 5 cm/2 inches cinnamon stick
- 3 medium (450 grams) potatoes
- 4 medium (250 grams) carrots
- 1 teaspoon (6 grams) salt
- Freshly squeezed lemon juice

INSTRUCTIONS

Peel and dice the potatoes in cubes of approximately 1.5 cm/0.6 inch thick.

Peel and dice the carrots into small pieces approximately 1 cm/0.4 inch thick.

Add the water and chicken in a large pot and bring to a boil at high heat. Allow to boil for an additional 10 minutes.

Remove the chicken from the broth and pass the broth through a sieve tube. Collect the broth and discard anything in the sieve tube.

Pour the broth back into the pot and add the chicken, cloves, cinnamon stick and freshly ground black pepper.

Cook at medium heat for 15 minutes or until the chicken is half cooked.

Add the diced carrots and potatoes and cook over medium heat for 30-40 minutes, until the potatoes are cooked and tender.

Once the soup is ready, **remove** the chicken, shred it and return it to the pot.

Add salt and serve the soup with freshly squeezed lemon juice and more freshly ground black pepper if desired.

Nutrition Facts	
Per serving: 200 kcal	14 grams carbohydrates
17 grams protein	3 grams fiber
9 grams total fat	High in vitamin A, niacin, vitamin B6, phosphorous, selenium, and manganese
2.5 grams saturated fat	

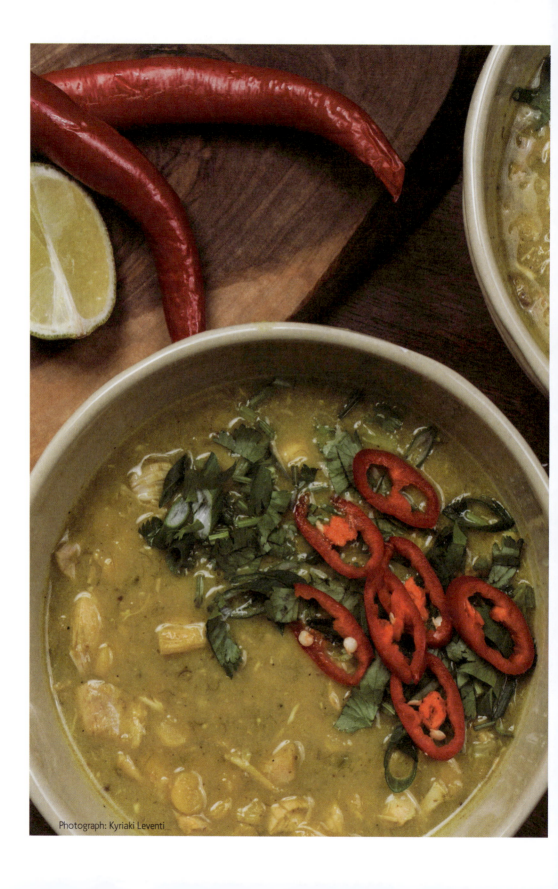

Photograph: Kyriaki Leventi

Thai Chicken Soup

PREPARATION 15 MINS	COOKING 60 MINS	SERVES 8 (363 GRAMS, 12.8 OZ)

INGREDIENTS

- 8 skinless chicken thighs with the bone (1.4 kilograms/3 pounds)
- 2 tablespoons (30 ml) of extra-virgin olive oil
- 6 spring onions (green parts only)
- 1 ½ tablespoon (9 grams) finely chopped fresh ginger
- 2 medium sized red (hot) chili peppers, deseeded and chopped finely (optional, only if tolerated)
- 1 teaspoon (2.2 grams) ground turmeric
- ½ teaspoon (1 gram) ground cumin
- ½ teaspoon (0.3 grams) ground coriander
- 330 grams canned and drained cooked chickpeas/preferably from a carton
- 4 ½ cups water (1.2 liters)
- 1 ¾ cups (400 ml) light coconut milk
- 2 tablespoons (30 ml) freshly squeezed lemon juice
- Salt and pepper
- For garnish: chopped cilantro, chopped green parts of spring onions, finely sliced red chili pepper (optional), roughly chopped roasted peanuts

INSTRUCTIONS

Heat the extra-virgin olive oil in a large pan over medium-high heat. Season chicken with salt and pepper and sauté for 5-7 minutes, until brown on all sides. Remove the chicken and set aside in a bowl.

Lower heat, add the chopped green onions, ginger and chili peppers and sauté until they turn soft.

To the pan mixture add the spices (turmeric, cumin and coriander), chickpeas and the browned chicken pieces.

Add the water and more salt and bring to a boil. Then, cover and cook on low heat for 45 minutes, stirring once or twice. The soup is ready when the chicken meat is coming off the bone.

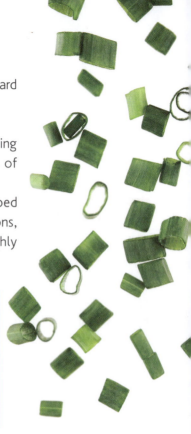

Remove the chicken pieces from the soup and on a board get the meat off the bone, discarding the bone.

Shred the chicken meat and return it to the pan.

Pour in the coconut milk and bring soup to a boil, adding more salt (only if desired) and 2 tablespoons of freshly squeezed lemon juice.

Serve the soup in bowls and garnish with chopped cilantro, the chopped green parts of spring onions, finely sliced red chili pepper (optional) and roughly chopped roasted peanuts.

Nutrition Facts	
Per serving: 410 kcal	4 grams fiber
34 grams protein	High in iron, riboflavin, niacin, folate, pantothenic acid, magnesium, zinc, copper, selenium, and vitamins A, C, and B6
24 grams total fat	
12 grams saturated fat	
16 grams carbohydrates	

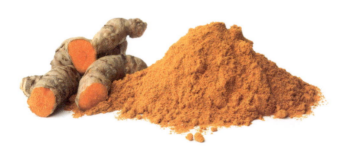

Fish Soup

PREPARATION 5 MINS	COOKING 40 MINS	SERVES 2

INGREDIENTS

- 1 tablespoon (15 ml) olive oil
- 5 cups (1200 ml) low FODMAP stock
- 2 medium (120 grams) carrots, chopped into cubes
- 3 medium (450 grams) potatoes, chopped into cubes

- 453 grams/1 pound sustainable white fish filet
- 1 bay leaf
- 1 sprig rosemary
- 1 star anise
- Freshly squeezed lemon juice

INSTRUCTIOINS

Heat a large pot over medium heat.

Add the oil and stir the carrots and potatoes.

Stir all the remaining ingredients except fish. For low FODMAP stock **see page 362**.

Heat to boiling.

Reduce heat; cover and simmer 20-30 minutes.

Add the fish.

Cook uncovered 5 to 7 minutes, stirring occasionally, until fish flakes easily with fork and vegetables are tender.

Served with lemon juice.

Nutrition Facts	
Per serving: 450 kcal	42 grams carbohydrates
45 grams protein	7 grams fiber
11 grams total fat	High in thiamin, niacin, phosphorous, magnesium, selenium, copper, manganese, and vitamins A, B6, B12, C, D, and K
1.5 grams saturated fat	

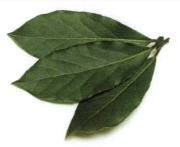

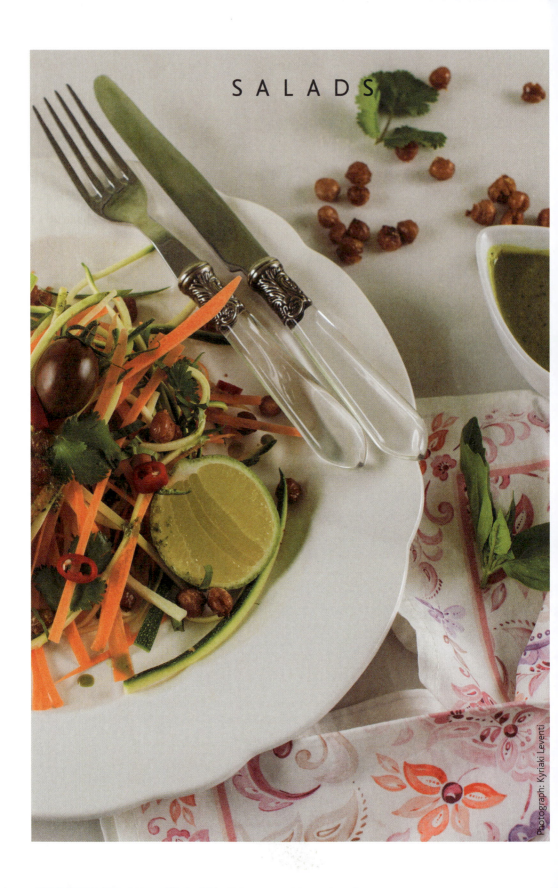

Photograph: Kyriaki Leventi

Chickpea Noodle Salad

PREPARATION 15 MINS	COOKING 35 MINS	SERVES 4 (SERVING SIZE: 267 GRAMS, 9.4 OZ

INGREDIENTS

Chickpeas

- 1 cup (152 grams) canned and drained cooked chickpeas, preferably in carton packaging
- 2 tablespoons (30 ml) extra-virgin olive oil
- ½ (3 grams) teaspoon salt

Thai orange dressing with olive oil

- ¼ cup (60 ml) extra-virgin olive oil
- ¼ cup (60 ml) freshly squeezed orange juice
- 1 tablespoon (6 grams) fresh ginger, finely chopped
- 1 tablespoon (15 ml) **gluten-free tamari (a variety of naturally fermented soy sauce)**
- 1 tablespoon (15 ml) 100% pure maple syrup
- ½ cup (12 grams) fresh basil
- ½ cup (12 grams) fresh cilantro

Salad

- 8 medium (480 grams) carrots
- 2 medium (260 grams) zucchini
- 1 cup (25 grams) cilantro leaves
- ½ cup (12 grams) basil leaves
- 1 cup roasted chickpeas

INSTRUCTIONS

Step 1: Chickpeas

Preheat oven to 204°C/400°F.

Drain and thoroughly **rinse** the chickpeas.

Pat them dry with a paper towel.

Spread them on parchment-lined rimmed baking sheet.

Toss chickpeas with oil and salt.

Roast the chickpeas for 30-35 minutes, until they are golden in color and crispy on the outside.

Step 2: Thai orange dressing

Blend all ingredients together until smooth or whisk all ingredients together until well combined.

Step 3: Salad

Cut your vegetables using a spiralizer.

If you do not have a spiralizer, use a vegetable peeler to create long ribbons.

Add vegetables to a mixing bowl.

Toss the vegetable noodles with the dressing.

Sprinkle salad with chopped cilantro and basil.

Serve with roasted chickpeas on top.

Nutrition Facts	
Per serving: 280 kcal	27 grams carbohydrates
5 grams protein	7 grams fiber
18 grams total fat	High in riboflavin, folate, manganese, potassium, and vitamins A, B 6, C, and K
2.5 grams saturated fat	

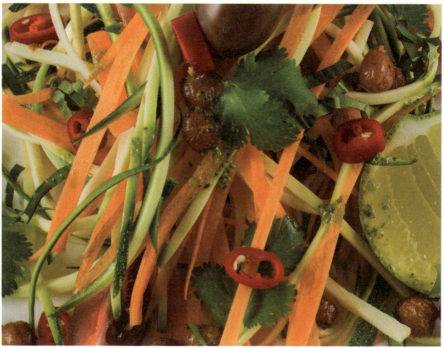

Photograph: Kyriaki Leventi

Tofu Pineapple Salad

PREPARATION 10 MINS	COOKING 15 MINS	PRESS TIME FOR TOFU: 30 MINS	SERVES 4 (SERVING SIZE: 420 GRAMS, 14.8 OZ)

INGREDIENTS

Tofu

- 450 grams/1 pound extra-firm tofu, drained, pressed and then cubed (2.5 x 0.6 cm/1 x ¼ inch)
- 2 tablespoons (30 ml) of extra-virgin olive oil

Peanut orange sauce

- 3 tablespoons (48 grams) peanut butter
- 1 ½ tablespoons (22.5 ml) freshly squeezed orange juice
- ½ teaspoon orange zest (organic)
- ½ tablespoon (7.5 ml) lime juice
- 1 tablespoon (15 ml) **gluten-free tamari (a variety of naturally fermented soy sauce)**
- ½ tablespoon (7.5 ml) 100% pure maple syrup
- 1 teaspoon (2 grams) grated ginger
- ¼ teaspoon (0.5 grams) crushed red pepper flakes (optional)

Salad

- Tofu
- 4 cups (440 grams) shredded carrot
- 3 cups (108 grams) lettuce
- 2 cups (280 grams) fresh pineapple
- 16 cherry (272 grams) tomatoes
- Peanut orange sauce

INSTRUCTIONS

Step 1: Press firm tofu

Drain the tofu.

Lay a dish towel and then a paper towel on a surface.

Add the tofu and another paper towel.

Place something heavy on top.

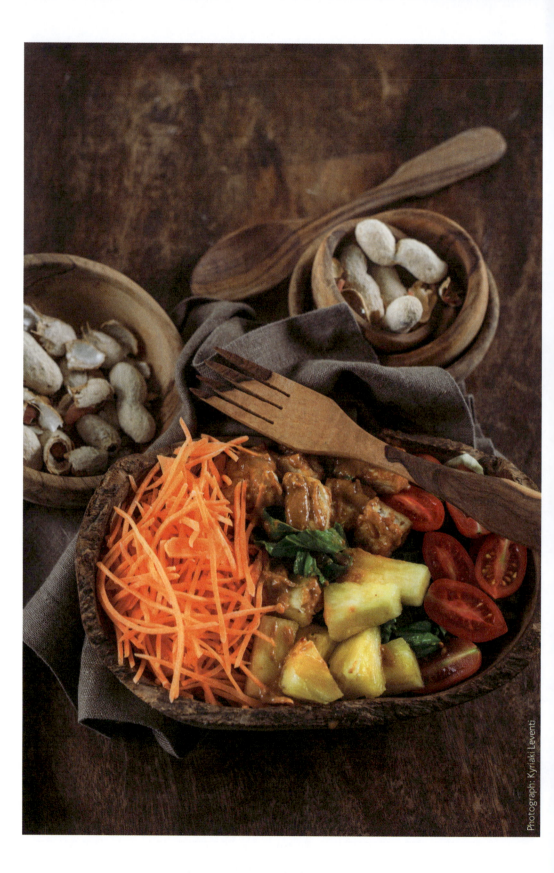

Press for 30 minutes.

Step 2: Cook tofu

Heat oil in a large pan over medium-high heat.

Fry tofu, stirring occasionally, until brown on each side.

Step 3: Peanut orange sauce

Blend all the ingredients of the peanut orange sauce together until smooth.

Step 4: Salad

Toss lettuce, carrots, tomatoes and pineapple with half the dressing.

Top with the warm tofu.

Add the remaining dressing.

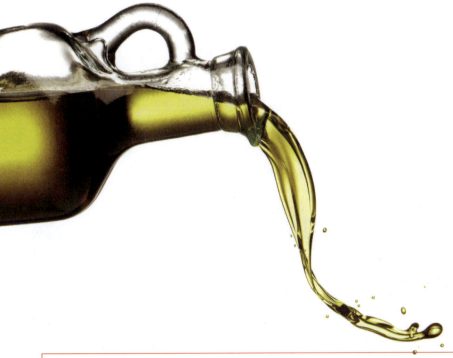

Nutrition Facts	
Per serving: 340 kcal	32 grams carbohydrates
16 grams protein	7 grams fiber
19 grams total fat	High in calcium, riboflavin, niacin, folate, potassium, phos-
2.5 grams saturated fat	phorous, manganese, and vitamins A, C, D, and K

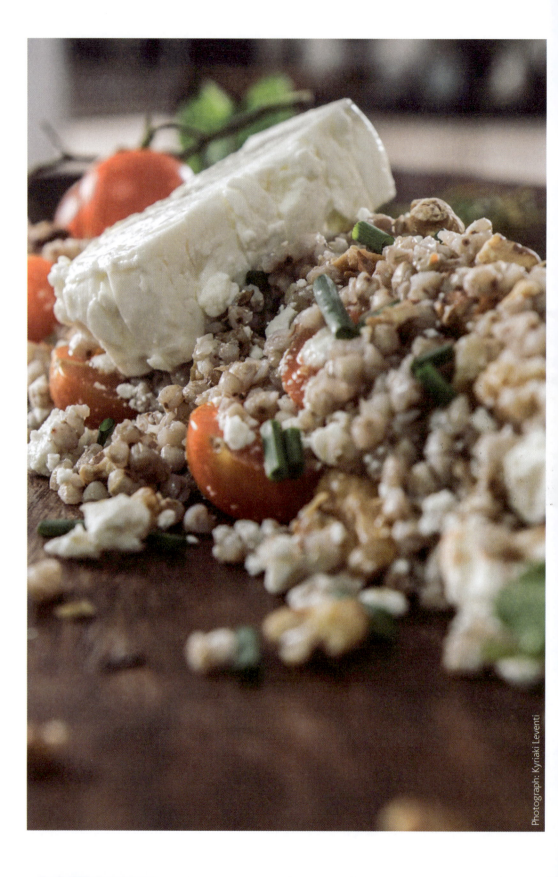

Buckwheat Salad

PREPARATION 15 MINS	COOKING 20 MINS	SERVES 4 (SERVING SIZE: 356 GRAMS, 12.6 OZ)

INGREDIENTS

Buckwheat

- 2 cups (480 ml) low FODMAP vegetable stock **(page362)** or use water
- 2 bay leaves
- 1 cup (180 grams) buckwheat groats
- 2 teaspoons (10 ml) extra-virgin olive oil

Classic French vinaigrette

- ½ cup (120 ml) garlic infused olive oil **(see recipe page 363)**
- 2 tablespoons (30 ml) red wine vinegar
- ½ teaspoon (2.5 grams) Dijon mustard
- Pinch of salt to taste

Salad

- 4 small common tomatoes (440 grams), finely cut
- ½ cup (70 grams) reduced fat feta, crumbled
- 1 cup (25 grams) fresh coriander leaves
- ½ cup (60 grams) roasted chopped walnuts

INSTRUCTIONS

Step 1: Buckwheat

Place groats in dry pan over medium heat, stirring for five minutes, until browned.

Add the stock and bay leaves and bring to a boil.

Add the oil, cover pan and reduce heat to low; simmer for 15 minutes.

Remove from heat and leave, covered, 10 minutes.

Uncover and **fluff** with a fork.

Season with salt to taste and allow to cool.

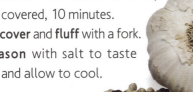

Step 2: Dressing

Blend all ingredients together until smooth or whisk all ingredients together until well combined.

Step 3: Salad

Toss salad with enough dressing to coat the ingredients.

Divide mixture among four plates and top with feta cheese.

Nutrition Facts	
Per serving: 430 kcal	38 grams carbohydrates
12 grams protein	7 grams fiber
28 grams total fat	High in niacin, phosphorous,magnesium, copper, riboflavin, and vitamins A, B6, C, E, and K
6 grams saturated fat	

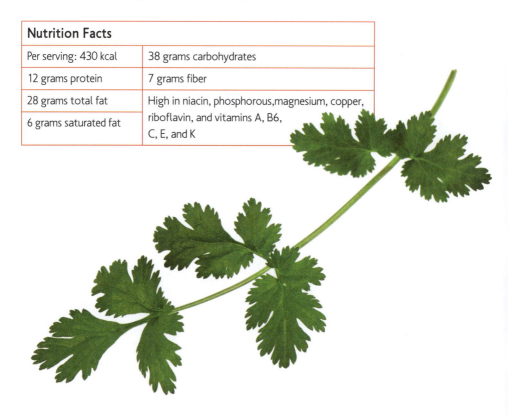

Arugula Salad with Quinoa

PREPARATION 5 MINS	COOKING TIME 15 MINS	SERVES 4 (SERVING SIZE: 213 GRAMS, 7.5 OZ)

INGREDIENTS

Raspberry vinaigrette

- 4 tablespoons (60 ml) of extra-virgin olive oil
- 2 tablespoons (30 ml) of raspberry champagne vinegar or white wine vinegar
- 4 fresh or frozen raspberries
- 2 teaspoons (10 ml) 100% pure maple syrup
- 1 teaspoon (5 grams) Dijon mustard
- Pinch of salt to taste

Salad

- 1 cup (180 grams) cooked quinoa, (⅓ cup (65 grams) dry quinoa; **page 364**)
- 8 cups (160 grams) baby arugula
- ½ cup (120 ml) raspberry vinaigrette
- 1 cup (140 grams) feta cheese, crumbled
- 20 strawberries (300 grams)

INSTRUCTIONS

Step 1: Raspberry vinaigrette

Vigorously shake all the ingredients in a jar.

Step 2: Salad

Toss salad with enough dressing to coat the ingredients.

Divide mixture among four plates and top with feta cheese.

Nutrition Facts	
Per serving: 330 kcal	20 grams carbohydrates
9 grams protein	3 grams fiber
25 grams total fat	High in folate, phosphorous, riboflavin, manganese, calcium, and vitamins A, C, and K
8 grams saturated fat	

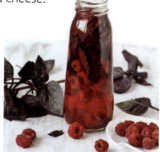

Salmon Salad

PREPARATION 10 MINS	COOKING TIME 10 MINS	SERVES 4 (SERVING SIZE: 310 GRAMS, 10.9 OZ)

INGREDIENTS

Salmon

- 4 pan-fried salmon fillets with crispy skin (170 grams each/6 oz)
- 2 tablespoon (30 ml) olive oil
- Salt and pepper

Vinaigrette

- 10 frozen or fresh raspberries (45 grams)
- 1 tablespoon (15 ml) lemon juice
- 1 tablespoon (15 ml) raspberry champagne vinegar
- 2 tablespoons (30 ml) of extra-virgin olive oil
- ½ teaspoon (2.5 ml) 100% pure maple syrup
- Pinch of salt to taste

Salad

- 8 cups (240 grams) salad greens
- 1 orange (130 grams), cut into wedges
- 20 blueberries (28 grams)
- 2 tablespoons (8 grams) almonds

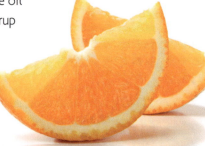

INSTRUCTIONS

Step 1: Pan-fried salmon

Bring the salmon to room temperature for a few minutes before cooking.

Dry salmon by pressing it between paper towels.

Remove any excess moisture from the skin by running the back of a knife through the skin.

Dry the salmon again with paper towels.

Heat a stainless steel or cast-iron skillet over medium-high heat. (To obtain a crispy fish skin, the skillet must be hot; to test it, splash a drop of water, and if it sizzles, the pan is ready.)

Season the fish with salt and pepper.

Oil the fish well and place it in the pan with the skin side down.

Lower the heat to medium to low.

Press gently on the back of the fillets with a spatula for 10 seconds. (If you are cooking multiple fillets, add them to the pan one at a time so you have time to press them.)

Continue to press occasionally; the fish is ready when it lifts easily.

Cook until an instant thermometer inserted in the center of the fillet registers 55°C/130°F (for medium), approximately 5-7 minutes total, depending on the thickness of the fillet. The salmon skin should be crisp and easy to lift and flip.

Turn the fish and cook for 15 seconds.

Transfer the fish on a serving plate and let it rest for a couple of minutes.

Step 2: Salad

Blend all ingredients for the vinaigrette together until smooth or whisk all ingredients together until well combined.

Toss salad with enough dressing to coat the ingredients.

Step 3

Divide mixture among four plates and top with 1 salmon fillet.

Drizzle each salmon with more dressing if desired.

> ❗ *The safe fish temperature recommended by USDA is an internal temperature of 62.8°C/145°F. The temperature will continue to rise during rest, achieving the ideal safe temperature.*

Nutrition Facts	
Per serving: 440 kcal	12 grams carbohydrates
36 grams protein	4 grams fiber
28 grams total fat	High levels of selenium, niacin, and vitamins A, B6, B12, C, and K
4 grams saturated fat	

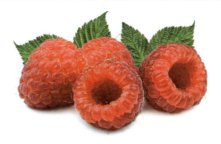

Pineapple Chicken Salad

PREPARATION 15 MINS	COOKING 12-15 MINS	SERVES 4 (SERVING SIZE: 316 GRAMS, 11.1 OZ)

INGREDIENTS

Chicken
- 2 chicken breast fillets (200 grams/7 oz each)
- 1 tablespoon (30 ml) extra-virgin olive oil

Passion fruit dressing
- ½ cup (120 grams) passion fruit pulp
- 2 tablespoons (30 ml) white wine vinegar or champagne vinegar
- 1 tablespoon (15 ml) 100% pure maple syrup
- 2 tablespoons (30 ml) extra-virgin olive oil
- Salt and pepper to taste

Salad
- Pan-fried chicken
- 2 cups (280 grams) fresh pineapple
- 8 cups (240 grams) green salad baby leaves
- 4 tablespoons (35 grams) toasted sunflower seeds
- Passion fruit dressing

INSTRUCTIONS

Step 1: Pan-fried chicken

Place the chicken in a resealable freezer bag or between two pieces of wrap or wax paper.

Flatten the chicken breasts (can be done with a meat mallet, rolling pin or a wide jar).

Pound first in the center and then move to the sides until the chicken is even in thickness.

Dry chicken with paper towels.

Season with salt and pepper.

Let the chicken rest.

Dry chicken again.

Heat the sauté pan over medium
heat.

Add the oil (1 tablespoon) in a
sauté pan when the pan is hot.

Lower heat to medium-low.

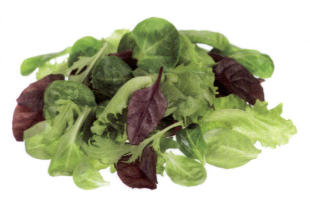

Add chicken and cook without
moving it for 3-4 minutes. The
sides should be pale golden
brown, and it should release
from the pan easily.

Add the remaining oil and combine so that the oil flows underneath. Cook 1
minute or until deep golden brown.

Turn chicken and cook 3-4 minutes.

Let chicken stand in the pan for 3 minutes.

Step 2: Passion fruit dressing

Mix together passion fruit pulp, olive oil, vinegar, and maple syrup.

Season to taste with salt and pepper. Set aside.

Step 3: Salad

Mix together the greens and the chicken. Top with fresh pineapple. Add passion
fruit dressing and toss.

> **!** *The chicken is cooked when there is no pink in the center of chicken*
> *breast or the internal temperature is 75°C/165°F. The meat or instant-read*
> *thermometer should be inserted into the center of breast.*

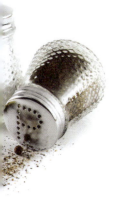

Nutrition Facts	
Per serving: 310 kcal	24 grams carbohydrates
27 grams protein	6 grams fiber
13 grams total fat	High in iron, phosphorous, manganese, selenium, niacin, and vitamins A, C, K, and B6
2 grams saturated fat	

Edamame Walnut Salad

PREPARATION 5 MINS	COOKING 12 MINS	SERVES 4 (SERVING SIZE: 226 GRAMS, 8 OZ)

INGREDIENTS

Strawberry vinaigrette

- 4 tablespoons (60 ml) olive oil
- 2 tablespoons (30 ml) raspberry champagne vinegar
- 2 teaspoons (10 ml) maple syrup
- 1 teaspoon (5 grams) Dijon mustard
- 4 frozen or fresh (56 grams) strawberries
- Salt and pepper

Maple walnuts

- 1 cup (125 grams) walnuts, chopped
- 2 tablespoons (30 ml) maple syrup
- ½ teaspoon (3 grams) salt

Salad

- 8 cups (250 grams) mix greens
- 40 raspberries (190 grams)
- 2 cups (310 grams) edamame (frozen soybeans)
- 2 tablespoons (21 grams) pomegranate seeds
- Strawberry vinaigrette
- Maple walnuts

INSTRUCTIONS

Step 1: Edamame

Steam edamame until tender (approximately 2 minutes).

Step 2: Maple walnuts

Toast walnuts over medium-low heat for 10 minutes or until the walnuts smell fragrantly toasted.

Add the maple syrup and sea salt to the pan. Stir vigorously combine, and turn the heat off after the liquid is absorbed by the walnuts.

Step 3: Strawberry vinaigrette

Vigorously shake all the ingredients in a jar.

Step 4: Salad

Toss salad with enough dressing to coat the ingredients.

Garnish with pomegranate seeds and maple walnuts

Nutrition Facts	
Per serving: 390 kcal	25 grams carbohydrates
18 grams protein	10 grams fiber
27 grams total fat	High in iron, phosphorus, riboflavin, magnesium, manga-
2 grams saturated fat	nese, copper, folate, potassium, and vitamins A, C, and K

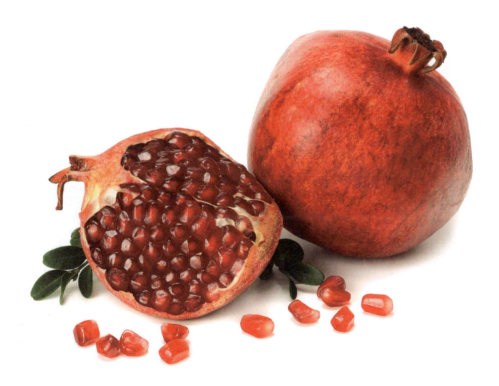

Carrot Ribbons Salad

PREPARATION 10 MINS	COOKING 6 MINS	SERVES 4 (SERVING SIZE: 171 GRAMS, 6 OZ)

INGREDIENTS

- 8 medium carrots, (480 grams) cut with a vegetable peeler into carrot ribbons
- 1 teaspoon (2 grams) cumin seeds
- 3 tablespoon (45 ml) extra-virgin olive oil
- 1 tablespoon (15 ml) sherry vinegar
- 1 teaspoon (5 ml) 100% pure maple syrup
- 4 tablespoons (35 grams) toasted macadamia nuts, roughly chopped
- ½ cup (70 grams) feta cheese
- 1 cup (25 grams) mint leaves
- Salt and pepper
- Juice from half a lemon

INSTRUCTIONS

Step 1: Toast macadamias on the stovetop
Heat a small nonstick frying pan over medium heat.
Add the nuts.
Cook, stirring, for 3-4 minutes or until golden.

Step 2
Heat a frying pan over medium heat.
Reduce heat to low.
Cook the cumin seeds, stirring, for 1-2 minutes or until aromatic and popping.
Transfer to a bowl.
In a small bowl, whisk together the oil, vinegar, lemon juice, maple syrup, cumin, salt and pepper (for the dressing).
Use a vegetable peeler to **slice** the carrots into long, thin ribbons.
Place the carrot ribbons in a large salad bowl.
Add the mint and pour the dressing.

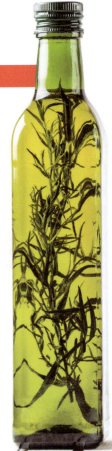

Toss to combine.

Add the feta and the toasted macadamias.

Top with extra mint leaves.

Nutrition Facts	
Per serving: 260 kcal	16 grams carbohydrates
5 grams protein	5 grams fiber
21 grams total fat	High in vitamins A and K
5 grams saturated fat	

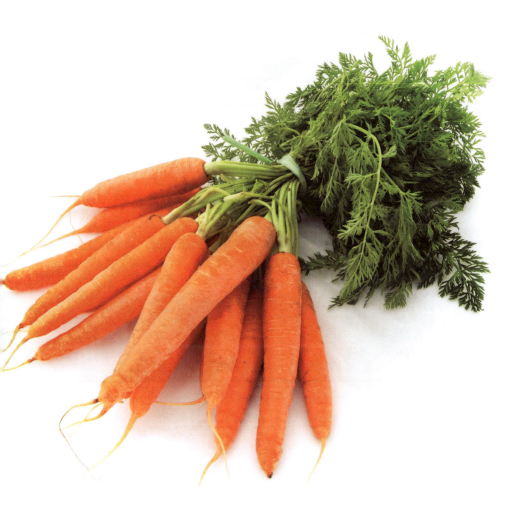

Pumpkin Salad

PREPARATION 15 MINS	COOKING 25 MINS	SERVES 4 (SERVING SIZE: 148 GRAMS, 5.2 OZ)

INGREDIENTS

Roasted pumpkin

- 2 cups (220 grams) Japanese pumpkin, cut into small pieces
- ⅛ teaspoon (0.3 grams) cumin
- ⅛ teaspoon (0.3 grams) sweet paprika
- 1 teaspoon (5 ml) olive oil
- Salt and pepper

Tahini dressing

- 3 tablespoons (42 grams) tahini paste
- 1 tablespoon (15 grams) lemon juice
- 3 tablespoon (45 ml) warm water
- ½ teaspoon (1.2 grams) cumin
- ½ teaspoon (1.2 grams) sweet paprika
- ½ teaspoon (3 grams) salt
- ¼ teaspoon (0.6 grams) pepper to taste

Salad

- Roasted pumpkin
- 20 toasted macadamia nuts
- 4 tablespoons (32 grams) toasted pumpkin seeds
- 8 cups (160 grams) baby arugula leaves
- Tahini dressing
- Poppy seeds to garnish

INSTRUCTIONS

Step 1: Roasted pumpkin

Preheat oven to 250°C/482°F.

Line 1 baking tray with baking paper.

Place pumpkin in a single layer.

Toss with oil and season with salt and spices and turn to coat both sides.

Roast pumpkin, turning once until golden and tender (about 20 minutes).

Set aside to cool to room temperature.

Step 2: Tahini dressing

Blend all the ingredients except water together until smooth. Whisk in 1 tablespoon of water at a time until the desired consistency is reached.

Step 3: Toast nuts and seeds

Heat a small, nonstick frying pan over medium heat.

Add nuts and seeds on separate positions in the pan.

Cook, stirring, for 3-4 minutes or until golden. The macadamia nuts will need a longer period of time to toast than the seeds.

Step 4: Salad

Mix together the arugula and roasted pumpkin. Top with nuts. Add tahini dressing and toss.

Nutrition Facts	
Per serving: 240 kcal	10 grams carbohydrates
7 grams protein	4 grams fiber
22 grams total fat	High in manganese, magnesium, phosphorous, copper, thiamin, and vitamins A, C, and K
3.5 grams saturated fat	

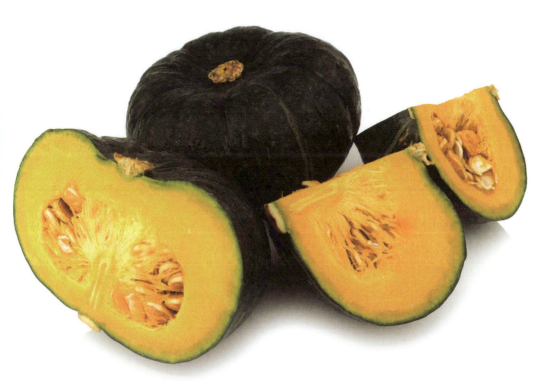

Quinoa Tabbouleh

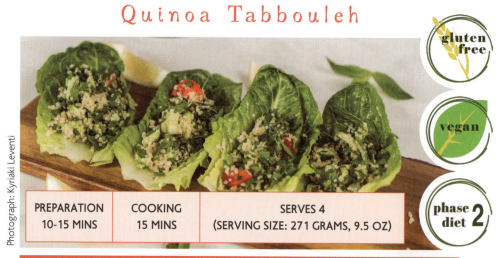

Photograph: Kyriaki Leventi

gluten free

vegan

phase diet 2

PREPARATION 10-15 MINS	COOKING 15 MINS	SERVES 4 (SERVING SIZE: 271 GRAMS, 9.5 OZ)

INGREDIENTS

Salad

- 2 cups (360 grams) cooked quinoa (¾ cup (130 grams) dry quinoa; **see recipe page 364**)
- 12 cherry tomatoes (204 grams/7.2 oz), chopped in quarters
- Green leaves of 4 spring onions, chopped (24 grams/0.8 oz)
- 1 large or (2 small) cucumber (300 grams/10.6 oz), peeled and diced into cubes
- 1 cup (25 grams) chopped parsley
- 2 tablespoons (30 ml) of olive oil
- Juice of 1-2 lemons
- 2-3 tablespoons of fresh mint leaves chopped
- Salt and pepper to taste

INSTRUCTIONS

Mix all ingredients in a bowl and chill for an hour before serving.

Nutrition Facts	
Per serving: 200 kcal	27 grams carbohydrates
6 grams protein	5 grams fiber
9 grams total fat	High in manganese, phosphorus, magnesium, iron, folate, and vitamins A, C, and K
1 gram saturated fat	

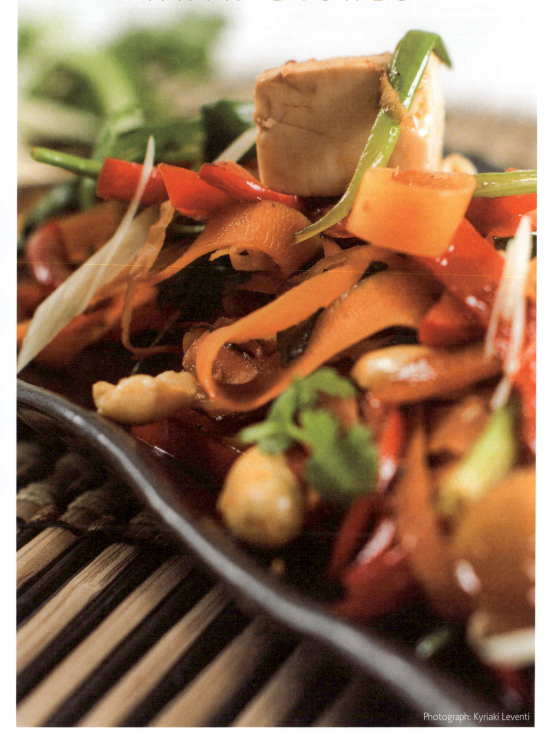

VEGETARIAN
MAIN DISHES

Arugula and Walnut Pesto Pasta

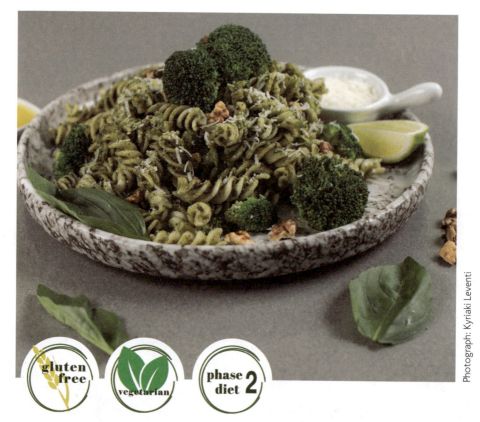

Photograph: Kyriaki Leventi

PREPARATION 10 MINS	COOKING 12 MINS	SERVES 5 (250 GRAMS, 8.8 OZ)

INGREDIENTS

Pesto

- 1 cup (20 grams) arugula leaves
- 1½ cups (38 grams) fresh basil leaves
- ⅓ cup (40 grams) walnuts
- 1 teaspoon (2 grams) finely grated organic lemon zest
- 1 tablespoon (15 ml) lemon juice
- ⅓ cup (33 grams) finely grated Parmesan
- ¼ cup (60 ml) garlic olive oil or olive oil

Pasta

- 300 grams/13.7 oz dry 100% quinoa pasta **(choose gluten-free, low FODMAP pasta)**
- ½ tablespoon (9 grams) salt
- 3 cups (300 grams) broccoli, heads only
- ½ cup (50 grams) grated Parmesan cheese
- ½ cup (60 grams) walnuts, toasted, coarsely chopped

INSTRUCTIONS

Step 1: Toast walnuts on the stovetop

Heat a small nonstick frying pan over medium heat.

Add the nuts.

Cook, stirring, for 3-4 minutes or until golden.

Step 2: Make the pesto

In a food processor, pulse the arugula, basil, nuts, lemon zest, lemon juice, cheese and 1 tablespoon of the oil until roughly chopped.

Add the remaining olive oil.

Season the pesto with salt and pepper.

Step 3: Pasta

Cook pasta according to packaging directions.

Add broccoli in the last 2 minutes of cooking.

Drain well.

Mix the pasta with pesto sauce.

Serve pasta topped with Parmesan and nuts.

Nutrition Facts
Per serving: 530 kcal
18 grams protein
30 grams total fat
5 grams saturated fat
51 grams carbohydrates
7 grams fiber
High in iron, calcium, phosphorous, copper, manganese, thiamin, and vitamins A, C, and K

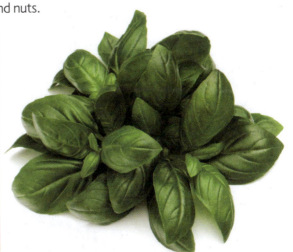

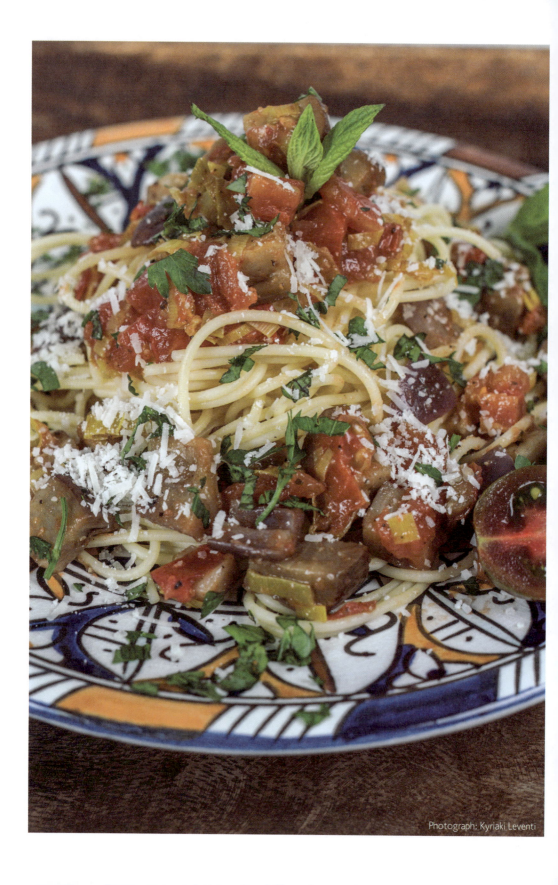

Lemony Eggplant Pasta

PREPARATION 15 MINS	COOKING 30-35 MINS	SERVES 6 (276 GRAMS, 9.7 OZ)

INGREDIENTS

- 4 tablespoons garlic extra-virgin olive oil **(See recipe page 363)**
- 2 medium eggplants (453 grams/1 pound), cut into ½-inch cubes
- 1 cup (50 grams) spring onions (the green part only), chopped
- 1 cup leeks (50 grams), the soft green part only, chopped
- 4 small tomatoes, common (440 grams), diced in ½-inch cubes
- 2 tablespoons (30 ml) lemon juice
- 2 tablespoons (12 grams) organic lemon zest
- 360 grams/12 ounces dry 100% **quinoa pasta (or choose any gluten-free, low FODMAP pasta)**
- ½ cup (12 grams) chopped fresh parsley
- ½ cup (12 grams) chopped fresh mint leaves
- 1 cup (100 grams) Parmesan cheese
- Salt and freshly ground pepper
- 2 tablespoons mint leaves and parsley leaves for garnish

INSTRUCTIONS

Bring a large pot of salted water to a boil.

Add quinoa pasta to the boiling water and cook according to the package directions.

Heat the oil in a large nonstick skillet over medium heat.

Add eggplant and cook, stirring occasionally, until just softened, approximately 15 minutes.

Add spring onions and leeks and cook, stirring, until fragrant (2 to 3 minutes).

Add tomatoes, salt, pepper; stir and cook for 10 minutes more.

Add the herbs, lemon juice and lemon zest and stir. Remove from the heat.

Drain the pasta, mix it with the sauce and toss to coat the pasta well.

Divide the pasta among 6 plates.

Sprinkle with parsley and mint leaves.

Top with Parmesan cheese.

Nutrition Facts
Per serving: 410 kcal
13 grams protein
15 grams total fat
4.5 grams saturated fat
59 grams carbohydrates
11 grams fiber
High in calcium, manganese, magnesium, and vitamins A, C, and K

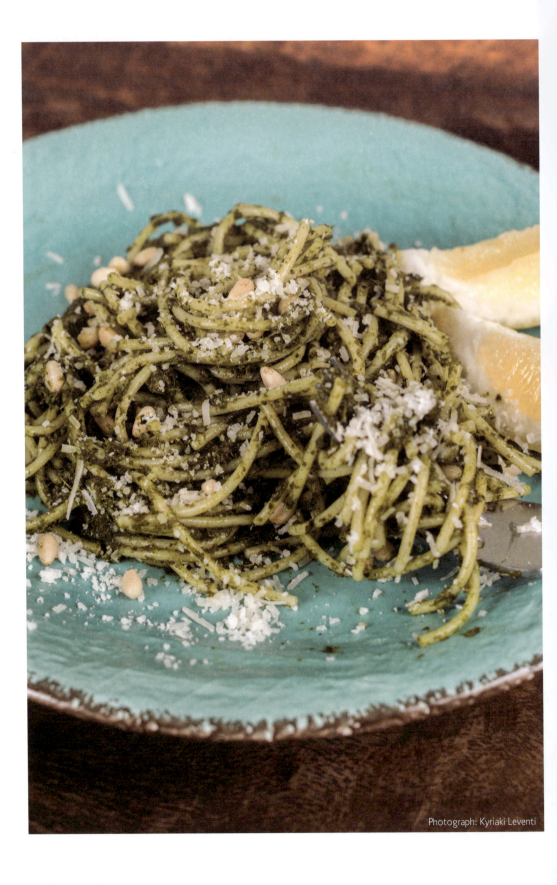

Photograph: Kyriaki Leventi

Kale Quinoa Pasta

PREPARATION 5 MINS	COOKING 15 MINS	SERVES 5 (260 GRAMS/9.1 OZ)

INGREDIENTS

- 2 tablespoons (30 ml) garlic olive oil or extra-virgin olive oil **(see the recipe for garlic oil page 363)**
- 1 pound/453 grams kale, thick ribs removed
- 300 grams/10.6 oz dry 100% **quinoa pasta (gluten-free/low FODMAP)**
- ½ cup (50 grams) grated low-fat Parmesan cheese
- ½ cup (67 grams) toasted pine nuts
- 2 tablespoons (30 ml) extra-virgin olive oil
- 1 teaspoon organic lemon zest
- 1 ½ tablespoon (8 grams) lemon juice
- 1 teaspoon (6 grams) salt
- ½ teaspoon (1 gram) freshly ground black pepper, to taste

INSTRUCTIONS

Bring to a boil a large pot of salted water, approximately 10 cups water and ½ tablespoon salt.

Add kale and cook for 5 minutes.

Pull out the hot and dripping kale leaves with tongs and transfer to a blender.

Do not drain the pot.

Add quinoa pasta to the boiling water and cook according to package directions.

Add garlic oil, lemon juice to the blender with the boiled kale.

Blend until smooth puree.

Add more hot water if needed.

Taste and **adjust** seasoning with salt, lemon and freshly ground pepper.

Drain the pasta and add the kale purée, grated Parmesan cheese, lemon zest and toasted pine nuts.

Toss until all the pasta is well coated.

Drizzle the pasta with extra-virgin olive oil and Parmesan cheese.

Nutrition Facts	
Per serving: 490 kcal	10 grams fiber
14 grams protein	High in calcium, magnesium, manganese, potassium, thiamin, phosphorous, copper, folate, and vitamins A, C, E, K, and B6
25 grams total fat	
4 grams saturated fat	
58 grams carbohydrates	

Buckwheat Risotto

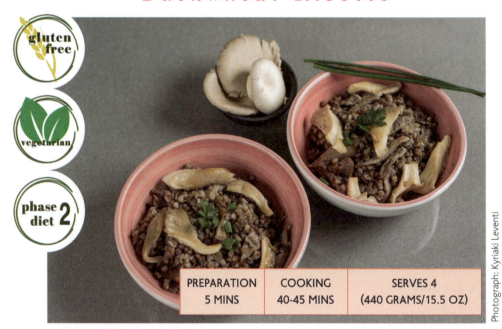

Photograph: Kyriaki Leventi

PREPARATION 5 MINS	COOKING 40-45 MINS	SERVES 4 (440 GRAMS/15.5 OZ)

INGREDIENTS

- 480 grams/16 ounces oyster mushrooms, sliced
- 2 cups leeks (100 grams) (the green part only), sliced
- 1 cup (50 grams) spring onions, the green part only, sliced
- 1 cup (180 grams) buckwheat groats

- 1 cup (240 ml) red wine
- 2 ½ cups (600 ml) warmed low FODMAP vegetable broth **(page 362)**
- 2 tablespoons (30 ml) of extra-virgin olive oil
- 2 bay leaves
- ½ cup (50 grams) grated Parmesan cheese
- 1 teaspoon (6 grams) salt
- ¼ teaspoon (0.5 grams) freshly ground black pepper
- Dill for garnish

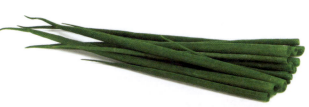

INSTRUCTIONS

Heat 1 tablespoon of olive oil in a sauté pan over medium-low heat.

Add the mushrooms, season with salt and cook for approximately 10 minutes, until all the liquid has evaporated.

Transfer to a plate and set aside.

Add the other tablespoon of oil to the sauté pan.

Add the bay leaves and cook for a few seconds; add leeks and spring onion, stirring occasionally until softened and starting to brown.

Add buckwheat groats to toast for 1-2 minutes.

Add the wine into the pan; stir and allow to cook until it is completely absorbed.

Continue to gradually add the vegetable broth approximately ½ cup at a time until all of the liquid has been absorbed. This process will take 30 minutes.

Keep the mixture at a low simmer while stirring occasionally.

Turn off the heat.

Stir the mushrooms and the Parmesan to combine.

Serve with dill and extra Parmesan.

Nutrition Facts	
Per serving: 360 kcal	8 grams fiber
16 grams protein	High in riboflavin, niacin, pantothenic acid, folate, iron, calcium, magnesium, manganese, and vitamins A and K
12 grams total fat	
3.5 grams saturated fat	
49 grams carbohydrates	

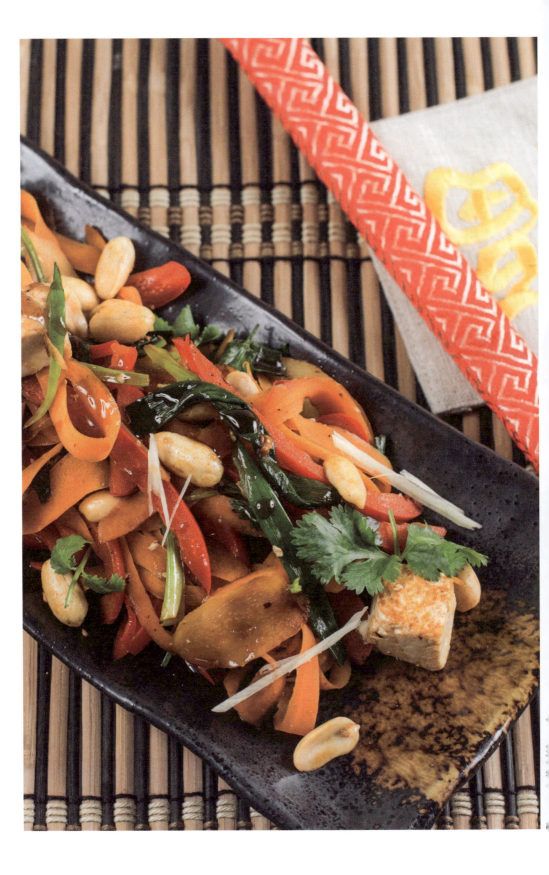

Tofu and Vegetable Stir Fry

PREPARATION 5 MINS	COOKING 10-15 MINS	PRESS TIME FOR TOFU 30 MINS	SERVES 5 (250 GRAMS, 8.8 OZ)

INGREDIENTS

- 1 block, 450 grams/1 pound extra-firm tofu, drained, pressed and cubed (2.5 x 0.6 cm/1 x ¼ inch)
- 4 tablespoons (60 ml) extra-virgin olive oil (use garlic infused oil for more intense taste) **(see recipe page 363)**
- 1 large (164 grams) red pepper, seeded and cut into strips
- 1 large (72 grams) carrot, peeled and cut with a vegetable peeler into carrot ribbons
- 3 tablespoons (18 grams) fresh ginger, grated
- 3 tablespoons (45 ml) **gluten-free tamari (a variety of naturally fermented soy sauce)**
- 2 tablespoons (30 ml) fresh lime juice
- 3 tablespoons (27 grams) toasted peanuts
- 4 tablespoons (8 grams) fresh basil
- 4 tablespoons (8 grams) fresh cilantro
- 2 cups (60 grams) baby spinach leaves
- ½ cup (25 grams) spring onions (the green parts only), chopped

INSTRUCTIONS

Step 1: Pressing the firm tofu

Drain the tofu.

Lay a dish towel and then a paper towel on a surface.

Add the tofu and again a paper towel.

Place something heavy on top.

Press for 30 minutes.

Step 2: Toast nuts

Place nuts in a dry skillet and place the skillet on the stovetop.

Cook over moderate heat until the nuts start to show color.

Step 3: Cook the tofu

Heat 2 tablespoons oil in wok over high heat.

Fry tofu, stirring occasionally, until brown on each side and set aside.

Add the remaining 2 tablespoons of oil.

Add pepper, carrot and ginger and sauté until softened (about 2 minutes).

Add tamari and lime juice; toss to blend.

Add spinach, tossing for 1 to 2 minutes until it begins to wilt.

Add herbs.

Season with salt and pepper.

Sprinkle with peanuts and green onions and serve.

Nutrition Facts	
Per serving: 300 kcal	3 grams fiber
16 grams protein	High in calcium, iron, folate, phosphorous, magnesium, manganese, selenium, copper, and vitamins A, C, E, and K
24 grams total fat	
3 grams saturated fat	
11 grams carbohydrates	

Tofu Broccoli Soba Noodles

PREPARATION 5 MINS	COOKING 15 MINS	PRESS TIME FOR TOFU 30 MINS	SERVES 4 (340 GRAMS, 12 OZ EACH)

INGREDIENTS

- 3 cups (300 grams) broccoli heads only, chopped
- 2 tablespoons (30 ml) extra-virgin olive oil
- 1 block, 450 grams/ 1 pound extra-firm tofu, drained, pressed and cubed (2.5x 0.6 cm/1 x ¼ inch)
- 2 tablespoons (12 grams) fresh ginger, grated
- ¼ cup (60 ml) cherry vinegar
- ¼ cup (60 ml) maple syrup
- ⅓ cup (80 ml) **gluten-free tamari (a variety of naturally fermented soy sauce)**
- 3 cups (342 grams) cooked soba noodles **(100% buckwheat)** (following the package directions, approximately 180 grams/6.3 oz dry)
- 1 teaspoon (3 grams) black or white sesame seeds

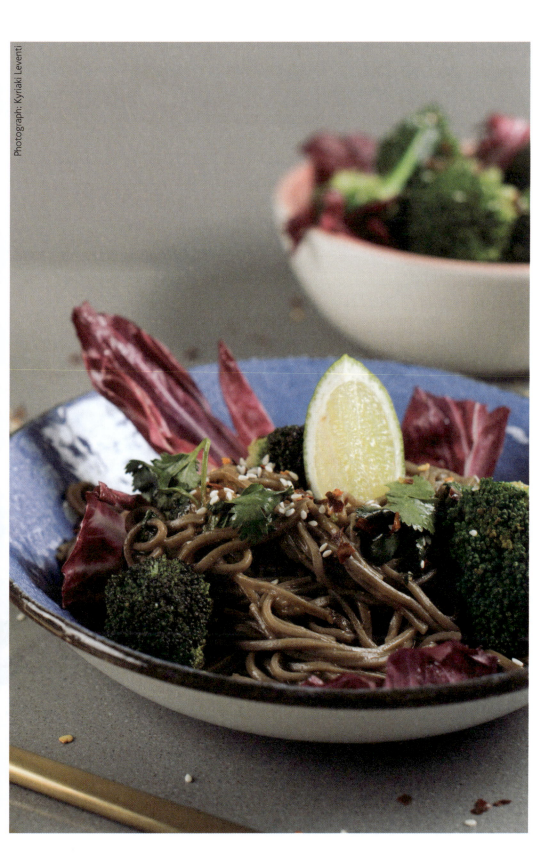

- 1 tablespoon (2 grams) fresh basil
- 1 tablespoon (2 grams) fresh cilantro
- Garnish with fresh radicchio
- Chili flakes optional only if tolerated

INSTRUCTIONS

Step 1: Blanch the broccoli florets

Wash the broccoli and cut off only the florets.

Blanch them in salted boiling water until crisp-tender (1 to 1 ½ minutes).

Remove with a slotted spoon.

Plunge immediately in ice water.

Step 2: Press the firm tofu

Drain the tofu.

Lay a dish towel and then a paper towel on a surface.

Add the tofu and again a paper towel.

Place something heavy on top.

Press for 30 minutes.

Step 3: Cook the tofu

Heat 2 tablespoons oil in a large pan over medium-high heat.

Fry tofu, stirring occasionally, until brown on each side.

Add ginger and continue cooking for a few seconds.

Add broccoli and the remaining ingredients and toss
     for a few seconds to combine.

Serve with soba noodles and sesame seeds and herbs.

Garnish with radicchio leaves.

Nutrition Facts	
Per serving: 340 kcal	2 grams fiber
20 grams protein	High in calcium, iron, riboflavin, folate, phosphorous, magnesium, manganese, selenium, and vitamins A and C
14 grams total fat	
1.5 grams saturated fat	
40 grams carbohydrates	

Tofu Mushroom Soba Noodles

PREPARATION 5 MINS	COOKING 15 MINS	PRESS TIME FOR TOFU 30 MINS	SERVES 4 (405 GRAMS, 14.3 OZ)

INGREDIENTS

- 6 cups (½ kilo) of oyster mushrooms chopped in 1 cm/0.4 inch pieces
- 2 tablespoons (30 ml) extra-virgin olive oil
- 1 block, 450 grams/1 pound extra-firm tofu, drained, pressed and cubed (2.5 x 0.6 cm/1 x ¼ inch)
- 2 tablespoon (12 grams) fresh ginger, grated
- 1 teaspoon (2.5 gram) red chili (if tolerated)
- ¼ cup (60 ml) cherry vinegar
- ¼ cup (60 ml) 100% pure maple syrup
- ⅓ cup (80 ml) **gluten-free tamari (a variety of naturally fermented soy sauce)**
- 3 cups (342 grams) cooked **gluten-free** soba noodles (**100% buckwheat**) (following the package directions, approximately 180 grams/6.3 oz dry)
- ½ cup (25 grams) green onions (the green parts only), chopped
- 1 tablespoon (9 grams) sesame seeds
- Garnish with fresh radish and chili pepper, only if tolerated

INSTRUCTIONS

Step 1: Pressing the firm tofu
Drain the tofu.
Lay a dish towel and then a paper towel on a surface.
Add the tofu and drain with a paper towel again.
Place something heavy on top.
Press for 30 minutes.

Step 2: Cook the tofu
Heat 2 tablespoons oil in a large pan over medium-high heat and
Fry tofu, stirring occasionally, until brown on each side. Set aside.

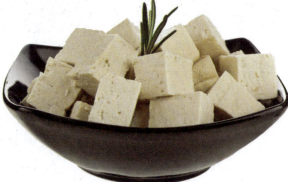

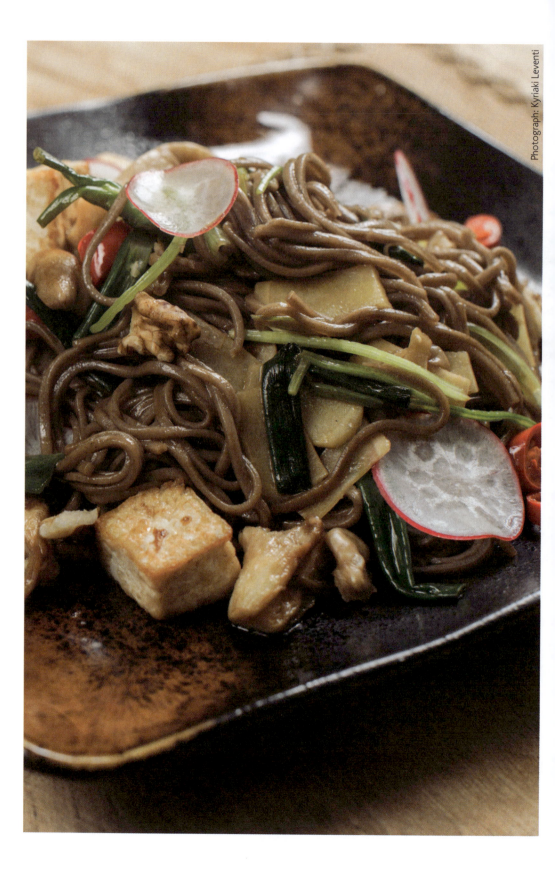

Photograph: Kyriaki Leventi

Heat the remaining 2 tablespoons oil.

Add mushrooms and cook for 5-7 minutes.

Add ginger and continue cooking for 2 minutes.

Toss until tender.

Add the remaining ingredients and toss for a few seconds.

Serve with soba noodles.

Garnish with sesame seeds and the green parts of the spring onions.

Nutrition Facts	
Per serving: 380 kcal	6 grams fiber
23 grams protein	High levels of vitamin K, thiamin, riboflavin, niacin, folate, pantothenic acid, manganese, copper, selenium, zinc, calcium, and potassium
15 grams total fat	
2 grams saturated fat	
45 grams carbohydrates	

Fennel and Chickpea Stew

PREPARATION 15 MINS	COOKING 65 MINS	SERVES 4 (340 GRAMS, 12 OZ)

INGREDIENTS

- 1 cup (152 grams) canned and drained cooked chickpeas, preferably in carton packaging
- 2 cups (174 grams) fennel, sliced
- 3 medium potatoes (450 grams), cut into cubes
- 4 spring onions, green parts only, chopped into 1-cm pieces
- 4 medium carrots (240 grams) cut in half lengthwise and then chopped into 1-cm thick pieces
- 1 cup fresh tomatoes (158 grams), cut into cubes
- 1 tablespoon rosemary leaves

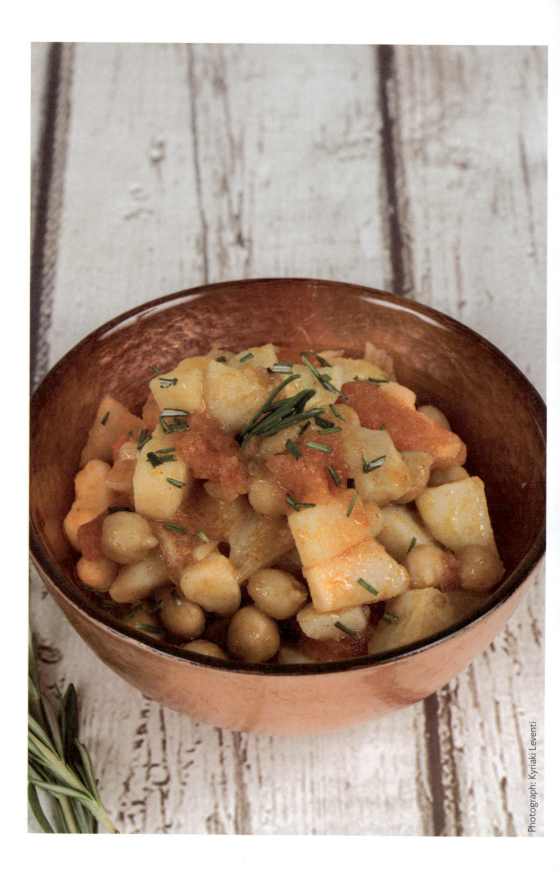

- 2 bay leaves
- 3 tablespoons (45 ml) extra-virgin olive oil
- Zest of one organic orange
- Zest of one organic lemon
- 2 cloves
- Juice of two medium oranges
- 4 teaspoons (6 grams) freshly grated Parmesan cheese, for garnish
- Salt and pepper

INSTRUCTIONS

Preheat oven to 180°C/356°F.

Drain and thoroughly rinse the chickpeas.

Pat them dry with a paper towel.

Wash and cut vegetables.

Boil vegetables (potatoes, carrots and fennel) for 15-20 minutes until soft.

Spoon all the ingredients into a baking dish and mix.

Bake for 50-60 minutes until crisp and golden.

Serve with sprinkled Parmesan cheese.

Nutrition Facts	
Per serving: 290 kcal	7 grams fiber
7 grams protein	High in folate, manganese, and vitamins A, C, K, and B6
12 grams total fat	
2 grams saturated fat	
41 grams carbohydrates	

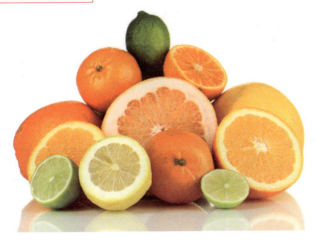

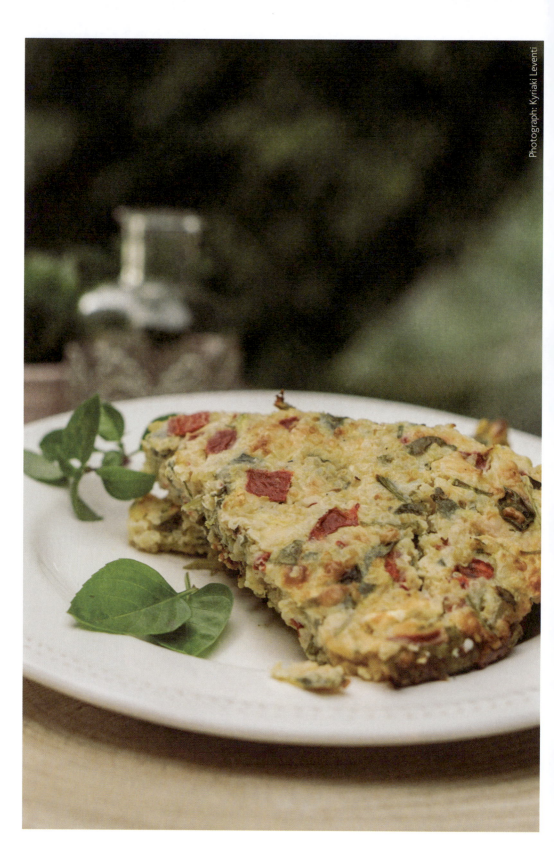

Quinoa Pie
with Cheese and Vegetables

PREPARATION 15 MINS	COOKING 40-45 MINS FOR THE PIE	COOKING QUINOA 15 MINS	SERVES 4 (300 GRAMS, 10.6 OZ)

INGREDIENTS

- 4 pastured eggs
- 3 cups (90 gram) fresh baby spinach
- 1 cup (95 grams) shredded unpeeled zucchini (after excess moisture is squeezed out)
- 2 ½ cup (450 grams) cooked quinoa (1 cup (180 grams) dry quinoa; **page 364**)
- 1 cup (100 grams) Parmesan cheese, grated
- 1 cup (240 ml) lactose-free milk
- ¾ cup (90 grams) feta cheese, crumbled
- 150 grams oven-roasted red bell pepper, cut into small pieces (you can use readymade roasted peppers) **or see recipe on page 188, step 1)**
- Salt and pepper

INSTRUCTIONS

Preheat oven to 180°C/356°F.

Shred the unpeeled zucchini.

Gather shredded zucchini in a clean kitchen tower and squeeze to remove as much moisture as possible.

Stir in the remaining ingredients.

Add salt and pepper (adjust salt according to your cheese).

Spoon in to a lightly greased 23 cm/9 in nonstick pan.

Place in the oven and bake for 40-45 minutes or until golden.

Nutrition Facts	
Per serving: 330 kcal	24 grams carbohydrates
20 grams protein	3 grams fiber
17 grams total fat	High in riboflavin, manganese, magnesium, zinc, selenium, folate, calcium, phosphorus, and vitamins A, C, K, B12, and B6
10 grams saturated fat	

Quinoa Spinach Mushroom Pie

PREPARATION 15 MINS	COOKING 40-45 MINS FOR THE PIE	COOKING QUINOA 15 MINS	SERVES 6 (300 GRAMS, 10.6 OZ)

INGREDIENTS

- 4 pastured eggs
- 3 ⅓ cups (100 grams) baby fresh spinach
- 6 cups (500 grams) of oyster mushrooms, cut into small pieces
- 1 teaspoon (5 ml) olive oil
- 2 ½ cups (450 grams) cooked quinoa (1 cup (180 grams) dry quinoa; **see recipe page 364**)
- 1 cup (100 grams) Parmesan cheese, grated
- 1 cup (240 ml) lactose-free milk
- ⅔ cup (90 grams) feta cheese, crumbled
- 150 grams oven-roasted red bell pepper, cut into small pieces (you can used readymade in the jar or **see recipe on page 188, step 1**)
- Salt and pepper

INSTRUCTIONS

Preheat the oven to 180°C/356°F.

Sauté the mushrooms to a non-skillet with 1 teaspoon olive oil until all moisture evaporates (5-7 minutes) and season with salt.

Coat a pie dish (23 cm/9 inches) with olive oil thoroughly.

Whisk together eggs, milk and feta cheese.

Add quinoa and roasted red peppers.

Add mushroom and spinach into the pie dish and cover with the egg mixture.

Top with Parmesan cheese.

Season with salt and pepper.

Bake for 40-45 minutes until the top is golden brown.

Nutrition Facts	
Per serving: 310 kcal	27 grams carbohydrates
21 grams protein	5 grams fiber
14 grams total fat	High in thiamin, riboflavin, niacin, folate, pantothenic acid, calcium, iron, phosphorus, magnesium, and vitamins A, C, K, B6, and B12
7 grams saturated fat	

VEGGIE BURGERS

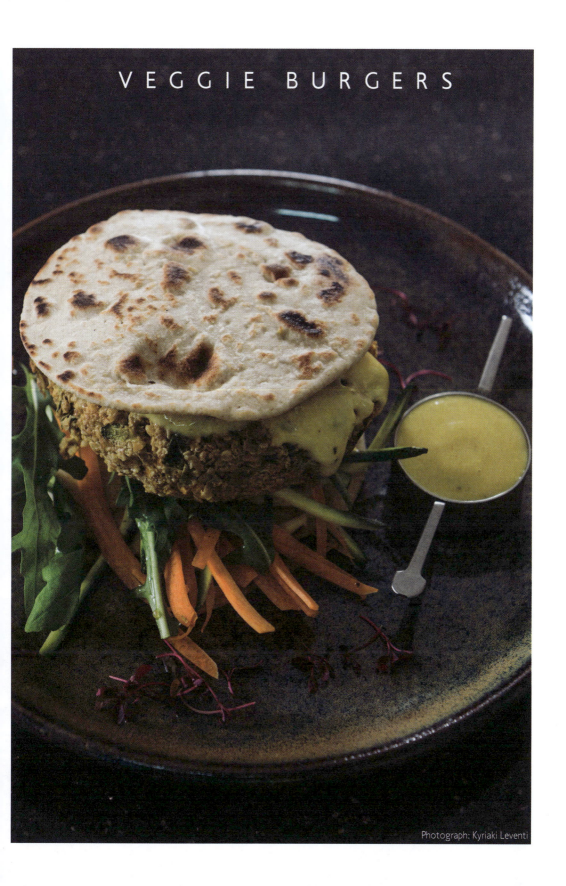

Quinoa Green Lentil Burger

Served with low FODMAP tzatziki page 358

PREPARATION 15 MINS	COOKING 40 MINS	COOKING LENTILS (IF NOT USING CANNED) 10-20 MINS	SERVES 6 (SERVING SIZE 150 GRAMS, 5.4 OZ EACH)

INGREDIENTS

Flaxseed gel
- 3 tablespoons (31,5 grams) freshly ground golden flaxseeds
- 9 tablespoons (135 ml) warm water

Spring onion leek mixture
- 2 cups (100 grams) leeks (the green part only), thinly sliced
- 1 cup (50 gram) spring onion (the green part only), thinly sliced
- 2 tablespoons (30 ml) olive oil
- 2 tablespoons (30 ml) white wine vinegar

Burger mixture
- Spring onion and leek mixture
- Flaxseed gel
- 1 medium (160 gram) parsnip, cooked and mashed
- ½ cup (60 grams) toasted walnuts, chopped
- 1 cup (180 grams) cooked quinoa (⅓ cup (65 grams) dry quinoa; **page 364**)
- ½ cup (92 grams) boiled green lentils or canned and drained
- 1 teaspoon (1,6 grams) dry thyme
- 1 teaspoon (1,6 grams) dry oregano
- 3 tablespoons (6 grams) fresh basil, chopped
- ½ teaspoon (3 grams) salt
- ¼ teaspoon ground black pepper
- ½ cup (50 grams) quinoa flakes or ground **gluten-free** oats

INSTRUCTIONS

Step 1: Cook lentils

Lentils cook quite fast, so they do not necessarily need soaking. You can just boil, cook for 10-20 minutes, drain and then add lemon juice.

1 part dry lentils makes 2 ½ parts cooked lentils.

Rinse lentils in a colander under cold running water.

Pour lentils into a pot and cover them with warm water.

Add a large strip of dried kombu (an edible seaweed) to the pot. Alternatively, use ginger or a few fennel or cumin seeds.

Cover and bring to a boil until the lentils are tender.

Skim and discard the foam during boiling.

Remove from the heat and add salt.

Let the lentils cool.

Step 2: Make the flaxseed gel

Mix together all the flaxseed gel ingredients until a gel is formed.

Step 3: Prepare the spring onion and leek mixture

Heat a sauté pan over medium heat.

Add the oil.

Cook leeks and spring onions for a few minutes until fragrant.

Deglaze the pan by adding the vinegar, turning up the heat to bring the liquid to a boil, and scraping up the sticky browned bits stuck to the pan.

Let it cool.

Step 4: Cook the parsnip

Peel and cut parsnip into evenly sized pieces.

Put it into a small pot and cover with water.

Bring to a boil and simmer until fork tender (approximately 20 minutes).

Mash coarsely with fork.

Step 5: Burgers

Preheat the oven to 190°C/375°F.

Drain and **rinse** the lentils well.

Pat them dry with a paper towel.

Mix all the ingredients together in a large mixing bowl.

Adjust seasoning if needed.

Fold in quinoa flakes; the mixture should be sticky but somewhat pliable.

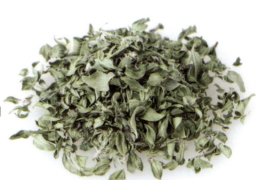

Add more quinoa flakes if too wet. **Add** one tablespoon at a time.

Shape into 6 patties.

Line a pan with parchment paper.

Cook in the oven for 12-15 minutes until firm and cooked through.

Nutrition Facts	
Per serving: 230 kcal	24 grams carbohydrates
6 grams protein	3 grams fiber
13 grams total fat	High in vitamin K, folate, and manganese
1.5 grams saturated fat	

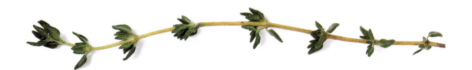

Sweet Potato Burger

PREPARATION 15 MINS	COOKING 45 MINS	SERVES 6 (SERVING SIZE 150 GRAMS, 5.4 OZ EACH)

INGREDIENTS

Flaxseed gel
- 3 tablespoons (31.5 grams) freshly ground golden flaxseeds
- 9 tablespoons (135 ml) warm water

Spring onion carrot mixture
- 2 cups (100 grams) spring onion (the green part only), thinly sliced
- 2 tablespoons (30 ml) extra-virgin olive oil
- 3 ½ cups (400 grams) grated carrot
- 1 tablespoon (6 grams) grated fresh ginger

- 1 tablespoon grated fresh turmeric (6 grams) or 1 teaspoon (6.8 grams) ground turmeric
- 1 teaspoon (2 grams) cumin
- ¾ teaspoon (1.5 grams) ground cardamom
- 1 tablespoon (15 ml) lemon juice

Burger mixture

- Spring onion mixture
- Flaxseed gel
- 1 small (70 grams) cooked sweet potato
- ½ cup (60 grams) toasted walnuts, chopped
- 1 teaspoon (5 grams) salt
- ½ cup (12 grams) finely chopped fresh basil
- 1 tablespoon (15 ml) lemon juice
- 1 tablespoon (16 grams) peanut butter
- ¼ teaspoon (0.5 grams) freshly ground black pepper
- ½ cup (50 grams) quinoa flakes or ground **gluten-free** oats

INSTRUCTIONS

Step 1: Make the flaxseed gel

Mix together all the flaxseed gel ingredients until a gel is formed.

Step 2: Make the spring onion carrot mixture

Heat a sauté pan over medium heat.

Add the oil.

Cook spring onions for a few minutes until fragrant.

Add ginger and turmeric and cook for a few seconds more.

Add carrots and spices and cook until soft (5 minutes).

Do not overcook.

Let it cool.

Step 3: Toast nuts

Heat a dry, heavy skillet over medium heat.

Add a single layer of chopped nuts when the pan is hot.

Stir frequently until the nuts turn golden brown with a rich, toasty fragrance.

Step 4: Cook the sweet potato

Peel and cut the sweet potato into evenly sized pieces.

Put it into a small pot and cover with water.

Bring to a boil and simmer until fork-tender, approximately 15-20 minutes

Mash coarsely with fork.

Step 5: Burgers

Preheat the oven to 190°C/375°F.

Mix all the ingredients together in a large mixing bowl.

Adjust seasoning if needed.

Fold in quinoa flakes, the mixture should be sticky but somewhat pliable.

Add more quinoa flakes if too wet. **Add** one tablespoon at a time.

Shape into 6 patties.

Line a pan with parchment paper.

Cook in the oven for 12-15 minutes until firm and cooked through.

Nutrition Facts	
Per serving: 200 kcal	17 grams carbohydrates
5 grams protein	6 grams fiber
14 grams total fat	High in manganese and vitamins A, C, and K
1.5 grams saturated fat	

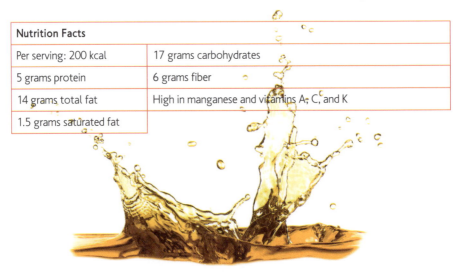

Mexican Carrot Burger

Served with pineapple salsa page 288

PREPARATION 15 MINS	COOKING 45 MINS	SERVES 7 (SERVING SIZE 150 GRAMS, 5.4 OZ EACH)

INGREDIENTS

Flaxseed gel

- 3 tablespoons (31.5 grams) freshly ground golden flaxseeds
- 9 tablespoons (135 ml) warm water

gluten free

vegan

phase diet **2**

Spring onion carrot mixture

- 2 cups (100 grams) spring onion (the green part only), thinly sliced
- 2 tablespoons (30 ml) of extra-virgin olive oil
- 3 ½ cups (400 grams) grated carrot
- 1 cup (95 grams) shredded unpeeled zucchini (after the excess moisture is squeezed out)
- 1 teaspoon (1.6 grams) coriander
- 1 teaspoon (2.5 grams) chili (if tolerated)
- ½ teaspoon (1 gram) cumin
- ¼ teaspoon (0.5 grams) oregano
- ¼ teaspoon (0.5 grams) cinnamon

Burger mixture

- Spring onion carrot mixture
- Flaxseed gel
- 1 small (125 grams) cooked potato
- ½ cup (60 grams) toasted walnuts, ground
- 1 teaspoon (6 grams) salt
- ½ cup (12 grams) finely chopped fresh cilantro
- 2 tablespoons (30 ml) lime juice
- ½ cup (50 grams) quinoa flakes or ground **gluten-free** oats (if tolerated)

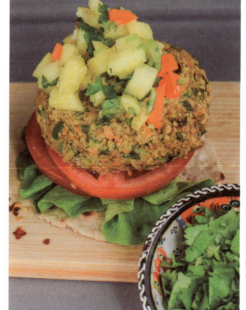

Photograph: Kyriaki Leventi

INSTRUCTIONS

Step 1: Make the flaxseed gel

Mix together all the flaxseed gel ingredients until a gel is formed.

Step 2: Make the spring onion vegetable mixture

Heat a sauté pan over medium heat.

Add the oil.

Cook spring onions for a few minutes until fragrant.

Add carrots, zucchini and spices and cook until soft, 5 minutes.

Do not overcook.

Let it cool.

Step 3: : Toast nuts

Heat a dry, heavy skillet over medium heat.

Add a single layer of nuts when the pan is hot.

Stir frequently until the nuts turn golden brown with a rich, toasty fragrance.

Step 4: Cook the potato

Peel and cut the potato into evenly sized pieces.

Put it into a small pot and cover with water.

Bring to a boil and simmer until fork-tender, approximately 20 to 30 minutes.

Mash coarsely with fork.

Step 5: Burgers

Preheat the oven to 190°C/375°F.

Mix all the ingredients together in a large mixing bowl.

Adjust seasoning if needed.

Fold in quinoa flakes; the mixture should be sticky but somewhat pliable.

Add more quinoa flakes if too wet. **Add** one tablespoon at a time.

Shape into 7 patties.

Line a pan with parchment paper.

Cook in the oven for 12-15 minutes until firm and cooked through.

Nutrition Facts	
Per serving: 190 kcal	17 grams carbohydrates
5 grams protein	5 grams fiber
12 grams total fat	High in manganese and vitamins A and K
1 gram saturated fat	

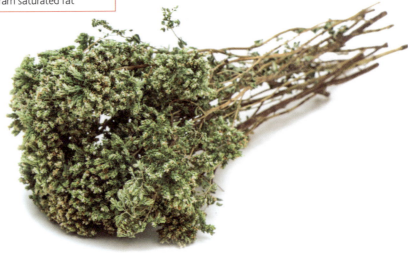

Indian Burger

Served with low FODMAP raita page 359

PREPARATION 15 MINS	COOKING 30 MINS	SERVES 7 (SERVING SIZE 150 GRAMS, 5.4 OZ EACH)

INGREDIENTS

Flaxseed gel
- 3 tablespoons (31.5 grams) freshly ground golden flaxseeds
- 9 tablespoons (135 ml) warm water

Spring onion carrot mixture
- 2 cups (100 grams) spring onion, the green part only thinly sliced
- 2 tablespoons (30 ml) of extra-virgin olive oil
- 5 ½ cups (600 grams) grated carrot
- 1 tablespoon (6 grams) grated fresh ginger
- 1 tablespoon (6 grams) grated fresh turmeric or 1 teaspoon (2.4 grams) ground turmeric
- ½ teaspoon (1 gram) ground coriander
- ½ teaspoon (1 gram) ground cumin
- ¼ teaspoon (0.5 grams) ground cardamom
- ¼ teaspoon (0.5 grams) ground cinnamon

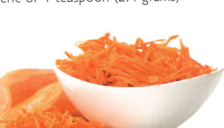

Burger mixture
- Spring onion carrot mixture
- Flaxseed gel
- ½ cup (70 grams) toasted sunflower seeds, ground
- 1 tablespoon (16 grams) peanut butter
- 1 teaspoon (6 grams) salt
- 2 tablespoons (30 ml) lime juice
- ½ cup (50 grams) quinoa flakes or ground **gluten-free** oats

INSTRUCTIONS

Step 1: Make the flaxseed gel
Mix together all the flaxseed gel ingredients until a gel is formed.

Step 2: Make the spring onion vegetable mixture

Heat a sauté pan over medium heat.

Add the oil.

Cook spring onions for a few minutes until fragrant.

Add carrots and spices and cook until soft (5 minutes).

Do not overcook.

Let it cool.

Step 3: Toast nuts

Heat a dry, heavy skillet over medium heat.

Add a single layer of seeds when the pan is hot.

Stir frequently until the seeds turn golden brown with a rich, toasty fragrance.

Step 4: Burgers

Preheat the oven to 190°C/375°F.

Mix all the ingredients together in a large mixing bowl.

Adjust seasoning if needed.

Fold in quinoa flakes; the mixture should be sticky but somewhat pliable.

Add more quinoa flakes if too wet. **Add** one tablespoon at a time.

Shape into 7 patties.

Line a pan with parchment paper.

Cook in the oven for 12-15 minutes until firm and cooked through.

Nutrition Facts	
Per serving: 190 kcal	17 grams carbohydrates
5 grams protein	5 grams fiber
13 grams total fat	High in thiamin, manganese and vitamins A, E, and K
1.5 grams saturated fat	

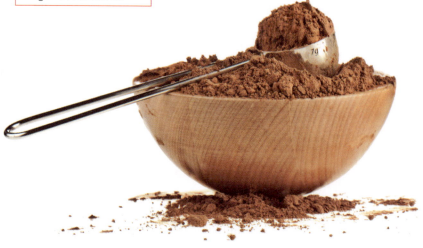

Spinach Carrot Burger

Served with tahini sauce page 361

PREPARATION 15 MINS	COOKING 40 MINS	COOKING POTATOES 20 MINS	SERVES 7 (SERVING SIZE 150 GRAMS, 5.4 OZ EACH)

INGREDIENTS

Flaxseed gel
- 3 tablespoons (31.5 grams) freshly ground golden flaxseeds
- 9 tablespoons (135 ml) warm water

Spring onion carrot mixture
- 2 cups (100 grams) spring onion (the green part only), thinly sliced
- 2 tablespoon (30 ml) extra-virgin olive oil
- 3 ½ cups (400 gram) grated carrot
- 1 tablespoon (6 grams) grated fresh ginger

Burger mixture
- Spring onion, carrot mixture
- Flaxseed gel
- 2 cups (60 grams) spinach
- 1 teaspoon (5 ml) olive oil
- 1 small potato (125 grams), cooked and mashed
- 1 teaspoon (6 grams) salt
- 3 tablespoons (6 grams) chopped fresh parsley
- 3 tablespoons (6 grams) chopped fresh basil
- 3 tablespoons (6 grams) chopped fresh chives
- ½ cup (60 grams) toasted walnuts, chopped
- ¼ teaspoon (0.5 grams) freshly ground black pepper
- ½ cup (50 grams) quinoa flakes or ground gluten-free oats (if tolerated)

INSTRUCTIONS

Step 1: Make the flaxseed gel
Mix together all the flaxseed gel ingredients until a gel is formed.

Step 2: Make the spring onion carrot mixture
Heat a sauté pan over medium heat.

Add the oil

Cook spring onions for a few minutes until fragrant.

Add ginger and cook for a few seconds more.

Add carrots and cook until soft for 5 minutes.

Do not overcook.

Let it cool.

Step 3: Cook the potato

Peel and **cut** potato into evenly sized pieces.

Put it into a small pot, **cover** with water.

Bring to a boil and simmer until fork-tender (approximately 20 to 30 minutes).

Mash coarsely with a fork.

Step 4: Toast nuts

Heat a dry, heavy skillet over medium heat.

Add a single layer of chopped nuts when the pan is hot.

Stir frequently until the nuts turn golden brown with a rich, toasty fragrance.

Step 5: Cook the spinach

Heat a large sauté pan over medium heat.

Add spinach and cook until wilted for 2 minutes.

Allow to cool.

Squeeze out any excess liquid.

Finely chop the spinach.

Step 6: Burgers

Preheat the oven to 190°C/375°F.

Mix all the ingredients together in a large mixing bowl.

Adjust seasoning if needed.

Fold in quinoa flakes; the mixture should be sticky but somewhat pliable.

Add more quinoa flakes if too wet. **Add** one tablespoon at a time.

Shape into 7 patties.

Line a pan with parchment paper.

Cook in the oven for 12-15 minutes until firm and
    cooked through.

Nutrition Facts	
Per serving: 190 kcal	18 grams carbohydrates
4 grams protein	5 grams fiber
13 grams total fat	High in thiamin and vitamins A, E, and K
1.5 grams saturated fat	

Carrot Ginger Burger

Served with peanut orange sauce page 233

PREPARATION 15 MINS	COOKING 25 MINS	SERVES 6 (SERVING SIZE 150 GRAMS, 5.4 OZ EACH)

INGREDIENTS

Flaxseed gel

- 3 tablespoons (31.5 grams) freshly ground golden flaxseeds
- 9 tablespoons (135 ml) warm water

Spring onion carrot mixture

- 2 cups (100 grams) spring onion (the green part only), thinly sliced
- 2 tablespoons (30 ml) extra-virgin olive oil
- 4 ⅓ cups (480 gram) grated carrot
- 1 tablespoon (6 grams) grated fresh ginger
- 1 tablespoon (6 grams) grated fresh turmeric or 1 teaspoon (6.8 grams) ground turmeric

Burger mixture

- Spring onion mixture
- Flaxseed gel
- 4 tablespoons (8 grams) chopped fresh cilantro
- ½ cup (60 grams) toasted walnuts, chopped
- 2 tablespoons (30 ml) lime juice
- 1 tablespoon (16 grams) peanut butter
- ¼ teaspoon (0.5 grams) freshly ground black pepper
- 1 teaspoon (6 grams) salt
- ½ cup (50 grams) quinoa flakes or ground **gluten-free** oats

INSTRUCTIONS

Step 1: Make the flaxseed gel

Mix together all the flaxseed gel ingredients until a gel is formed.

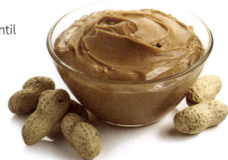

Step 2: Make the spring onion carrot mixture

Heat a sauté pan over medium heat.

Add the oil.

Cook spring onions for a few minutes until fragrant.

Add ginger and turmeric and cook for a few seconds more.

Add carrots and cook until soft for 5 minutes.

Do not overcook.

Let it cool.

Step 3: Toast nuts

Heat a dry, heavy skillet over medium heat.

Add a single layer of the chopped nuts when the pan is hot.

Stir frequently until the nuts turn golden brown with a rich, toasty fragrance.

Step 4: Burgers

Preheat the oven to 190°C/375°F.

Mix all the ingredients together in a large mixing bowl.

Adjust seasoning if needed.

Fold in quinoa flake; the mixture should be sticky but somewhat pliable.

Add more quinoa flakes if too wet.

Add one tablespoon at a time.

Shape into 6 patties.

Line a pan with parchment paper.

Cook in the oven for 12-15 minutes until firm and cooked through.

Nutrition Facts	
Per serving: 210 kcal	16 grams carbohydrates
5 grams protein	6 grams fiber
15 grams total fat	High in manganese and vitamins A and K
2 grams saturated fat	

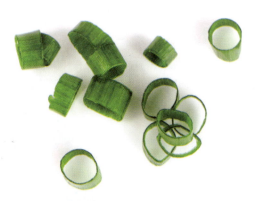

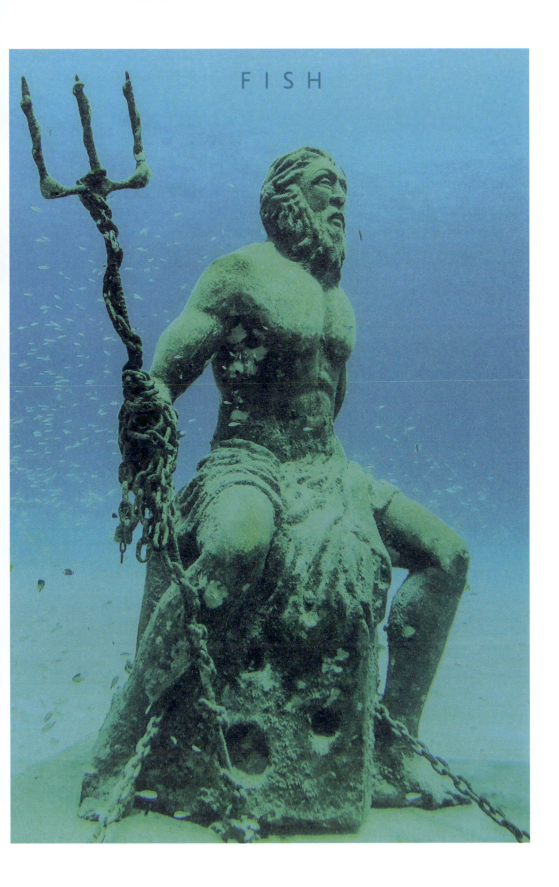

FISH

Pan-Fried Salmon Fillets with Pineapple Salsa

PREPARATION 10 MINS	WAITING TIME FOR SALSA 2 HOURS	COOKING 10 MINS	SERVES 4 (SERVING SIZE 170 GRAMS, 6 OZ)

INGREDIENTS

Salsa

- 1 ½ cup (248 grams) pineapple, cut into small cubes
- ½ cup (75 grams) red bell pepper, cut into small cubes
- 2 tablespoons (30 ml) freshly squeezed lime juice
- 5 tablespoons (10 grams) thinly cut cilantro leaves
- 2 tablespoons (10 grams) thinly sliced spring onions (the green part only)
- Salt and pepper

Salmon

- 4 salmon fillets with skin on (170 grams/6 oz each)
- 2 tablespoon (30 ml) olive oil
- Salt and pepper

INSTRUCTIONS

Step 1: Salsa

Combine all ingredients in the bowl.

Adjust seasoning to taste.

Let sit for 2 hours to allow flavors to blend.

Step 2: Pan-fried salmon

See page 240 (Salmon salad step 1).

Step 3

Serve salmon with salsa.

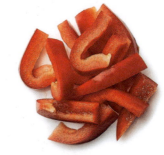

Nutrition Facts	
Per serving: 340 kcal	10 grams carbohydrates
34 grams protein	1 gram fiber
18 grams total fat	High in pantothenic acid, thiamin, riboflavin, selenium, potassium, copper, manganese, and vitamins C, B6, and B12
2.5 grams saturated fat	

Baked Maple Salmon

PREPARATION 5 MINS	COOKING 25 MINS	SERVES 5 (SERVING SIZE 200 GRAMS, 7 OZ)

INGREDIENTS

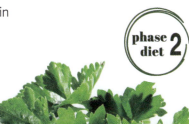

- 700 grams/1.5 pounds side of salmon without skin
- ½ cup (120 ml) 100% pure maple syrup
- 4 tablespoons (60 ml) **gluten-free tamari sauce (a variety of naturally fermented soy sauce)**
- 2 tablespoons (12 grams) grated fresh ginger
- Juice of 4 limes plus 1 lime, thinly sliced
- 2 tablespoons (30 ml) olive oil
- ½ teaspoon (2.5 ml) hot chili sauce (optional, only if tolerated)
- Salt and pepper

For garnish

- 2 tablespoons (4 grams) chopped cilantro
- 1 green onion (the green part only), thinly sliced
- 1 teaspoon (3 grams) toasted sesame seeds

INSTRUCTIONS

Preheat oven to 177°C/350°F.

Line a large baking sheet with foil and a sheet of parchment paper.

Lay salmon on parchment paper and season to taste with salt and pepper on both sides.

Place lime slices underneath the salmon.

Mix maple syrup, olive oil, tamari sauce, ginger and hot sauce, if using, in a small bowl; whisk well to mix.

Pour mixture over salmon.

Fold the sides of the foil over the salmon, sealing the packet closed.

Bake for 15-20 minutes. Adjust cooking time according to the thickness of the salmon.

Uncover and broil for 5 more minutes.

Garnish with cilantro, green onion and sesame seeds.

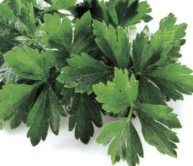

> **!** *The safe fish temperature recommended by USDA is an internal temperature of 62.8°C/145°F. Remove your salmon from the oven immediately after the temperature reaches 55°C/130°F. The temperature will continue to rise during the 5-minute rest time, achieving the ideal safe temperature.*

Nutrition Facts	
Per serving: 340 kcal	24 grams carbohydrates
29 grams protein	0 gram fiber
14 grams total fat	High in phosphorus, niacin, selenium, manganese, thiamin,
2 grams saturated fat	riboflavin, pantothenic acid, potassium, and vitamins B6 and B12

Grilled Butterflied Sardines

PREPARATION 10 MINS	COOKING SARDINES 5-10 MINS	SERVES 4 (SERVING SIZE 2 SARDINES)

INGREDIENTS

Sardines
- 8 whole sardines (720 grams/1.6 pound), butterflied, scaled, gutted, backbone removed (ask your fishmonger to do this for you)
- 2 tablespoons (30 ml) lemon juice
- Olive oil for brushing the sardines
- Salt and pepper

Chermoula sauce
- ¼ teaspoon (0.4 grams) coriander seeds
- ¼ teaspoon (0.5 grams) cumin seeds
- 2 tablespoons (30 ml) garlic olive oil
- ⅛ teaspoon finely grated lemon zest

- 1 tablespoon (15 ml) fresh lemon juice
- ¼ teaspoon (0.6 grams) smoked paprika
- ½ teaspoon (3 grams) salt
- ¼ cup cilantro (6 grams) leaves
- ¼ cup parsley (6 grams) leaves
- 1 tablespoon (2 grams) mint leaves

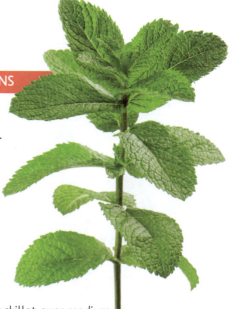

INSTRUCTIONS

Step 1 Sardines

Heat the griddle pan or barbecue on high heat.

Season the sardines with salt, pepper
and lemon juice and leave for 5 minutes.

Brush the sardines with extra-virgin olive oil
and cook on high heat.

Cook for 2 minutes on each side
until just cooked through.

Remove and **allow** to rest for 2 minutes.

Step 2: Chermoula sauce

Toast coriander and cumin seeds in a small dry skillet over medium
heat until fragrant.

Let cool.

Blend everything except the herbs in a food processor until smooth.

Add the herbs and process until combined while still retaining some texture.

Step 3: Assembled the plate

Arrange potatoes **(see recipe oven roasted baby potatoes page 339)** in a
plate.

Top with the sardines.

Serve with the sauce.

Nutrition Facts	
Per serving: 550 kcal	22 grams carbohydrates
41 grams protein	3 grams fiber
34 grams total fat	High in calcium, iron, and vitamins A, C, K, and B6
6 grams saturated fat	

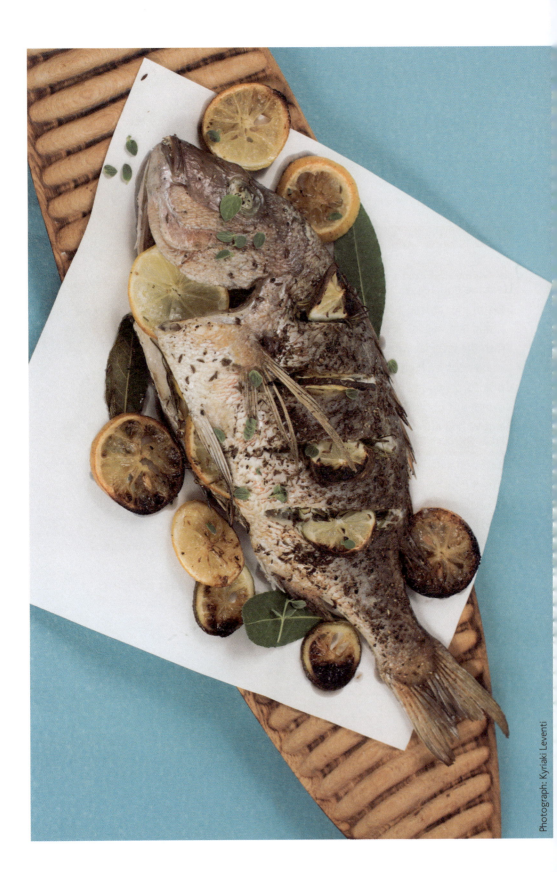

Whole Roasted Fish

PREPARATION 5 MINS	COOKING 20 MINS	SERVES 4 (SERVING SIZE 272 GRAMS OF FISH, 9.6 OZ)

INGREDIENTS

- 1 kilo/2.2 pounds cleaned and scaled sustainable whole fish
- 2 tablespoons (30 ml) of extra-virgin olive oil
- 1 lemon thinly sliced
- 5 sprigs of rosemary
- 5 sprigs of thyme
- 5 sprigs of oregano
- ¼ cup (58 grams) fennel bulb, thinly sliced
- 1 teaspoon (1.6 grams) fennel seeds
- 1 teaspoon (1.6 grams) oregano
- Salt and pepper

INSTRUCTIONS

Preheat the oven to 220°C/428°F.

Line a baking sheet with a parchment paper.

Make 3 crosswise slashes on each side of the fish, but do not cut too deep.

Rub fish with olive oil and season it well with salt, pepper, fennel seeds and oregano.

Stuff the cavity with herbs, fennel and lemon slices.

Stuff the crosswise slashes with lemon slices and some herbs.

Roast for approximately 20 minutes, until the flesh is opaque and separates easily from the backbone.

> **!** *The safe internal temperature for cooked fish is 62,8°C/145°F, or until the fish is opaque and flakes easily with a fork. When cooking fish, cook it until the center reaches 62,8°C/145°F on an instant-read or meat thermometer.*

Nutrition Facts	
Per serving: 310 kcal	2 grams carbohydrates
46 grams protein	‹ 1 gram fiber
12 grams total fat	High in thiamin, niacin, riboflavin, phosphorus, selenium, panto-thenic acid, and vitamins D and B6
2 grams saturated fat	

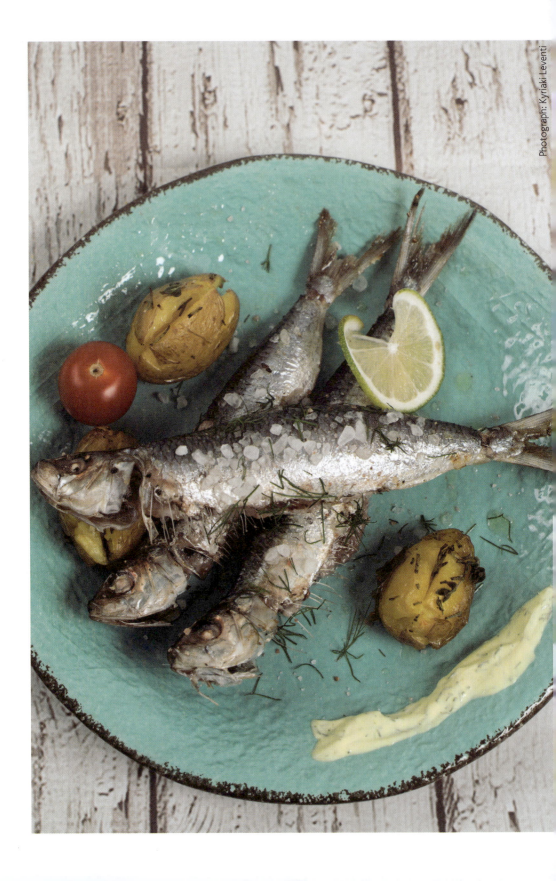

Photograph: Kyriaki Leventi

Oven Baked Sardines

PREPARATION 5 MINS	COOKING SARDINES 10-15 MINS	SERVES 4 (SERVING SIZE 225 GRAMS OF FISH, 7.9 OZ)

INGREDIENTS

- 8 whole fresh sardines (720 grams/1.6 pound), cleaned
- 6 cherry tomatoes (100 grams), halved
- 2 tablespoons (30 ml) lemon juice
- 1 tablespoon (6 grams) organic lemon zest
- ½ teaspoon (1.2 grams) paprika
- 2 tablespoons (30 ml) garlic olive oil
- 2 tablespoons (4 grams) flat-leaf parsley, chopped

INSTRUCTIONS

Heat the oven to 180°C/356°F.

Grease a large roasting pan.

Mix lemon juice and zest, paprika, parsley and garlic olive oil.

Season with salt and pepper.

Fill the cavity of the sardines with some of the mixture.

Place sardines in the roasting pan and scatter over the remainder of the mixture.

Place tomatoes in between the sardines.

Roast for 10-15 minutes or until cooked through.

Serve immediately.

Nutrition Facts	
Per serving: 470 kcal	3 grams carbohydrates
44 grams protein	0 grams fiber
31 grams total fat	High in calcium and iron
7 grams saturated fat	

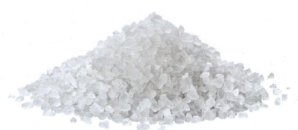

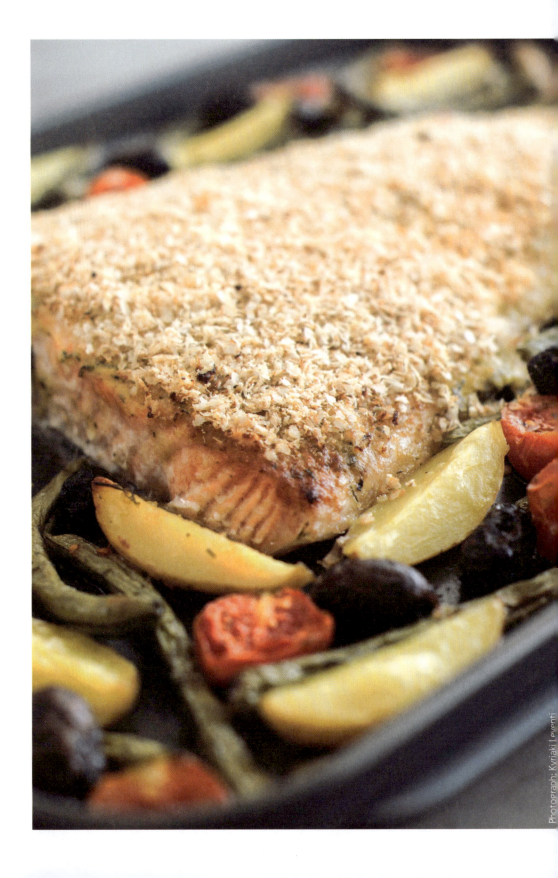

Baked Salmon and Vegetables with Cream Cheese Crust

gluten free

PREPARATION 15 MINS	COOKING 45 MINS	SERVES 5 (SERVING SIZE 368 GRAMS, 13 OZ)

phase diet 2

INGREDIENTS

Vinaigrette
- 4 tablespoons (60 ml) olive oil
- 2 tablespoons (30 ml) red wine vinegar
- 1 teaspoon (5 grams) Dijon mustard
- 2 tablespoons (4 grams) fresh tarragon
- 2 tablespoons (4 grams) fresh dill
- Salt and pepper

Salmon
- 700 grams/1.5 pounds side of salmon without skin
- 2 tablespoons (40 grams) cream cheese
- 2 teaspoons (10 grams) Dijon mustard
- 1 teaspoon (1 gram) fresh dill, finely chopped
- 1 teaspoon (2 grams) organic lemon zest
- ¼ cup (25 grams) quinoa flakes
- ¼ cup (25 grams) grated Parmesan cheese

Vegetables
- 20 mini potatoes (510 grams), cooked and halved (boiled for 20 minutes)
- 50 green beans (250 grams), trimmed
- 15 cherry (225 grams) tomatoes, halved
- ½ cup black Kalamata olives

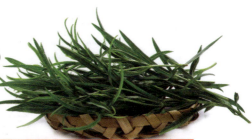

INSTRUCTIONS

Preheat oven to 218°C/425°F.

Line a large baking sheet with foil and a sheet of parchment paper.

Lay salmon on parchment paper and season to taste with salt and pepper on both sides.

Mix olive oil, mustard, vinegar, salt, pepper and herbs in a small bowl; whisk well to mix.

Brush salmon with 1 tablespoon of the vinaigrette.

Mix cream cheese, mustard, lemon zest and herbs.

Spoon cream cheese mixture over salmon.

Mix quinoa flakes and Parmesan.

Top salmon with Parmesan quinoa flakes.

Toss together, the vegetables and the vinaigrette.

Arrange vegetables around salmon.

Bake for 18-22 minutes. Adjust cooking time according to the thickness of the salmon.

> **!** *The safe fish temperature recommended by USDA is an internal temperature of 62.8°C/145°F. Remove your salmon from the oven immediately after the temperature reaches 55°C/130°F. The temperature will continue to rise during the 5-minute rest time, achieving the ideal safe temperature.*

Nutrition Facts	
Per serving: 500 kcal	31 grams carbohydrates
34 grams protein	5 grams fiber
27 grams total fat	High in copper, magnesium, selenium, potassium, thiamin, niacin, riboflavin, and vitamins A, C, K, B6, and B12
5 grams saturated fat	

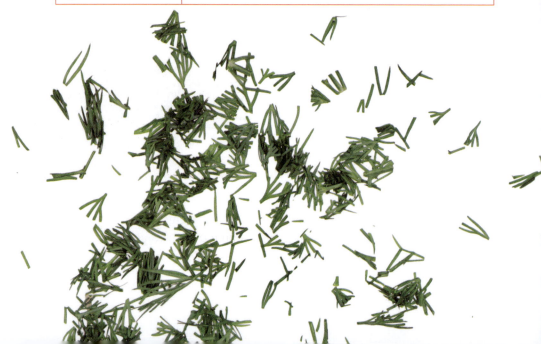

Steamed Fish with Fennel and Leeks and Yogurt Dressing

PREPARATION 5 MINS	COOKING 15-20 MINS	SERVES 4 (SERVING SIZE 292 GRAMS, 10.3 OZ)

INGREDIENTS

phase diet **2**

Fish

- 4 sustainable thick fish fillets, approximately 175 grams/6 oz each
- 1 cup (100 grams) leek (the green part only)
- ½ bulb fennel (192 grams), finely sliced
- 1 tablespoon (2 grams) fresh dill
- 1 tablespoon (15 ml) olive oil
- 2 teaspoons (8 grams) capers
- 1 teaspoon (2 grams) organic lemon zest
- 1 cup (240 ml) dry wine
- 1 cup (240 ml) water
- Salt and pepper

Yogurt fish dressing

- ½ cup **lactose-free** yogurt
- 2 teaspoons vinegar
- 2 teaspoons Dijon mustard
- 4 teaspoons finely chopped dill

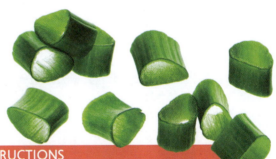

INSTRUCTIONS

Step 1: Yogurt fish dressing

Mix everything together.

Step 2: Fish

Heat 1 tablespoon oil in a large pan over medium-high heat.

Fry fennel and leeks until soften, stirring occasionally for a few minutes.

Pour the wine, the dill, the lemon zest, capers and **season** with salt and pepper.

Pour in 1 cup (240 ml) hot water.

Sprinkle the fish with salt and pepper and lay it on top of the vegetables.

Lower the heat so that the mixture simmers.

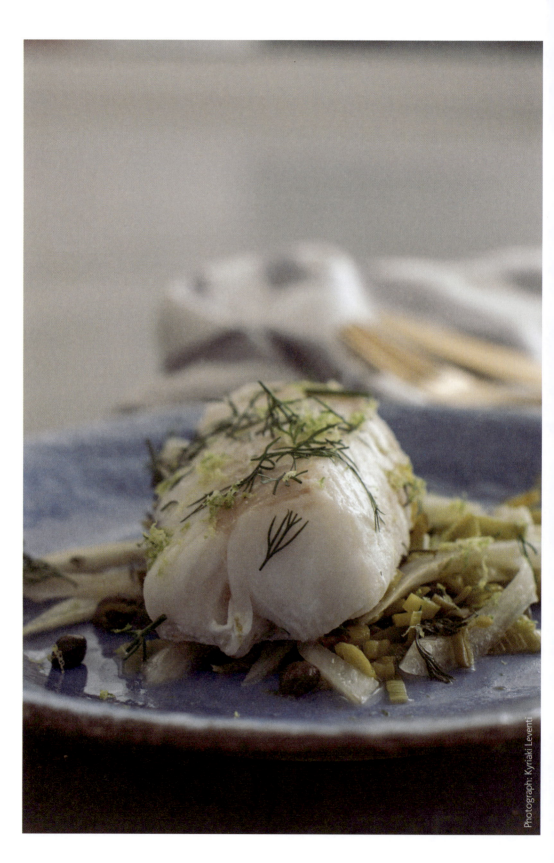

Cover and **cook**. Cooking will take 5 to 12 minutes, depending on the thickness of the fish.

Serve with yogurt fish dressing.

> ❗ *The safe internal temperature for cooked fish is 62,8°C/145°F, or until the fish is opaque and flakes easily with a fork. When cooking fish, cook it until the center reaches 62,8°C/145°F on an instant-read or meat thermometer.*

Nutrition Facts	
Per serving: 230 kcal	9 grams carbohydrates
31 grams protein	2 grams fiber
7 grams total fat	High in phosphorus, selenium, potassium, niacin, and vitamins A, K, B6, and B12
2.5 grams saturated fat	

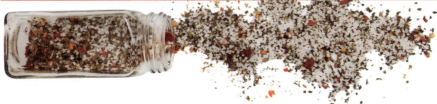

Baked Trout in a Bag

PREPARATION 5 MINS	COOKING 40-45 MINS	SERVES 1 (SERVING SIZE 466 GRAMS, 16.4 OZ)

INGREDIENTS

- 1 sustainable fish fillet (such as trout), approximately 175 grams/6 oz (skinned and without the bone)
- 1 tablespoon (15 ml) olive oil
- 48 grams/1.7 oz fennel bulb, finely sliced
- 1 small potato (125 grams), boiled and sliced
- ¼ cup leek (12.5 grams), finely sliced (only the green part)
- 1 teaspoon (1 gram) chopped dill
- 2 tablespoons (30 ml) white wine

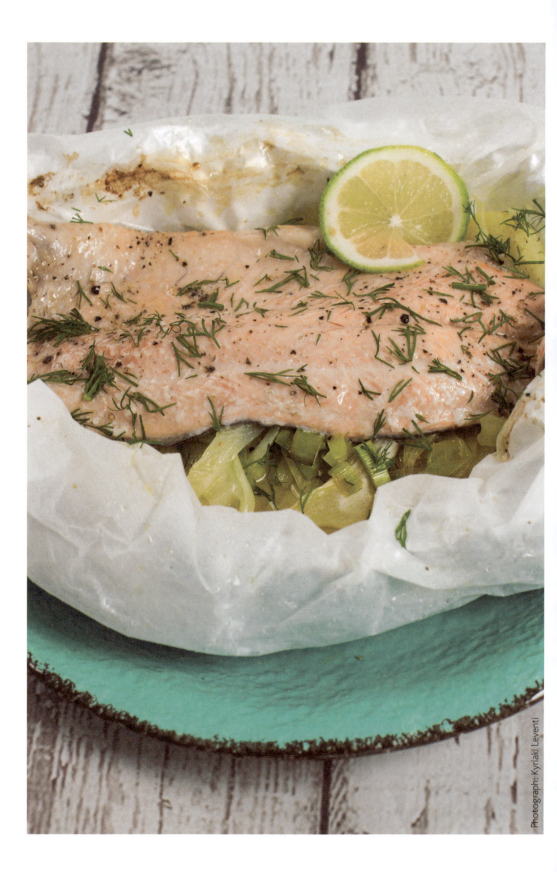

Photograph: Kyriaki Leventi

- Olive oil, drizzled
- Squeezed lemon juice
- Salt and freshly ground black pepper

INSTRUCTIONS

Preheat the oven to 180°C/356°F.

Cut out one square of baking paper and one square of tin foil double the size of the fish fillet.

Lay the baking paper on top of the tin foil.

Boil the potatoes until soft (approximately 20 minutes).

Let them cool; then slice them.

Heat 1 tablespoon oil in a large pan over medium-high heat.

Fry fennel and leeks until softened, stirring occasionally for a few minutes.

Lay the fennel, leeks and potatoes on one side of the baking paper and put the fish on top.

Drizzle with some oil and lemon juice.

Season with salt and pepper and sprinkle with dill.

Fold the foil over the vegetables and the fish.

Double fold the edges to make a parcel.

Pour the wine before the final edge is sealed.

Bake on a baking tray for 12-18 minutes, depending on the fillet size; the fish should be opaque and break easily into flakes when you nudge it with a fork in the thickest part.

Take the parcel out of the oven and carefully open the parcel. **Be careful,** as the steam will be hot.

> ! *The safe internal temperature for cooked fish is 62,8°C/145°F, or until the fish is opaque and flakes easily with a fork. When cooking fish, cook it until the center reaches 62,8°C/145°F on an instant-read or meat thermometer.*

Nutrition Facts	
Per serving: 390 kcal	40 grams carbohydrates
34 grams protein	7 grams fiber
11 grams total fat	High in folate, phosphorus, copper, magnesium, manganese, potassium, thiamin, niacin, riboflavin, pantothenic acid, and vitamins A, C, K, B6, and B12
2.5 grams saturated fat	

Baked Fish in a Bag

PREPARATION 5 MINS	COOKING 40-45 MINS	SERVES 1 (SERVING SIZE 365 GRAMS, 12.9 OZ)

INGREDIENTS

- 1 sustainable white fish fillet (cod), approximately 175 grams/6 oz (skinned and without the bone)
- 1 teaspoon (5 ml) olive oil
- 1 medium (60 grams) carrot, finely sliced
- 1 small potato (125 grams), cut into small cubes
- 2 tablespoons low FODMAP stock **(see recipe page 362)** or water
- Olive oil, drizzled
- Squeeze of lemon juice
- Salt to taste
- Chopped dill to sprinkle on top

INSTRUCTIONS

Preheat the oven to 180°C/356°F.

Cut out one square of baking paper and one square tin foil double the size of the fish fillet.

Lay the baking paper on top of tin foil.

Boil the potatoes and carrots until soft for approximately 20 minutes.

Let them cool.

Lay the carrots and the potatoes on one side of the baking paper and put the fish on top.

Drizzle with some oil and lemon juice.

Season with salt and sprinkle with the dill.

Fold the foil over the vegetables and the fish.

Double fold the edges to make a parcel.

Pour the low FODMAP stock before the final edge is sealed.

Bake on a baking tray for 20-30 minutes depending on the fillet size, the fish should be opaque and break easily into flakes when you nudge it with a fork in the thickest part.

Take the parcel out of the oven and carefully open the parcel. **Be careful,** as the steam will be hot.

> **!** *The safe internal temperature for cooked fish is 62,8°C/145°F, or until the fish is opaque and flakes easily with a fork. When cooking fish, cook it until the center reaches 62,8°C/145°F on an instant-read or meat thermometer.*

Nutrition Facts	
Per serving: 320 kcal	31 grams carbohydrates
34 grams protein	4 grams fiber
6 grams total fat	High in folate, phosphorus, magnesium, selenium, potassium, thiamin, niacin, and vitamins A, C, B6, and B12
1.5 grams saturated fat	

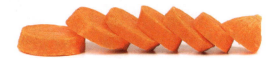

Polenta Crusted Fish Fillets

PREPARATION 15 MINS	COOKING 10-15 MINS	SERVES 5 (SERVING SIZE 208 GRAMS, 7.3 OZ)

INGREDIENTS

- 1 kilo/2.2 pounds sustainable fish fillets
- ½ cup (120 grams) **lactose-free low-fat** Greek yogurt
- ¾ cup (100 grams) finely ground polenta (cornmeal)
- 2 teaspoons (4.6 grams) sweet paprika
- 2 teaspoons (1.6 grams) finely chopped fresh thyme
- ¼ teaspoon (0.5 grams) ground black pepper
- 3 tablespoons (45 ml) olive oil
- ½ teaspoon (3 grams) salt

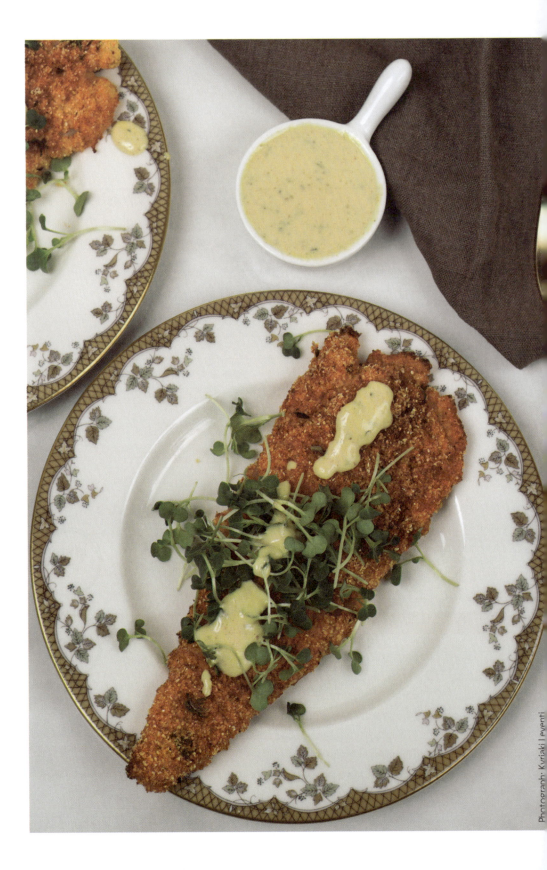

INSTRUCTIONS

Preheat oven to 246°C/475°F.

Line with a sheet of parchment paper and coat with olive oil.

Brush the fish with yogurt.

Combine the polenta, salt, pepper, paprika and the finely chopped thyme.

Coat the fish with the polenta mixture.

Drizzle with olive oil.

Bake for 10-15 minutes or until crisp and golden.

Sprinkle with salt and pepper.

Cooking time depends on the thickness of the fish.

> ❗ *The safe internal temperature for cooked fish is 62,8°C/145°F, or until the fish is opaque and flakes easily with a fork. When cooking fish, cook it until the center reaches 62,8°C/145°F on an instant-read or meat thermometer.*

Nutrition Facts	
Per serving: 310 kcal	12 grams carbohydrates
40 grams protein	2 grams fiber
11 grams total fat	High in potassium, niacin, phosphorus, selenium, and vitamins B6 and B12
2.5 grams saturated fat	

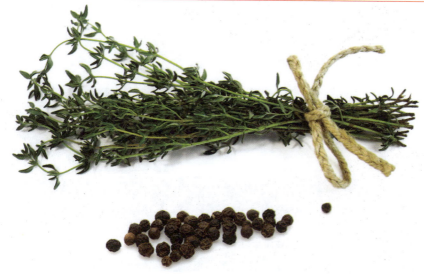

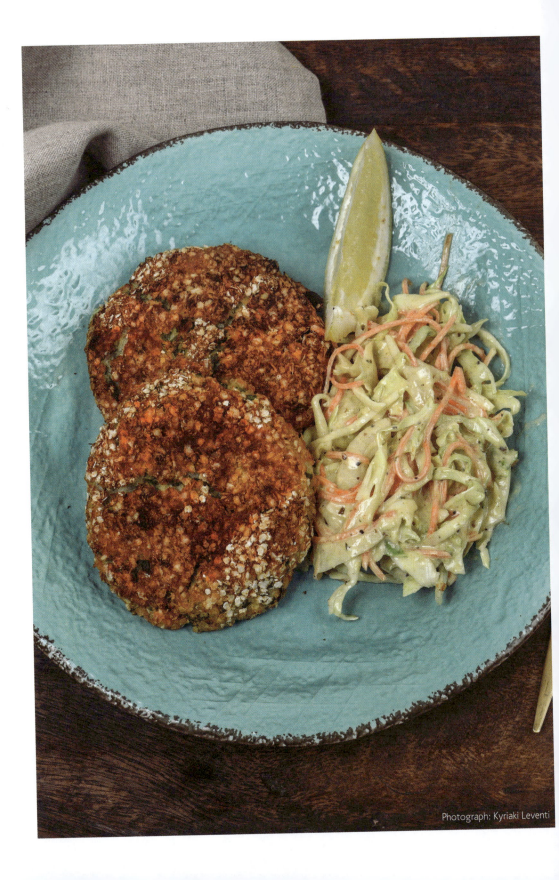

Photograph: Kyriaki Leventi

Fish cakes

Served with coleslaw page 344

PREPARATION 10 MINS	COOKING 45 MINS	WAITING TIME 20 MINS	SERVES 4 (SERVING SIZE 217 GRAMS, 7.6 OZ)

INGREDIENTS

- 2 medium potatoes (300 grams), cut into cubes
- 400 grams/0.9 pounds sustainable white fish fillet
- 2 bay leaves
- 1 organic lime, finely zested
- 1 cup (50 grams) spring onions (the green part only), finely sliced
- 1 cup (60 grams) finely sliced chives
- Olive oil, for drizzle
- 1 pastured egg
- ½ cup (50 grams) quinoa flakes
- 1 teaspoon (2.3 grams) paprika

INSTRUCTIONS

Boil the potatoes until soft.

Lay the fish fillet and bay leaves in a saucepan.

Cover the fish with water.

Cover, bring to a boil, then lower the heat and simmer for 4 minutes.

Take the pan off the heat and leave the fish to stand for 5 minutes.

Drain the potatoes and mash them.

Season the mash with salt and pepper.

Drain the fish in a colander and break it into large chunks.

Add the fish to the mash potatoes and stir the lime zest, spring onions and chives.

Let the mixture sit in the refrigerator for 20 minutes.

Line a baking tin with parchment paper and coat it with olive oil.

Beat the egg in a shallow bowl.

Mix the quinoa flakes with the paprika in another shallow bowl.

Dip the fishcakes into the egg, coating well.

Allow any excess egg to drip off.

Place the fish cake in the quinoa flakes, turning it and pressing firmly to get an even coating on all sides.

Preheat the oven to 220°C/428°F.

Drizzle with olive oil and bake the fish cakes on a baking tray for 15 to 20 minutes until crisp and golden brown.

Nutrition Facts	
Per serving: 200 kcal	21 grams carbohydrates
23 grams protein	3 grams fiber
2.5 grams total fat	High in phosphorus, magnesium, manganese, selenium, and vitamins A, C, K, and B6
0.5 grams saturated fat	

Polenta Crusted Oven Baked Calamari

PREPARATION 15 MINS	COOKING 10-15 MINS	SERVES 3 (SERVING SIZE 236 GRAMS, 8.3 OZ)

INGREDIENTS

- 453 grams/1 pound calamari rings
- ¼ cup (45 grams) potato flour
- 1 teaspoon (6 grams) salt
- 2 pastured eggs
- 1 teaspoon (5 ml) water
- ¾ cup (100 grams) finely ground polenta (cornmeal)
- ¼ cup (25 grams) quinoa flakes
- 1 teaspoon (2.3 grams) paprika
- 1 teaspoon (1 gram) finely chopped fresh thyme
- Freshly ground pepper

INSTRUCTIONS

Preheat oven to 246°C/475°F.

Line with a sheet of parchment paper and coat with olive oil.

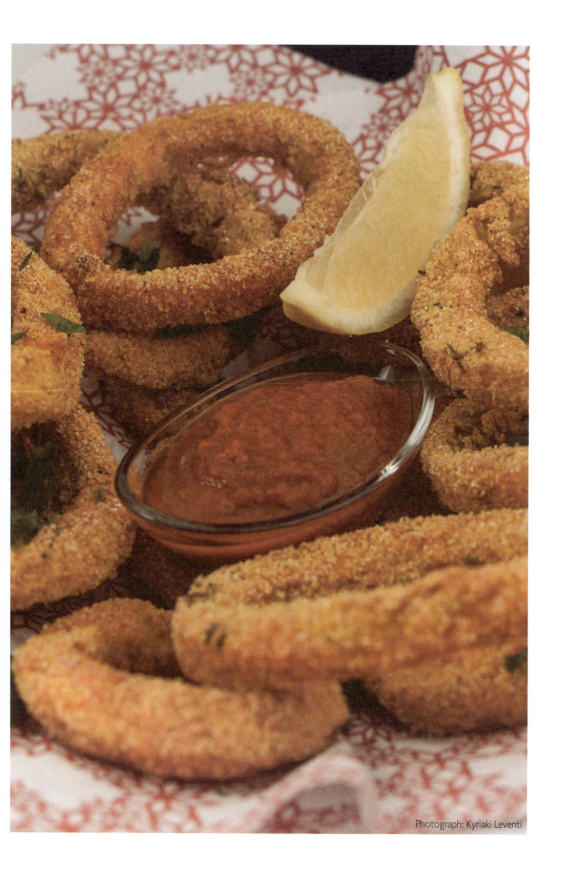

Combine the potato flour with ½ teaspoon salt and pepper in a flat dish.

Beat the eggs with the water.

In another flat dish, **combine** the polenta, ½ teaspoon salt, paprika and thyme.

Working in batches, dip the calamari in the flour mixture.

Shake off any excess flour.

Dip calamari into the egg and then coat them in the polenta mixture.

Shake off any excess polenta mixture.

Drizzle with olive oil.

Bake for 10-15 minutes or until nicely golden.

Sprinkle with salt and pepper.

Served with lemon juice.

To cook the calamari safely, cook until the flesh is pearly and opaque.

Nutrition Facts	
Per serving: 370 kcal	45 grams carbohydrates
32 grams protein	6 grams fiber
7 grams total fat	High in riboflavin, niacin, phosphorus, zinc, copper, vitamin B12, and selenium
1.5 grams saturated fat	

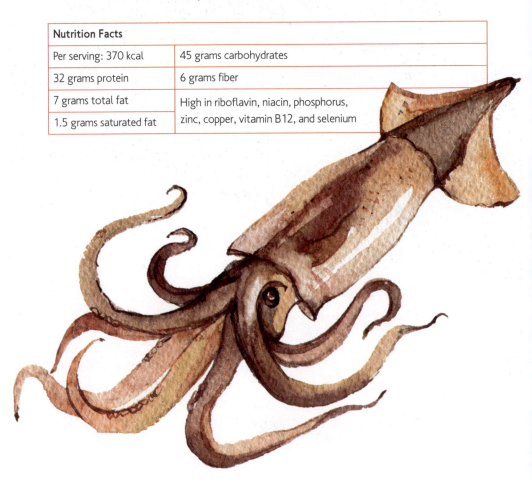

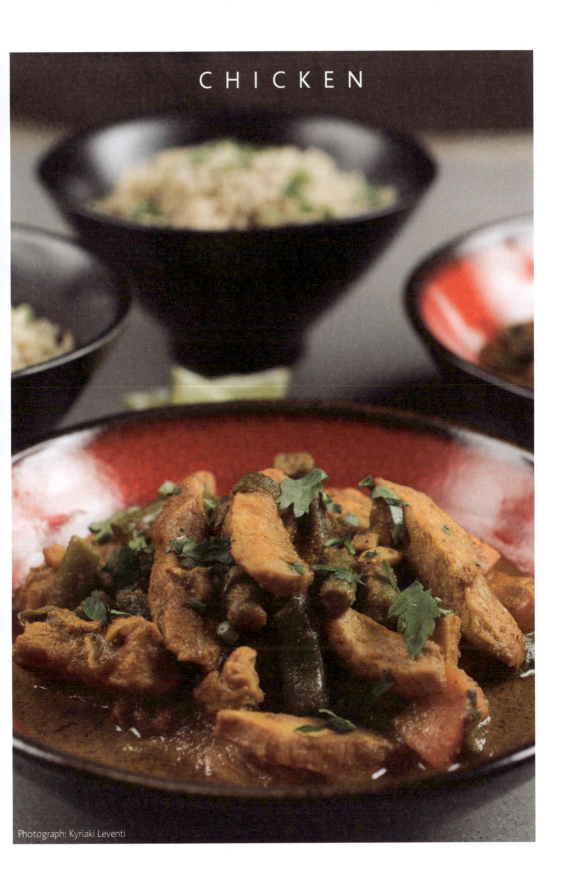

CHICKEN

Chicken Curry

PREPARATION 20 MINS	COOKING 35 MINS	SERVES 6 (SERVING SIZE 421 GRAMS, 14.9 OZ)

INGREDIENTS

Curry mix

- 3 tablespoons (14.5 grams) coriander powder
- 2 tablespoons (12 grams) cumin powder
- The seeds only from ½ teaspoon (1 gram) cardamom
- 1 teaspoon (2 grams) cloves powder
- ½ teaspoon (1 gram) cinnamon powder
- ½ teaspoon (1 gram) freshly ground black pepper
- 1 teaspoon (1.8 grams) cayenne powder
- 2 tablespoons (2.2 grams) turmeric powder
- 1 teaspoon (2 grams) dry mustard powder
- ½ teaspoon (1 gram) ginger powder

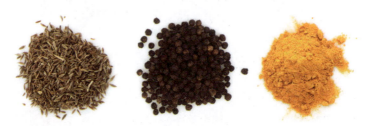

Chicken curry

- 1 kilo/2.2 pounds chicken breast cut into small pieces (approximately 2.5 cm/1 inch long and 1 cm/0.4 inch thick)
- 2 cups (224 grams) green beans cut into approximately 2 cm/0.8 inch long pieces
- 2 medium (90 grams) size green chilis, deseeded and chopped into small pieces
- 4 tablespoons (24 grams) finely chopped fresh ginger
- 5 spring onions, green parts only, chopped into 1 cm/0.4 inch long pieces
- 6 carrots (300 grams) cut in half lengthwise and then chopped into 2 cm/0.8 inch thick pieces
- 3 tomatoes (350 grams), cut into small cubes

- 2 tablespoons (30 ml) sesame oil
- 3 tablespoons (45 ml) of extra-virgin olive oil
- 15 curry leaves
- 400 ml (13.5 fluid ounces) light coconut milk (long life from a can)
- All of the low FODMAP curry mix from above

INSTRUCTIONS

Step 1: Curry mix
Mix all the ingredients for the curry.

Step 2: Chicken curry
Heat a nonstick pan well and brown the chicken on all sides. Set aside the chicken and its juices in a bowl.

Sauté fresh ginger, the green parts of spring onions and the chilis in the same nonstick pan in 2 tablespoons extra-virgin olive oil and 2 tablespoons sesame seed oil for a few minutes on high heat.

Add the beans and stir for 2-3 minutes.

Add the tomatoes and carrots and reduce the heat to medium.

Cover the pot and cook until all the juices are absorbed, stirring occasionally. This process will take 5-10 minutes.

Cook 1 tablespoon olive oil and the low FODMAP curry mix over medium heat in another large nonstick pan, stirring for 2-3 minutes until the spices turn brown.

Add the vegetables, the chicken with its juices, the curry leaves and the coconut milk to the pan. **Let it** all simmer until the chicken is cooked through (approximately 15 minutes). Stir occasionally.

Nutrition Facts	
Per serving: 480 kcal	17 grams carbohydrates
38 grams protein	6 grams fiber
31 grams total fat	High in iron, riboflavin, pantothenic acid, selenium, manganese, vitamins A, C, K, and B6
15 grams saturated fat	

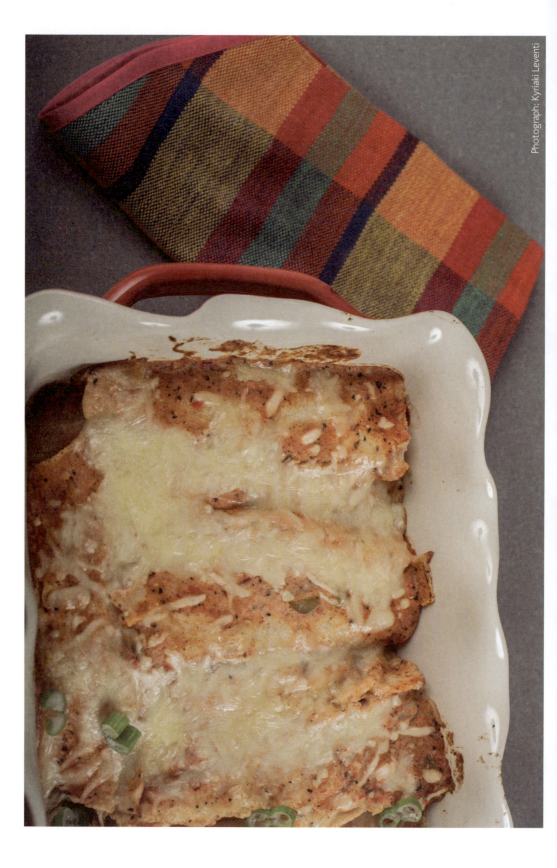

Chicken Enchiladas

PREPARATION 30 MINS	COOKING 1 HOUR 30 MINS	SERVES 4 (SERVING SIZE 2 ENCHILADAS)

INGREDIENTS

- 400 grams/14.1 oz skinless chicken breast
- 150 grams/5.9 oz bell peppers (½ green and ½ red bell pepper), chopped
- 2 bay leaves
- ½ teaspoon (1 gram) cumin
- Sprig of cilantro
- Salt and pepper to taste
- 3 small (330 grams) common tomatoes
- 1 medium-sized chili pepper
- 4 tablespoons (60 ml) extra-virgin olive oil
- ½ cup (120 grams) low-fat **lactose-free** yogurt
- ½ cup (60 grams) grated mozzarella cheese
- 8 corn tortillas

Based on the Monash FODMAP app, the low FODMAP serving size for corn tortillas with no gums or fiber added is 57 grams.

INSTRUCTIONS

Step 1: Chicken

Place the chicken in a deep pot and cover with water.

Add the cumin, bay leaves, sprig of cilantro and salt and pepper to the pot and bring to a boil. Boil at high heat for approximately 45 minutes until the chicken is cooked.

Remove the chicken and allow it to cool before shredding.

Step 2: Tomato sauce

While the chicken is boiling, **roast** the tomatoes and chili pepper on a grill or use the grill setting on your oven until charred (approximately 10 minutes).

Blend the tomatoes and pepper until smooth.

Heat 2 tablespoons olive oil in a large pan and sauté the tomato mixture for 10 minutes. Add salt to taste and remove from heat.

Add the yogurt to the tomato mixture once it has cooled and stir until it is incorporated.

Step 3: Peppers

Heat 2 tablespoons of olive oil in a pot and sauté the chopped peppers until soft.

Step 4: Enchiladas

Preheat the oven to 180°C/356°F.

Coat the bottom of a baking dish with 4 tablespoons of the tomato sauce. Make sure the baking dish fits 8 rolled corn tortillas.

Dip each one of the corn tortillas in the tomato sauce. They should be lightly covered.

Add 2 tablespoons of chicken and 1 teaspoon of the pepper mixture to each tortilla.

Roll the tortillas and place them in the baking dish.

Pour the remaining tomato sauce over the 8 rolled tortillas and sprinkle with cheese.

Cover with foil and bake in the oven for 20 minutes.

Nutrition Facts	
Per serving: 500 kcal	31 grams carbohydrates
31 grams protein	5 grams fiber
28 grams total fat	High in niacin, phosphorus, selenium, manganese, and vitamin A, C, K, and B6
7 grams saturated fat	

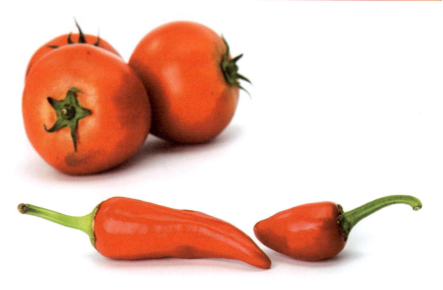

Polenta Crusted Chicken Tenders

PREPARATION 10 MINS	COOKING 20-25 MINS	SERVES 3 (SERVING SIZE 203 GRAMS, 7.2 OZ)

INGREDIENTS

- 453 grams/1 pound chicken tenderloins
- ½ cup (90 grams) potato flour
- 1 pastured egg
- 1 teaspoon (5 ml) water
- ½ cup (60 grams) finely ground polenta (cornmeal)
- 2 teaspoons (4.6 grams) paprika
- Salt and pepper to taste
- Olive oil

INSTRUCTIONS

Preheat oven to 218°C/425°F.

Line with a sheet of parchment paper and coat with olive oil.

Lay 3 bowls in a row.

Add the potato flour with 1 teaspoon of paprika, salt and pepper in the first bowl.

Beat the egg with water in the second bowl.

Add the polenta with 1 teaspoon paprika and salt and pepper in the third bowl.

Working in batches, dip the chicken tenderloins in the flour mixture.

Shake off any excess flour.

Dip them into the egg and then coat them in the polenta mixture.

Shake off any excess polenta mixture.

Place coated tenders on prepared baking sheets.

Drizzle with olive oil.

Bake for 20-25 minutes, turning once until crisp and golden.

Sprinkle with salt and pepper.

Serve immediately.

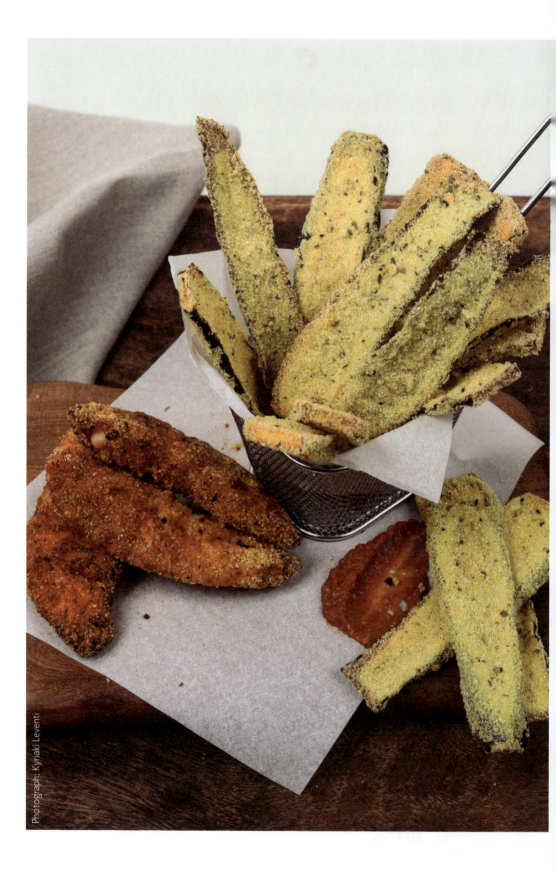

> **!** *The chicken is cooked when there is no pink in the center of chicken breast or the internal temperature is 75°C/165°F. The meat or instant-read thermometer should be inserted into the center of breast.*

Nutrition Facts	
Per serving: 340 kcal	39 grams carbohydrates
36 grams protein	4 grams fiber
6 grams total fat	High in niacin, vitamin B6, pantothenic acid, phosphorus, and selenium
1 gram saturated fat	

Stuffed Chicken

PREPARATION 30 MINS	COOKING 2 HOURS AND 40 MINS	SERVES 5

INGREDIENTS

Chicken
- 2 kilos/4.4 pounds chicken

For aromatic oil
- 3 tablespoons (45 ml) olive oil
- 1 tablespoon (15 grams) mustard
- 1 tablespoon (15 ml) 100% pure maple syrup
- 10 sprigs thyme (only the leaves)

For filling

- 1 ½ cup (75 grams) spring onions (the green part only)
- 2 tablespoons (30 ml) olive oil
- ½ cup (70 grams) chestnuts, boiled
- ¼ cup (33 grams) pine nuts, toasted
- 100 grams/3.5 oz chicken livers
- ¼ cup (60 ml) white wine
- 1 cup (180 grams) cooked quinoa (⅓ cup (60 grams) dry quinoa) (see recipe)
- 2 tablespoons (20 grams) raisins
- ½ cup (120 ml) water
- Grated zest of 1 organic orange
- Salt and pepper
- 1 tablespoon (1.6 grams) dill, finely chopped

INSTRUCTIONS

Step 1: For filling

Heat a deep pan over medium heat.

Add the olive oil and the spring onions.

Sauté for a few minutes.

Chop the chestnuts into small pieces and add them to the pan.

Chop the chicken livers into large pieces and add them to the pan.

Stir and sauté for 4-5 minutes until golden.

Add the wine and cook until all the juices evaporate.

Add the quinoa and raisins and stir to combine.

Season well with salt and pepper.

Add the water and the orange zest and cook until the juice is boiled.

Remove from heat and add the dill.

Add the toasted pine nuts.

Stir and **set** aside until needed.

Step 2: For the aromatic oil

Mix all the ingredients well.

Step 3: For the chicken

Preheat the oven to 190°C/374°F.

Wear disposable gloves.

Pull the chicken skin away from the flesh very carefully
    to avoid tearing the skin.

Rub the aromatic oil over the flesh.

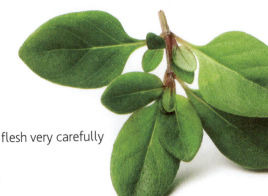

Spread the aromatic oil all over chicken.

Fill the chicken with the stuffing.

Tie the chicken legs together with kitchen twine.

Cover with parchment paper and aluminum foil and bake for 2 hours.

Remove the parchment and aluminum foil and bake for another 30 minutes until golden.

Let the chicken rest before cutting.

Use an instant-read thermometer inserted into the thickest part of the thigh (but not touching the bone) to check if the chicken is done.

 The safe internal temperature for cooked chicken is 75°C/165°F.

Nutrition Facts	
Per serving: 650 kcal	25 grams carbohydrates
45 grams protein	3 grams fiber
42 grams total fat	High in copper, selenium, iron, riboflavin, folate, manganese and vitamins A, C, K, B6, and B12
8 grams saturated fat	

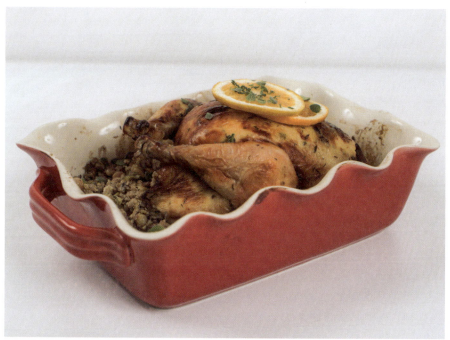

Photograph: Kyriaki Leventi

L A M B

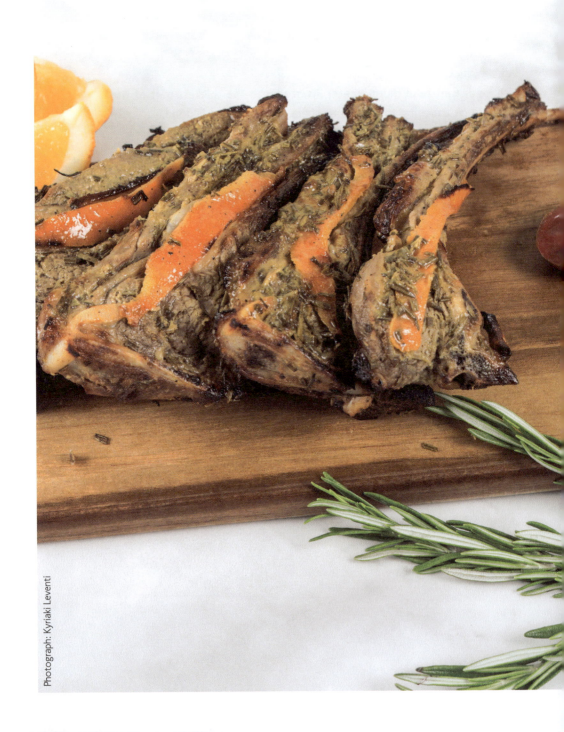

Photograph: Kyriaki Leventi

Lean Lamb Chops with Orange Sauce

PREPARATION 10 MINS	COOKING 15 MINS	MARINADE 3-4 HOURS	SERVES 4 (SERVING SIZE 2 SMALL LAMB CHOPS)

INGREDIENTS

- Juice of 4 oranges
- 8 strips of organic orange zest (use a vegetable peeler; avoid the white part of the orange)
- 4 tablespoons (8 grams) chopped fresh rosemary
- 8 lean lamb chops approximately, ½ inch thick (100 grams each with bone)
- 1 teaspoon (5 ml) extra-virgin olive oil
- 2 teaspoons (10 ml) 100% pure maple syrup
- ½ teaspoon (1 gram) freshly crushed black pepper
- ½ teaspoon (3 grams) salt

INSTRUCTIONS

Mix the orange juice, orange zest strips, rosemary, olive oil, and pepper to taste.

Trim all excess fat from lamb chops.

Spoon orange juice mixture over chops; cover and refrigerate 3-4 hours.

Coat a large skillet with olive oil.

Heat the skillet on medium-high heat.

Remove the chops from the marinade.

Reserve the marinade.

Cook the lamb for 3 minutes on each side or until cooked to medium.

Remove the chops to a plate to rest.

Add the marinade back to the pan and let it **bubble** and reduce until sticky (approximately 8 minutes).

Add maple syrup and stir until well combined.

Return lamb chops to skillet to cover with the sauce.

Serve with oven roasted rosemary potatoes and vegetables.

> **!** *The safe temperature for lamb chops recommended by USDA is an internal temperature of 62,8°C/145°F (medium rare), followed by 3 minutes of rest time.*

Nutrition Facts	
Per serving: 260 kcal	12 grams carbohydrates
29 grams protein	0 grams fiber
10 grams total fat	High in phosphorus, niacin, thiamin, riboflavin, and vitamins C and B12
4 grams saturated fat	

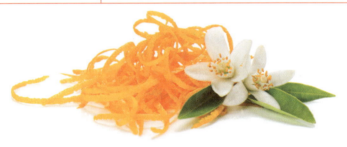

Lamb and Potato Stew

PREPARATION 15 MINS	COOKING 90 MINS	MARINADE 3-4 HOURS	SERVES 6 (SERVING SIZE 273 GRAMS, 9.6 OZ)

INGREDIENTS

- 600 grams/1.3 pounds leg of lamb chopped in large chunks of approximately 3 cm/1.2 inches
- 4 tablespoons (60 ml) of extra-virgin olive oil
- 6 spring onions (green parts only)
- ¾ teaspoon (1.5 grams) ground cinnamon
- ¾ teaspoon (1.5 grams) black pepper
- ¾ teaspoon (1.5 grams) cumin
- 2 ¼ cups (400 grams) fresh tomatoes chopped
- 3 small-sized peeled potatoes (400 grams/14.1 oz), cut into cubes
- 1 tablespoon (2 grams) fresh or dry basil

- ½ cup (12 grams) chopped parsley
- ½ cup (12 grams) chopped cilantro
- Juice of ½ lemon
- Salt
- 28 grams/1 oz pine nuts (to serve)

INSTRUCTIONS

Heat 2 tablespoons extra-virgin olive oil in a large casserole over high heat and sauté the lamb chunks until they are brown on all sides. It will take approximately 5 minutes.

Transfer the lamb to a bowl and reduce the heat to medium. In the same olive oil, sauté the chopped green parts of the spring onions until soft.

Return the lamb back to the casserole and add all the spices (cinnamon, pepper, cumin) and the fresh or dry basil. Finally, add the fresh chopped tomatoes.

Cook over low heat for one hour, until the lamb is soft.

Heat the remaining 2 tablespoons extra-virgin olive oil in a different pan over high heat and sauté the chopped potatoes until they turn brown (approximately 5 minutes). Once ready, put them aside.

When the lamb is ready, **add** the potatoes, the juice of half a lemon and salt to the stew. Cover and cook over low heat for an additional 15 minutes.

When ready, **remove** from the heat and add the fresh parsley and cilantro, mixing until the leaves are incorporated in the stew.

Add pine nuts to serve.

Nutrition Facts	
Per serving: 430 kcal	18 grams carbohydrates
20 grams protein	2 grams fiber
31 grams total fat	High in phosphorous, iron, niacin, zinc, selenium, and vitamins A, C, K, B6, and B12
11 grams saturated fat	

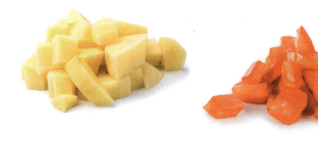

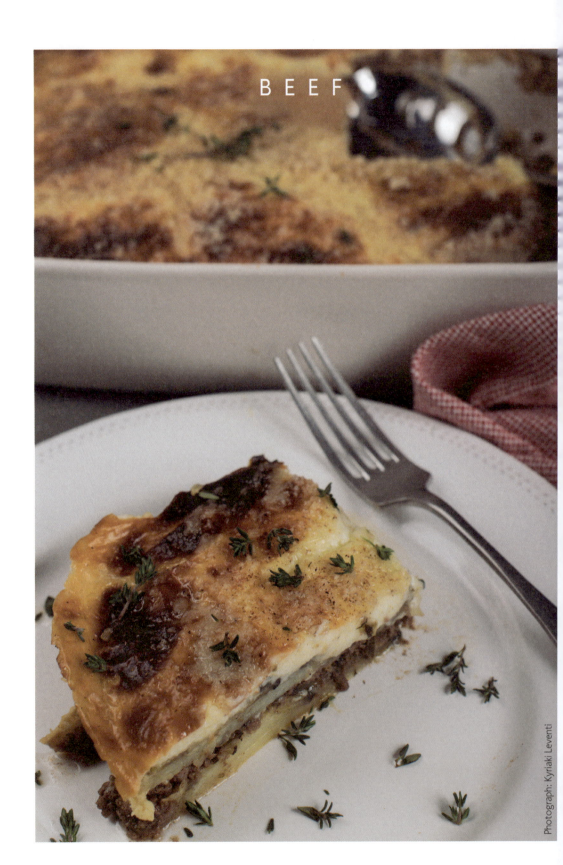

BEEF

Gluten-Free Moussaka

PREPARATION 20 MINS	COOKING 120 MINS	SERVES 8 (SERVING SIZE 490 GRAMS, 17.3 OZ)

INGREDIENTS

For the meat sauce

- 500 grams/17.6 oz lean ground meat of your choice (beef, lamb, chicken, pork, turkey)
- 2 medium tomatoes (220 grams) fresh crushed tomatoes, to puree
- 1 cup (50 grams) spring onions, finely chopped (the green parts only)
- 1 cup (50 grams) leeks, finely chopped (the green parts only)
- 4 fresh bay leaves
- ½ cup (120 ml) white wine
- 1 teaspoon (2 grams) ground cinnamon
- 1 teaspoon (2 grams) ground cloves
- ½ teaspoon (1 gram) freshly grated black pepper
- 3 cups (72 grams) of parsley, finely chopped
- ½ teaspoon (3 grams) salt

For the béchamel sauce

- 1 liter **lactose-free**, low-fat milk
- ¾ cup (120 grams) potato starch
- 4 tablespoons (60 ml) extra-virgin olive oil
- 2 pastured eggs
- 1 teaspoon (2 grams) nutmeg
- 1 teaspoon (6 grams) salt
- Pepper to taste

Vegetables

- ½ cup olive oil, for brushing the vegetables
- 8 medium (1200 grams) potatoes
- 1 large (550 grams) eggplant
- 1 cup (100 grams) Parmesan
- Salt and pepper

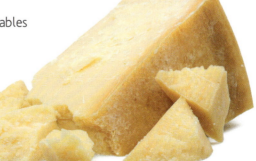

INSTRUCTIONS

Step 1: Cook the meat sauce

Place a pan over medium heat.

Add the ground meat and cook for few minutes until all the meat juice evaporates.

Add the spring onions and leeks and cook for a few minutes more.

Add the freshly made tomato puree and cook until the juice evaporates.

Add the bay leaves.

Add the wine and let the alcohol evaporate.

Add the freshly ground black pepper, nutmeg and cinnamon.

Add finely chopped parsley and **remove** from heat.

Discard the bay leaves and set aside until needed.

Step 2: Béchamel sauce

Heat the olive oil in a pot over medium heat.

Add the potato starch.

Stir continuously with a hand whisk and sauté the potato starch.

Scrape down the sides of any excess potato starch.

Remove from heat.

Add the milk a drizzle at a time, whisking continuously so that no lumps form in the mixture.

Put the pot back on the stove and heat the mixture, continuing to stir until the sauce becomes smooth and creamy.

Avoid boiling. Potato starch can lose its thickening power if brought to a boil for too long. Make sure to monitor the heat and simmer the sauce at no more than 80°C/176°F.

Remove from heat and add salt, pepper and nutmeg.

Beat the two eggs well with a hand whisker and add them to the béchamel, continuing to whisk hard and fast to incorporate.

Set aside until needed.

Step 3: Bake the vegetables

Preheat oven to 200°C/390°F.

Peel the potatoes and cut into thin slices (½ cm/0.2 in); coat them with olive oil.

Slice the eggplant thinly to ½ cm/0.2 inches pieces and coat them with olive oil.

Season the vegetables with salt and pepper.

Line 3 pans with parchment paper.

Spread the vegetables in a single layer on a baking sheet.

Bake the potatoes for 30 minutes, and bake the eggplant 20 minutes or until golden.

Step 4: Assembling the moussaka

Preheat the oven to 180°C/356°F.

Brush a baking pan (3 x 9 x 3 inch/33 x 23 x 7 cm) with olive oil.

Taste the vegetables and confirm that they are properly seasoned.

Lay out half of the potato slices into a layer, pressing gently into the pan.

Sprinkle with 3 tablespoons of the Parmesan cheese.

Place half the eggplant slices on top of the potatoes.

Sprinkle with another 3 tablespoons of the Parmesan cheese.

Mix ⅓ **of the** béchamel sauce into the meat sauce and spoon the meat sauce on top of the vegetable.

Lay out one more layer of potato slices.

Sprinkle with 3 tablespoons of the Parmesan cheese.

Place the rest of the eggplant slices on top of the potatoes.

Finish by **topping** with the béchamel and the last 5 tablespoons of Parmesan cheese.

Bake for 30-40 minutes, until the béchamel turns golden brown.

Nutrition Facts	
Per serving: 620 kcal	58 grams carbohydrates
31 grams protein	5 grams fiber
30 grams total fat	High in iron, riboflavin, niacin, phosphorus, magnesium, zinc, manganese, selenium, and vitamins A, E, C, K, B6, and B12
8 grams saturated fat	

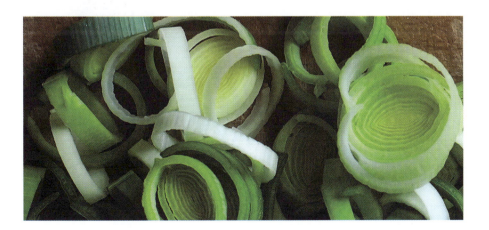

Gluten-Free Pastitsio Greek Baked Pasta

PREPARATION 20 MINS	COOKING 80 MINS	SERVES 8 (SERVING SIZE 390 GRAMS, 14.1 OZ)

INGREDIENTS

For the meat sauce

- 500 grams/17.6 oz lean ground meat of your choice (beef, lamb, pork, chicken, turkey)
- 2 medium tomatoes (220 grams) crushed fresh tomatoes, to puree
- 1 cup (50 grams) spring onions, finely chopped (the green parts only)
- 1 cup (50 grams) leeks, finely chopped (the green parts only)
- 4 fresh bay leaves
- ½ cup white wine (120 ml)
- 1 teaspoon (2 grams) ground cinnamon
- 1 teaspoon (2 grams) ground cloves
- ½ teaspoon (1 gram) freshly grated black pepper
- 3 cups (72 grams) of parsley, finely chopped

For the béchamel sauce

- 1 liter **lactose-free** milk (4.2 cups)
- 120 grams/4.2 oz potato starch
- ¼ cup (60 ml) olive oil
- 2 pastured eggs
- ½ teaspoon (1 gram) nutmeg
- 2 teaspoons (12 grams) salt
- Pepper to taste

For the pasta

- 400 grams/17.6 oz **gluten-free low FODMAP** long ziti pasta **(preferably 100% quinoa pasta)**
- 100 grams/3.5 oz low-fat cheese, grated (kasseri or Parmesan)

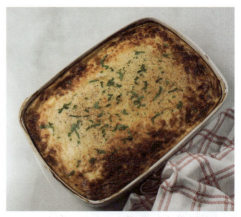

Photograph: Kyriaki Leventi

INSTRUCTIONS

Step 1: Meat sauce

Place a pan over medium heat.

Add the ground meat and cook for a few minutes until all the meat juice has evaporated.

Add the spring onions and leeks and cook for a few minutes more.

Add the freshly made tomato puree and cook until the juice evaporates.

Add the bay leaves.

Add the wine and let the alcohol evaporate.

Add the freshly ground black pepper, cloves and cinnamon.

Add finely chopped parsley and **remove** from heat.

Discard the bay leaves and set aside until needed.

Step 2: Béchamel sauce

Heat the olive oil in a pot over medium heat.

Add the potato starch.

Stir continuously with a hand whisk and sauté the potato starch.

Scrape down the sides of any excess potato starch. **Remove** from heat.

Add the milk a drizzle at a time, whisking continuously so that no lumps form in the mixture.

Put the pot back on the stove and heat the mixture, continuing to stir until the sauce becomes smooth and creamy.

Avoid boiling. Potato starch can lose its thickening power if brought to a boil for too long. Make sure to monitor the heat and **simmer the sauce** no more than **80°C/176°F**.

Remove from heat and add salt, pepper and nutmeg.

Beat the two eggs well with a hand whisker and add them to the béchamel, continuing to whisk hard and fast to incorporate.

Set aside until needed.

Step 3: Pasta

Boil the pasta in salted water for 2 minutes less than the time noted on the instructions on the box.

Drain the pasta.

Mix with the cheese (leave some cheese to sprinkle on top of the pastitsio).

Step 4: Assemble

Preheat oven to **180°C/356°F**.

Brush a baking pan (3 x 9 x 3 inch/33 x 23 x 7 cm) with olive oil.

Mix the meat sauce with one-third of the béchamel sauce.

Spread the pasta in the baking pan.

Add the meat sauce.

Finish with the béchamel sauce and sprinkle some cheese on top.

Bake for 30-40 minutes or until the béchamel turns golden brown.

Nutrition Facts	
Per serving: 430 kcal	52 grams carbohydrates
20 grams protein	4 grams fiber
16 grams total fat	High in calcium, riboflavin, phosphorus, magnesium, selenium, zinc, and vitamins A, C, K, and B12
6 grams saturated fat	

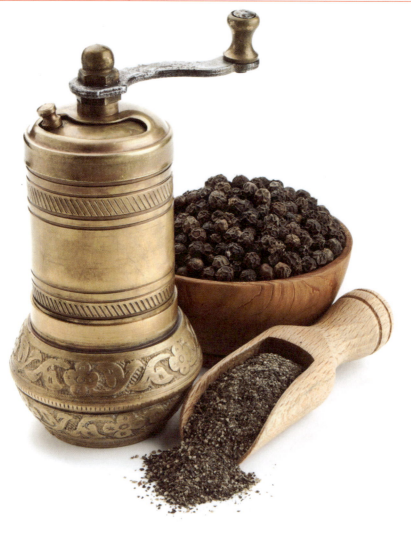

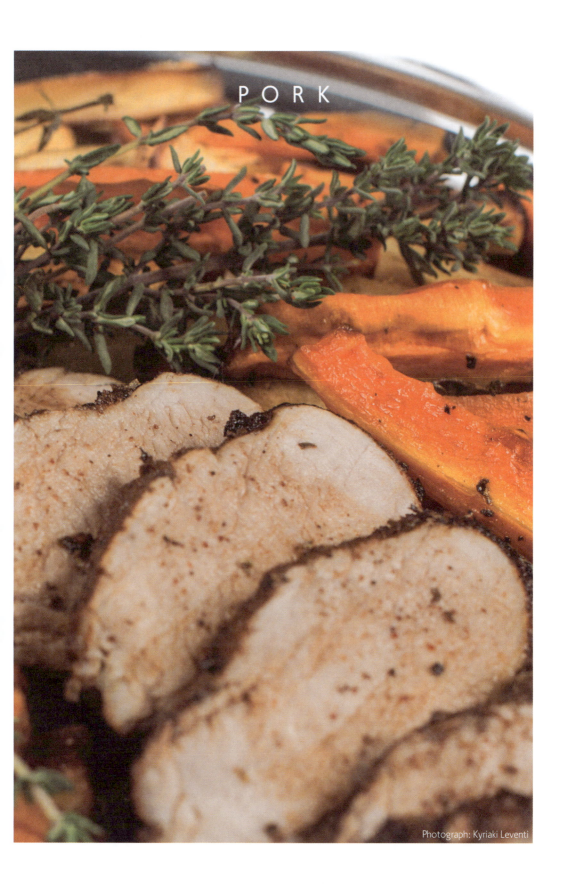

PORK

Photograph: Kyriaki Leventi

Pork Tenderloins with Paprika and Cocoa Rub

PREPARATION 10 MINS	COOKING 25 MINS	SERVES 5 (SERVING SIZE 150 GRAMS, 5.3 OZ)

gluten free

phase diet 2

INGREDIENTS

- 2 pork tenderloins (1 kilo/2.2 pounds)
- 2 tablespoons (30 ml) olive oil

For the dry rub

- 1 tablespoon (12.5 grams) brown raw sugar
- 1 tablespoon (5 grams) dry oregano
- 1 tablespoon (7 grams) sweet paprika
- 1 tablespoon (18 grams) salt
- 2 teaspoons (4 grams) unsweetened cocoa powder
- 1 teaspoon (2 grams) freshly ground black pepper
- 1 teaspoon (2 grams) cumin
- 1 teaspoon (2 grams) mustard seeds
- 1 teaspoon (1.6 grams) thyme
- 1 teaspoon (1.3 grams) chili pepper flakes (use only if tolerated)

INSTRUCTIONS

Preheat the oven to 180°C/356°F.

Mix all the ingredients for the dry rub either by hand or with a spice grinder. A spice grinder is recommended so that all the ingredients are mixed properly.

Apply the dry rub on the pork tenderloin by patting it down. The pork tenderloins should be covered completely.

Heat the 2-3 tablespoons of olive oil in an oven-proof pan at medium-high heat on the stovetop.

Once the oil is hot enough, **sear** the pork tenderloins on all sides and transfer the pan to the oven.

Roast for 20-22 minutes, depending on the thickness of the pork tenderloins.

Remove from the oven and let them rest for 15-20 minutes before slicing.

> **!** *The safe temperature for pork recommended by USDA is an internal temperature of 62,8°C/145°F. Cook pork to 62,8°C/145°F, which is medium rare, followed by 3 minutes of rest time for tender and juicy pork..*

Nutrition Facts	
Per serving: 190 kcal	2 grams carbohydrates
29 grams protein	0 grams fiber
7 grams total fat	High in phosphorus, thiamin, riboflavin, niacin, vitamin B6, and selenium
1.5 grams saturated fat	

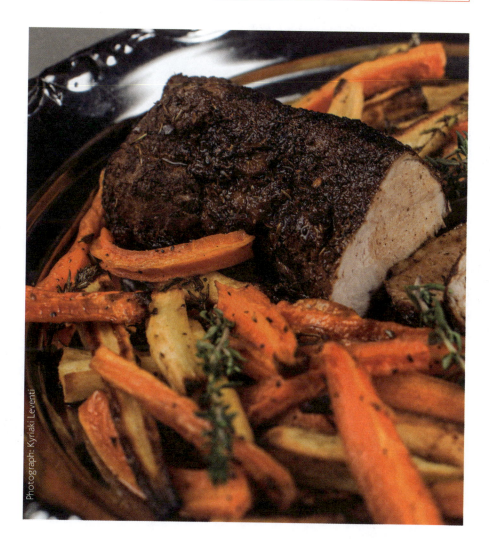

Photograph: Kyriaki Leventi

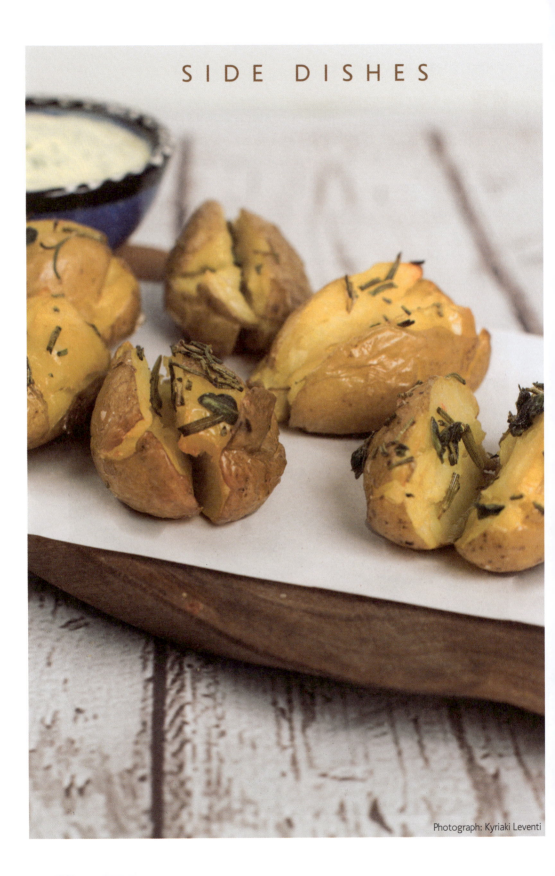

Photograph: Kyriaki Leventi

Oven Roasted Baby Potatoes with Herbs

PREPARATION 5 MINS	COOKING 45 MINS	SERVES 4 (4 SMALL POTATOES)

INGREDIENTS

- 16 small (400 grams) baby potatoes
- 3 tablespoons (45 ml) olive oil
- 2 sprigs of rosemary finely chopped
- 2 sprigs of thyme
- 2 sprigs of oregano

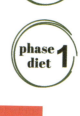

INSTRUCTIONS

Boil the potatoes for 15 minutes until soft.

Let them cool.

Use a knife to make a crisscross slit on top of each potato.

Squeeze them with your fingers to break them open.

Preheat the oven to 205°C/400°F.

Place them in a roasting pan.

Brush them well with olive oil.

Add the herbs on top of and in between the potatoes.

Season with salt and pepper.

Roast in the oven for 30 minutes.

Nutrition Facts	
Per serving: 190 kcal	21 grams carbohydrates
3 grams protein	2 grams fiber
10 grams total fat	High in vitamin B6
1.5 grams saturated fat	

How to Roast Vegetables

Use a sheet pan for roasting your vegetables.

Cut veggies into the same size.

Give your vegetables space.

Cut them into a ½-inch dice or ½-inch-thick slices, or, for starchy vegetables like potatoes, dice them into pieces (1 ½ inch–2inches), but when possible, roast smaller vegetables whole.

Coat vegetables with olive oil and herbs (use two tablespoons of olive oil per sheet pan of veggies).

Roast vegetables with a few sprigs of fresh rosemary, oregano, or thyme (or use a teaspoon dried).

Season your vegetables well.

Sprinkle with grated Parmesan 15 minutes before roasting is completed.

Toss the vegetables thoroughly by using a spatula every 10 minutes or so until they are tender with a nice color.

Roasting time depends on the vegetable; if vegetables with different roasting times are mixed, then slow-roasting vegetables, such as potatoes, carrots, and parsnip, should be cut into smaller pieces.

Toss your vegetables with fresh herbs after roasting.

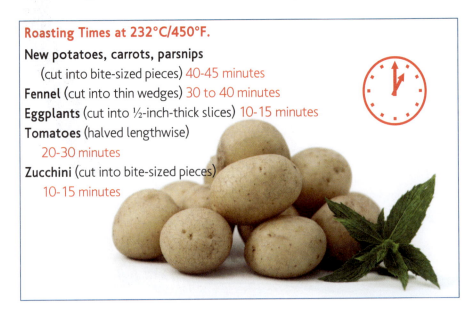

Roasting Times at 232°C/450°F.

New potatoes, carrots, parsnips
  (cut into bite-sized pieces) 40-45 minutes
Fennel (cut into thin wedges) 30 to 40 minutes
Eggplants (cut into ½-inch-thick slices) 10-15 minutes
Tomatoes (halved lengthwise)
  20-30 minutes
Zucchini (cut into bite-sized pieces)
  10-15 minutes

Carrot and Parsnip Puree

PREPARATION 10 MINS	COOKING 30 MINS	SERVES 6 (SERVING SIZE: 122 GRAMS, 4.3 OZ)

INGREDIENTS

- 1 pound (453 grams) carrots, peeled and cut into cubes
- 1 pound parsnips (453 grams), peeled and cut into cubes
- Low FODMAP vegetable stock **(page 362)** or water
- 1 tablespoon (8 grams) peeled fresh ginger
- 2 tablespoons (30 ml) of extra-virgin olive oil
- 1 teaspoon (5 ml) 100% pure maple syrup
- Salt
- Chopped chives, for garnish

INSTRUCTIONS

Add carrots, parsnips and ginger to a large pan.

Add enough low FODMAP stock or water to cover and bring to boil.

Adjust salt.

Simmer until the vegetables are tender (approximately 30 minutes).

Drain the vegetables but reserve 1 cup of liquid.

Blend the vegetables and liquid in a blender until smooth.

Add the olive oil, maple syrup and salt if needed.

Add more liquid if needed for a thinner pure.

Garnish with chives.

Nutrition Facts	
Per serving: 100 kcal	15 grams carbohydrates
1 gram of protein	3 grams fiber
4.5 grams total fat	High in manganese and vitamins C and K
0.5 grams saturated fat	

Roasted Root Vegetables

PREPARATION 5 MINS	COOKING 45 MINS	SERVES 4 (SERVING SIZE: 140 GRAMS, 4.9 OZ)

INGREDIENTS

- Three medium parsnips (225 grams), cut into pieces lengthwise
- 4 medium carrots (240 grams), cut into pieces lengthwise
- 3 tablespoons (45 ml) olive oil
- 1 tablespoon (15 ml) 100% pure maple syrup
- 3 small sprigs of fresh thyme
- Salt to taste
- Freshly ground black pepper to taste

INSTRUCTIONS

Preheat oven to 180°C/356°F.

Toss all the ingredients together make sure that the vegetables are coated with olive oil and maple syrup.

Roast on a baking tray for 45 minutes.

Nutrition Facts	
Per serving: 170 kcal	20 grams carbohydrates
1 gram of protein	4 grams fiber
11 grams total fat	High in manganese and vitamins A, C, and K
1.5 grams saturated fat	

Zucchini Oven Fries

PREPARATION 20 MINS	COOKING 20-30 MINS	SERVES 10 (SERVING SIZE: 86 GRAMS, 3 OZ)

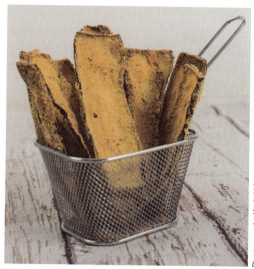

INGREDIENTS

- 4.5 medium (590 grams) zucchinis sliced lengthwise and not very thin (approximately 6 slices per zucchini)
- 2 pastured eggs (beaten)
- ¼ cup (60 ml) **lactose-free** milk
- 1 cup (120 grams) polenta (medium or coarsely ground cornmeal)
- 1 teaspoon (1.6 grams) dry oregano
- 1 teaspoon (2.3 grams) paprika

INSTRUCTIONS

Preheat the oven to 180°C/356°F.

Beat the eggs.

Add ¼ cup lactose-free milk to the eggs and mix with the polenta. Add salt, pepper, oregano and paprika and mix.

Dip each zucchini slice in the egg wash.

Coat with the polenta mixture.

Lay the zucchini slices on parchment paper and bake in the oven until golden and crispy.

Nutrition Facts
Per serving: 70 kcal
3 grams protein
1.5 grams total fat
11 grams carbohydrates
2 grams fiber
High in vitamin C

Photograph: Kyriaki Leventi

Coleslaw

PREPARATION 5 MINS	COOKING 0 MINS	SERVES 4 (SERVING SIZE: 1 CUP 128 GRAMS, 4.5 OZ)

INGREDIENTS

- 2 cups (200 grams) shredded cabbage
- 2 cups (200 grams) shredded carrot
- 2 tablespoons (30 grams) **lactose-free** yogurt
- 2 tablespoons (30 ml) extra-virgin olive oil
- 2 tablespoons (30 grams) yellow mustard
- 1 tablespoon (15 ml) 100% pure maple syrup
- ½ teaspoon (0.8 grams) dry oregano
- 1 teaspoon (5 ml) naturally aged balsamic vinegar
- ½ teaspoon (1 gram) cumin
- Salt and pepper to taste

INSTRUCTIONS

Mix all the ingredients (besides the shredded cabbage and carrot) together and whisk until they are well mixed.

Add the shredded cabbage and carrot and toss until they are well coated (see photo page 308).

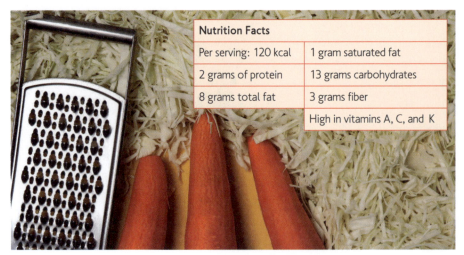

Nutrition Facts	
Per serving: 120 kcal	1 gram saturated fat
2 grams of protein	13 grams carbohydrates
8 grams total fat	3 grams fiber
	High in vitamins A, C, and K

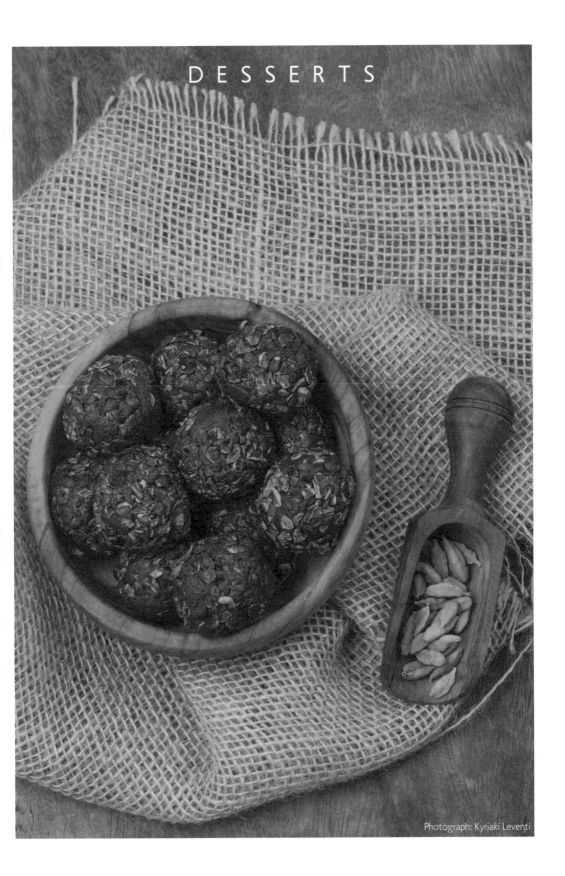

DESSERTS

Photograph: Kyriaki Leventi

Vegan Dark Chocolate Truffles

PREPARATION 30 MINS	COOKING 3 MINS	WAITING TIME OVERNIGHT	SERVES 40 (SERVING SIZE: 16 GRAMS, 0.6 OZ)

INGREDIENTS

- 400 grams/4 oz good-quality dark chocolate (70-85% cocoa solids)
- 200 grams/7 oz of almond milk (**see recipe page 171**)
- ½ teaspoon (2.5 ml) pure vanilla extract
- Cocoa nibs or cocoa for coating

Optional
- 1 tablespoon (15 ml) flavored orange liqueur
- 2 teaspoons orange zest

INSTRUCTIONS

Truffle mixture

Chop the chocolate very finely with a food processor or with a sharp knife.

Transfer the chocolate in a heatproof mixing bowl.

Warm the almond milk in a saucepan over medium heat until it reaches the boiling point.

Pour the almond milk over the chocolate and stir with a wire whisk until the chocolate is completely melted.

Stir in the vanilla (and the liqueur and zest if using).

Set aside to cool and chill overnight.

To shape the truffles

Spoon round balls of the mixture.

Roll the truffles between your hands to make it round.

Place them onto a large plate lined with parchment paper.

Refrigerate for two hours to set, if needed.

Roll the truffles between your hands to shape.

Roll in cocoa powder or cocoa nibs.

Keep refrigerated for up to 2 weeks.

Serve at room temperature.

Nutrition Facts		
Per serving: 70 kcal	4.5 grams total fat	6 grams carbohydrates
3 grams of protein	2.5 grams saturated fat	1 gram fiber

Buckwheat Brownie Cake

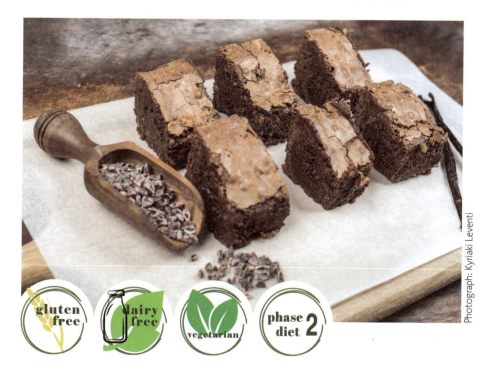

Photograph: Kyriaki Leventi

gluten free · dairy free · vegetarian · phase diet 2

PREPARATION 15 MINS	COOKING 30 MINS	SERVES 20 (SERVING SIZE: 40 GRAMS, 1.4 OZ)

INGREDIENTS

- 120 grams/4.2 oz buckwheat flour
- 300 grams/10.6 oz good-quality dark chocolate chips (70- 85% cacao solids)
- 160 grams/5.6 oz extra-virgin olive oil
- 4 pastured eggs
- 120 grams/4.2 oz raw sugar

INSTRUCTIONS

Preheat the oven to 160°C/320°F.

Coat a 23 x 13 x 8 cm (9 x 5 x 3 inch) loaf pan with olive oil.

Melt the chocolate in a heatproof bowl over a saucepan of simmering water.

Add the olive oil and mix.

Beat the eggs with a handheld mixer and add the sugar until the mixture becomes white and fluffy.

Mix in with the chocolate.

Add the sieved buckwheat flour slowly into the chocolate mixture and mix carefully. Do not overmix.

Pour the cake mix into the loaf pan and bake for 30 minutes.

Rotate the pan of brownies halfway through.

Be careful not to overbake.

The brownie is done when the edges of the brownie appear to be baked through and a toothpick inserted into the center of the brownie has a few moist crumbs but no wet batter sticking onto it after it comes out.

Nutrition Facts	
Per serving: 200 kcal	4.5 grams saturated fat
3 grams of protein	16 grams carbohydrates
14 grams total fat	2 grams fiber

Gluten-Free Vegan Banana Cake

PREPARATION 10 MINS	COOKING 50-60 MINS	SERVES 20 (SERVING SIZE: 60 GRAMS, 2.1 OZ)

INGREDIENTS

- 4 medium sugar bananas ripe (475 grams), mashed **(safe low FODMAP serving size 56 grams)**
- 2 tablespoons (21 grams) ground flaxseed
- ⅓ cup (80 ml) almond milk **(see recipe for nondairy milks page 171 or use unsweetened almond milk)**
- ⅓ cup (80 ml) olive oil
- 2 tablespoons (30 ml) 100% pure maple syrup
- 1 tablespoon (15 ml) pure vanilla extract
- 10 tablespoons (125 grams) of raw sugar

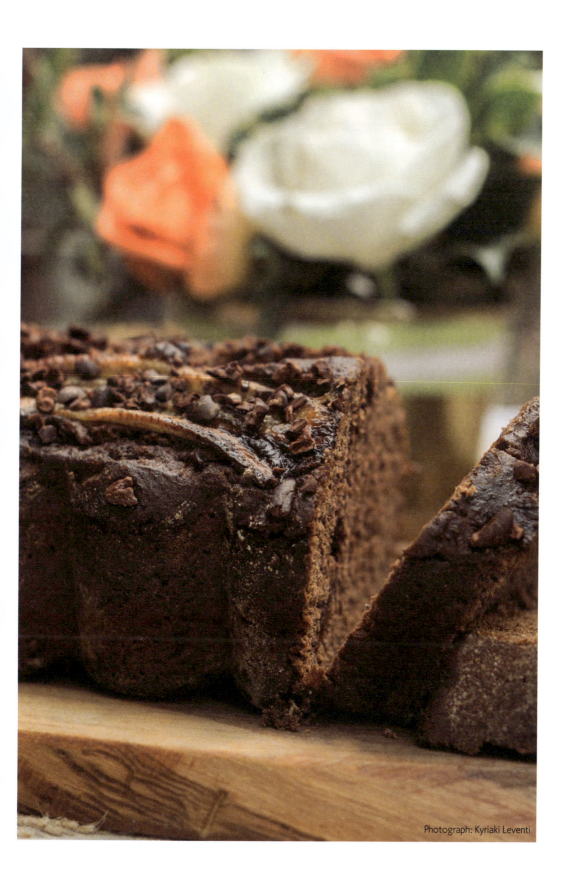

- 1 cup (112 grams) quinoa flour
- 1 teaspoon (4,6 grams) baking soda
- ½ teaspoon (2,4 grams) **gluten-free** baking powder
- ½ teaspoon (3 grams) salt
- 1 cup (135 grams) buckwheat flour
- 1 cup (165 grams) dark chocolate chips (70-85% cocoa solids)
- 2 tablespoons (12 grams) of raw cocoa

Cocoa nibs and banana for decoration

INSTRUCTIONS

Preheat the oven to 180°C/356°F.

Coat a 23 x 13 x 8 cm (9 x 5 x 3 inch) loaf pan lightly with olive oil.

Mash the bananas in a large bowl and mix it with all the wet ingredients (milk, oil, vanilla and maple syrup).

Stir until well combined.

Add the dry ingredients (flour, ground flaxseeds, sugar, quinoa flour, baking powder, baking soda and salt) one at a time until well combined.

Fold in the chocolate chips.

Decorate the cake with cocoa nibs and sliced banana.

Bake until golden and a toothpick or knife inserted into the center comes out clean (approximately 50-60 minutes).

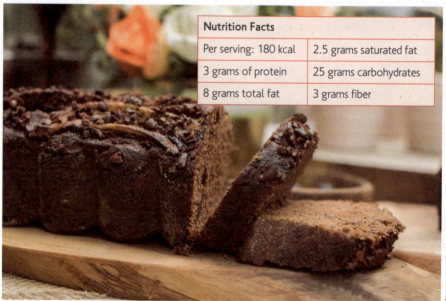

Nutrition Facts	
Per serving: 180 kcal	2.5 grams saturated fat
3 grams of protein	25 grams carbohydrates
8 grams total fat	3 grams fiber

Photograph: Kyriaki Leventi

Passion Fruit Pudding

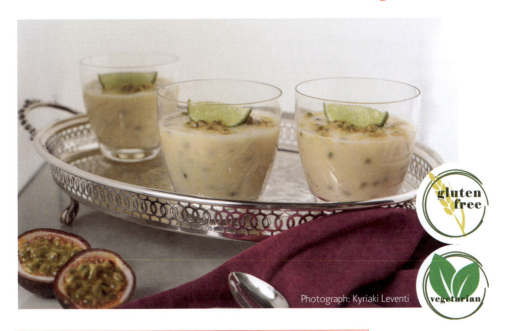

Photograph: Kyriaki Leventi

PREPARATION 2 MINS	COOKING 5-10 MINS	REFRIGERATE UNTIL IT SETS 1-2 HOURS	SERVES 6 (SERVING SIZE: 142 GRAMS, 5 OZ)

INGREDIENTS

- 2 cups (480 ml) of almond milk (**page 171**) or **lactose-free** low-fat milk
- 6 tablespoons (90 ml) maple syrup
- 2 tablespoon (30 ml) water
- 140 grams/4.9 oz fresh passion fruit pulp (6 passion fruits)
- 2 egg whites
- 3 tablespoons (30 grams) potato starch
- 1 teaspoon (5 ml) pure vanilla extract

INSTRUCTIONS

Heat the almond milk with passion fruit pulp gently to a simmer and stir in the maple syrup.

Mix the potato starch with 2 tablespoons water and the egg whites.

Pour ⅓ of the warm milk to the potato starch mixture, whisking constantly.

Pour the potato starch mixture back into the milk while whisking constantly over heat.

Add vanilla and stir until thickened.

Pour in a large bowl.

Refrigerate 1-2 hours until set.

Remove from the refrigerator and beat until smooth.

Arrange in individual bowls.

Nutrition Facts	
Per serving: 130 kcal	0 grams saturated fat
2 grams of protein	30 grams carbohydrates
1 gram total fat	3 grams fiber

Olive Oil Chocolate Polenta Cake

PREPARATION 10 MINS	COOKING 40 MINS	SERVES 20 (SERVING SIZE: 40 GRAMS, 1.4 OZ)

INGREDIENTS

- ½ cup plus 2 tablespoons (125 grams/4.4 oz) olive oil
- 225 grams/7.9 oz good-quality dark chocolate chips (70- 85% cacao solids)
- 5 pastured eggs
- ½ cup plus 2 tablespoons (120 grams/4.2 oz) raw sugar
- ½ cup plus 2 tablespoons (100 grams/3.5 oz) polenta (ground cornmeal)
- 25 ml Cognac or Bourbon
- 1 tablespoon (6 grams) organic orange zest
- 1 teaspoon (5 ml) pure vanilla extract

INSTRUCTIONS

Use a 35 cm/10 inch springform, deep-sided cake tin (avoid using a tin with lots of ridges because the cake tends to stick. Make sure you coat pan with olive oil and polenta well).

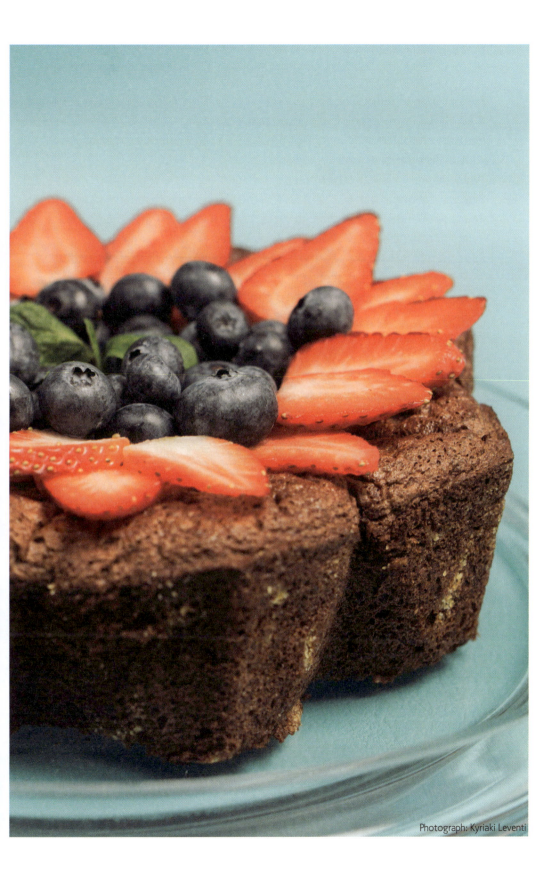

Photograph: Kyriaki Leventi

Preheat oven to 180°C/356°F.

Coat pan well with olive oil and polenta.

Melt the chocolate in a heatproof bowl over a saucepan of simmering water. Add the olive oil and mix.

Whisk the egg yolks with 60 grams sugar and slowly add to the chocolate oil mixture.

Beat the egg whites with 60 grams sugar with a handheld mixer until stiff peaks form.

Pour the polenta, cognac, vanilla extract and orange zest into the chocolate mixture and then slowly fold in the egg whites. Do not overmix.

Pour the mix into a cake pan and bake for approximately 30 minutes, until the knife comes out clean when inserted into the cake.

Remove from the oven and allow to cool (note: the cake will sink as it cools down).

You can garnish the cake with powdered sugar and fruit.

Nutrition Facts	
Per serving: 180 kcal	4 grams saturated fat
3 grams of protein	15 grams carbohydrates
12 grams total fat	2 grams fiber

Chocolate Mousse

PREPARATION 2 MINS	COOKING 10 MINS	REFRIGERATE UNTIL IT SETS 2-4 HOURS	SERVES 12 (SERVING SIZE: 100 GRAMS, 3.5 OZ)

INGREDIENTS

- 300 grams/10.6 oz good-quality dark chocolate (70- 85% cacao solids)
- 900 grams/1.9 pounds almond milk **(see recipe page 171)**
- 2 teaspoons (10 ml) orange liqueur (optional)

INSTRUCTIONS

Pour the almond milk into a small saucepan over medium-low heat and heat for a few minutes (needs to be hot).

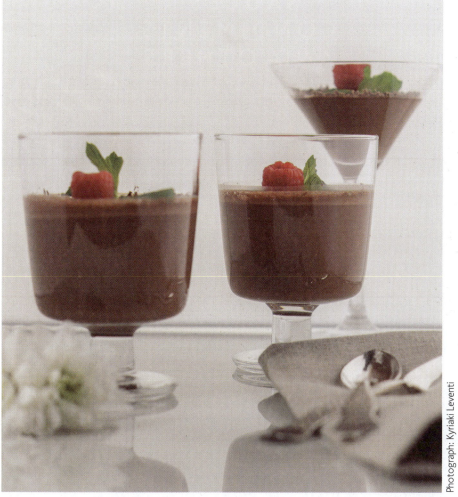

Photograph: Kyriaki Leventi

Finely chop the chocolate and place in a bowl.

Pour hot milk over the chocolate.

Wait 1 minute and stir gently to distribute the chocolate through the milk.

Add the liqueur and stir to combine.

Refrigerate until set, 2-4 hours.

Nutrition Facts	
Per serving: 180 kcal	6 grams saturated fat
2 grams of protein	16 grams carbohydrates
11 grams total fat	3 grams fiber

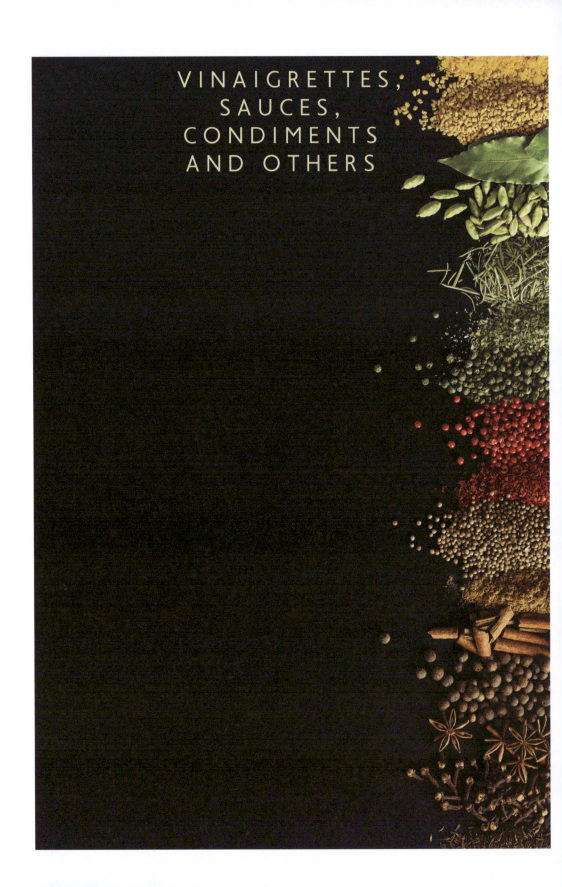

VINAIGRETTES; SAUCES, CONDIMENTS AND OTHERS

Balsamic Vinaigrette

PREPARATION 5 MINS	COOKING 0 MINS	SERVES 14 (SERVING SIZE: 1 TABLESPOON, 15 ml)

INGREDIENTS

- 1 cup (240 ml) extra-virgin olive oil
- ½ cup (120 ml) balsamic vinegar
- 1 ½ tablespoon (22 grams) Dijon mustard
- ½ tablespoon (1.5 grams) finely chopped fresh oregano
- ½ tablespoon (1.5 grams) finely chopped fresh thyme
- Pinch of salt to taste
- Freshly ground black pepper

INSTRUCTIONS

Blend all ingredients together until smooth or whisk all ingredients together until well combined.

Nutrition Facts	
Per serving: 140 kcal	2 grams saturated fat
0 grams of protein	1 gram carbohydrates
15 grams total fat	0 grams fiber

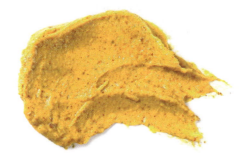

Low FODMAP tzatziki

PREPARATION 5 MINS	COOKING 0 MINS	SERVES 4 (SERVING SIZE: 116, 6 GRAMS, 4.1 OZ)

INGREDIENTS

- 1 medium (200 grams) cucumber, peeled, seeded and finely chopped
- 1 cup (227 grams) low-fat **lactose-free** Greek yogurt
- Small bunch mint, finely chopped
- 1 teaspoon (5 ml) garlic olive oil (**see recipe page 363**)
- A pinch of salt
- Juice of ½ lemon

INSTRUCTIONS

Combine all the ingredients.
Chill until ready to serve.

Nutrition Facts	
Per serving: 50 kcal	0 grams saturated fat
6 grams of protein	4 grams carbohydrates
1.5 grams total fat	1 gram fiber

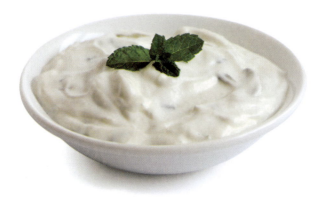

Low FODMAP Raita

PREPARATION 5 MINS	COOKING 1 MIN	SERVES 14 (SERVING SIZE: 2 TABLESPOONS, 30 GRAMS)

INGREDIENTS

- 2 teaspoons (10 ml) garlic olive oil (**see recipe page 363**)
- ½ teaspoon (1 gram) cumin seeds
- ½ teaspoon (1 gram) mustard seeds
- 1 medium (200 grams) cucumber
- 1 cup (240 grams**) lactose-free** Greek yogurt
- 1 tablespoon (15 ml) lime juice
- ⅓ cup (8 grams) finely chopped cilantro
- ½ teaspoon (1.2 grams) paprika

INSTRUCTIONS

Heat a dry saucepan over a medium heat.

Add cumin and mustard seeds and toast until fragrant.

Let them cool.

Reserve ¼ teaspoon for serving.

Grind them in a food processor or in a spice mill.

Grate cucumbers and squeeze out the excess moisture.

Mix everything together.

Garnish with cilantro leaves, paprika and spices.

Nutrition Facts	
Per serving: 30 kcal	1 gram saturated fat
‹1 gram protein	1 gram carbohydrates
2.5 grams total fat	0 grams fiber

Low FODMAP
Salsa Fresca/Pico de Gallo

PREPARATION 10 MINS	COOKING 0 MINS	SERVES 6 (SERVING SIZE: 146 GRAMS, 5.2 OZ)

INGREDIENTS

- ¾ cup (40 grams) spring onions chopped (green parts only)
- ½ cup (30 grams) chopped cilantro
- 2 cups (700 grams unpeeled) chopped tomatoes
  (use ripe but firm vine tomatoes; remove skin and most of the water and seeds before chopping)
- 1-2 finely chopped green chili peppers (only if tolerated)
- Juice of 1 lemon
- Salt and pepper to taste

phase diet 2

Chop all the ingredients and mix them together.
Add lemon, salt and pepper to taste and toss.

Nutrition Facts	
Per serving: 30 kcal	0 grams saturated fat
1 gram protein	7 grams carbohydrates
2.5 grams total fat	2 grams fiber

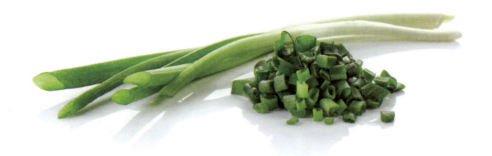

Tahini Orange Sauce

PREPARATION 5 MINS	COOKING 0 MINS	SERVES 11 (SERVING SIZE: 1 TABLESPOON, 15 GRAMS)

INGREDIENTS

- 3 tablespoons (45 ml) orange juice
- 3 tablespoons (45 grams) tahini paste
- 2 tablespoons (30 ml) lime juice
- 1 tablespoon (15 ml) **gluten-free tamari (a variety of naturally fermented soy sauce)**
- 1 tablespoon (15 ml) 100 % pure maple syrup
- 2 teaspoons (4 grams) orange zest
- 2 teaspoons (4 grams) grated ginger
- Salt and pepper to taste

INSTRUCTIONS

Blend all the ingredients together until smooth.

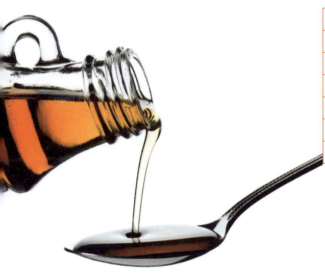

Nutrition Facts
Per serving: 30 kcal
‹1 gram protein
2 grams total fat
0 grams saturated fat
3 grams carbohydrates
0 grams fiber

Low FODMAP Vegetable Stock

PREPARATION 10 MINS	COOKING 55 MINS	12 SERVINGS

INGREDIENTS

- 1 tablespoon (15 ml) olive oil
- 2 cups (100 grams/3.6 oz), leeks (green part only)
- 2 carrots (330 grams/11.6 oz)
- 1 cup spring onions (50 grams/1.8 oz) (green part only)
- 10 sprigs fresh parsley
- 10 sprigs fresh thyme
- 2 bay leaves
- 1 teaspoon of salt
- 2 liters of water

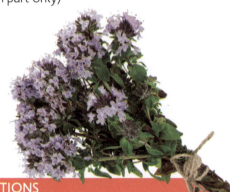

INSTRUCTIONS

Chop vegetables into small chunks.

Heat oil in a large pot.

Add the vegetables and herbs and cook over high heat for 5 to 10 minutes, stirring frequently.

Add salt and water and bring to a boil. Lower heat.

Simmer, uncovered, for 45 minutes.

Strain and discard vegetables.

How to Pan-Fry Haloumi Cheese

Slice the haloumi into ½-inch slices.

Add the haloumi to a hot frying pan.

Cook the first side for a minute or two until the haloumi begins to release some liquid.

Do not turn; wait until the liquid has evaporated and the haloumi has become golden brown.

Flip the haloumi and brown the other side.

BASIC RECIPES

Garlic Oil

PREPARATION	COOKING
2 MINS	35 MINS

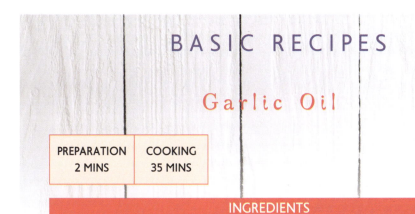

INGREDIENTS

- 10 to 12 cloves of garlic
- 2 cups (480 ml) of extra-virgin olive oil

INSTRUCTIONS

Peel the skin off the garlic cloves.
(Keep the garlic cloves whole; avoid rinsing or soaking the garlic in water.)
Place the garlic cloves and the oil into a small pot.
Heat the oil and garlic over low to medium heat until the oil bubbles gently.
(The temperature should be approximately 93°C/200°F.)
The garlic should not be frying; if it is, remove it from the heat for some time.
Continue to heat the oil for 30 minutes for a stronger garlic taste.
Adjust the time according to preference.
Remove and discard garlic with a strainer.
Store the oil in a glass jar for up to 2 weeks.
Do not keep the oil for a longer period of time to avoid botulism
   or salmonella contamination.

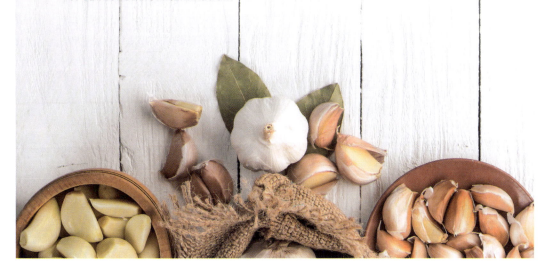

How to Cook Quinoa

1 part uncooked quinoa
(it will yield 3-3½ parts cooked quinoa)

Measure the quinoa and put it in a large bowl.

Cover the quinoa with fresh water.

Let it soak for a few minutes.

Stir the quinoa for a few minutes with a wire whisk until you see a soapy residue (saponin), which is responsible for the bitter flavor of quinoa.

Pour the quinoa into a fine mesh colander.

Rinse the quinoa well under cold water.

Drain well.

Put into a saucepan and add double the amount of salted water or low FODMAP vegetable stock.

Cover and bring to boil as soon as it starts to boil turn the heat over to a simmer.

Simmer for 10 to 15 minutes, or until tender and the liquid is absorbed.

Turn the heat off, put the lid on and let sit for 5 minutes.

Fluff with a fork and serve.

How to Cook Buckwheat and Millet

1 part uncooked buckwheat/millet
(it will yield 3-3½ parts cooked buckwheat/millet)

Toast buckwheat/millet for 4-5 minutes in a large, dry pan until golden brown.

Add double the amount of salted water or low FODMAP vegetable stock.

Bring to a boil; then lower the heat and simmer until almost all the liquid is absorbed (approximately 15 minutes).

Remove from heat and let it sit for a few minutes covered until all the liquid is absorbed.

Fluff and serve.

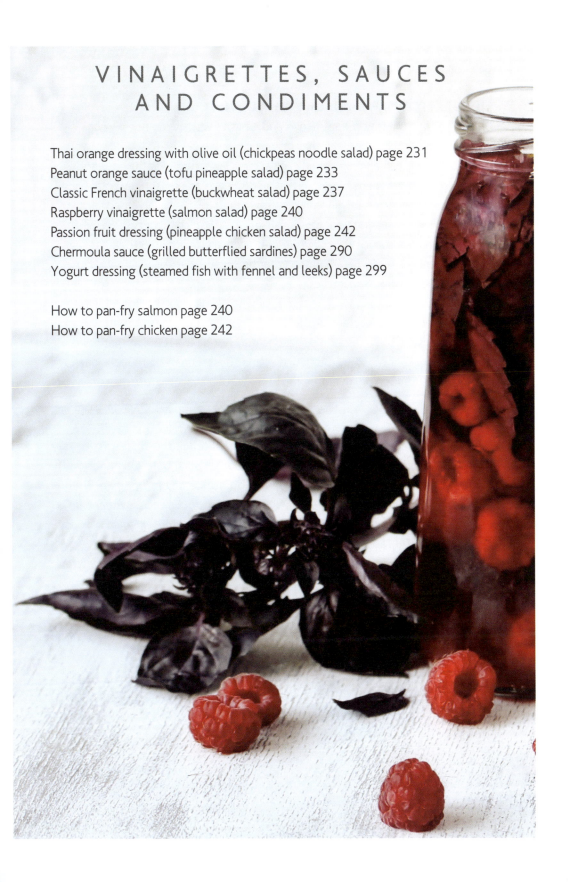

VINAIGRETTES, SAUCES AND CONDIMENTS

If the low FODMAP diet Doesn't Work, Do Not Give Up

If you've tried the low FODMAP diet and it hasn't worked, do not give up. There are several reasons why that may be so, and it is best to work with your gastroenterologist and registered clinical dietitian to look for the answer.

It may be that the cause of your digestive distress is an unidentified underlying organic disease. Alternatively, your distress could be due to increased air swallowing when eating your meals, a habit that would still persist even if you reduced the quantity of FODMAPs you consume. Other factors that might affect the response are gastroenteritis, levels of physical activity and menstruation in women.

More importantly, however, the timing of when you pursue the low FODMAP diet is particularly important. Anxiety and stress can increase gut sensitivity, so tackling symptoms through diet alone may not be adequate at that point. A combination of the low FODMAP diet and stress management techniques (mind-body connection) might be the best approach to symptom management.

The information provided in this book is not intended as a substitute for the advice and care of your healthcare provider. You should always consult your physician or health care provider if you notice any red flags or if you will be making changes to your diet, medication or current treatment. It is recommended that the low FODMAP diet is followed under the guidance and supervision of a registered dietitian. Nutritional needs and tolerances vary for each individual.

References

2015-2020 Dietary Guidelines for Americans.

2017 EPA-FDA Advice about Eating Fish and Shellfish
https: //www.consumerreports.org/cro/magazine/2014/10/can-eating-the-wrong-
fish-put-you-at-higher-risk-for-mercury-exposure/index.htm/

Academy of nutrition and dietetics
https: //www.eatright.org/

American Academy of Allergy, Asthma and Immunology (AAAAI)
https: //www.aaaai.org/

American Botanical Council. Peppermint Oil Capsules Reduce Irritable Bowel
Syndrome Symptoms.

American Cancer Society
https: //www.cancer.org/

An SY, Lee MS, Jeon JY, Ha ES, Kim TH, Yoon JY, Ok CO, Lee HK, Hwang WS,
Choe SJ et al. (2013) Beneficial effects of fresh and fermented kimchi in
prediabetic individuals. *Ann Nutr Metab*; 63: 111-119.

Anderson KE. (2011) Comparison of fatty acid, cholesterol, and vitamin A and
E composition in eggs from hens housed in conventional cage and range
production facilities. *Poult Sci*; 90 (7): 1600-1608.

Barbaro MR, Cremon C, Stanghellini V, Barbara G. (2018) Recent advances in
understanding non-celiac gluten sensitivity. Published online. *F1000Research*;
7: F1000
https: //doi.org/10.12688/f1000research.15849.1

Barrett J. (2017) Dietary Fibre Series - Resistant Starch.
http: //fodmapmonash.blogspot.com/2016/11/dietary-fibre-series-resistant-
starch.html. Updated November 14, 2016. Accessed February 28, 2017

Belkaid Y, Hand TW. (2014) Role of the microbiota in immunity and inflammation. *Cell*; 157: 121–141.

Beth Israel Deaconess Medical Center – Celiac Now

https: //www.bidmc.org/centers-and-departments/digestive-disease-center/
    services-and-programs/celiac-center/celiacnow

Bintsis T. (2018) Lactic Acid Bacteria: Their Applications in Foods. *J Bacteriol Mycol*; 5 (2): 1065.

Blake MR, Raker JM, Whelan K. (2016) Validity and reliability of the Bristol Stool Form Scale in healthy adults and patients with diarrhoea-predominant irritable bowel syndrome. *Aliment Pharmacol Ther.* 44 (7): 693-703.

Borresen EC, Henderson AJ, Kumar A, Weir TL, Ryan EP. (2012) Fermented foods: patented approaches and formulations for nutritional supplementation and health promotion. *Recent Pat Food Nutr Agric*; 4 (2): 134-140.

Bull MJ, Plumer NT. (2014) Part 1: The human gut microbiome in health and disease. *Integr Med (Encinitas)*; 13 (6): 17-22.

Camilleri M. (2014) Advances in understanding of bile acid diarrhea. *Expert Review of Gastroenterology & Hepatology*; 8: 49.

Camilleri M. (2015) Bile Acid Diarrhea: Prevalence, Pathogenesis, and Therapy. *Gut Liver*; 9 (3): 332-339.

Campbell K. Your guide to the difference between fermented foods and probiotics. Gut Microbiota News Watch website.

Celiac Disease Foundation
    https: //celiac.org/

Chassaing B, Koren O, Goodrich JK, Poole AC, Srinivasan S, Ley RE, Gewirtz AT. (2015) Dietary emulsifiers impact the mouse gut microbiota promoting colitis and metabolic syndrome. *Nature*; 5 (519):92-96.

Chen M, Sun Q, Giovannucci E, Mozaffarian D, Manson JE, Willett WC, Hu FB. (2014) Dairy consumption and risk of type 2 diabetes: 3 cohorts of US adults and an updated meta-analysis. *BMC Med*; 12: 215.

Chilton SN, Burton JP, Reid G. (2015) Inclusion of fermented foods in food guides around the world. *Nutrients*; 7 (1): 390-404.

Choi CH, Jo SY, Park HJ, Chang SK, Byeon J-S, Myung S-J. (2011) A randomized, double-blind, placebo-controlled multicenter trial of saccharomyces boulardii in irritable bowel syndrome: effect on quality of life. *J Clin Gastroenterol*; 45 (8): 679–83.

Christopher L, Gentile CL, Weir TL. (2018) The gut microbiota at the intersection of diet and human health. *Science;* 362 (6416): 776-780.

Chumpitazi BP, Cope JL, Hollister EB, Tsai CM, McMeans AR, Luna RA, Versalovic J, Shulman RJ. (2015) Randomised clinical trial: gut microbiome biomarkers are associated with clinical response to a low FODMAP diet in children with the irritable bowel syndrome. *Aliment Pharmacol Ther*; 42 (4): 418-27.

Clinical Guide to Probiotic Supplements Available in the United States and Canada

http: //usprobioticguide.com/

http: //www.probioticchart.ca/

http: //www.worldgastroenterology.org/guidelines/global-guidelines/diet-and-the-gut/diet-and-the-gut-english/

Costantini L, Molinari R, Farinon B, Merendino N. (2017) Impact of Omega-3 Fatty Acids on the Gut Microbiota. *Int J Mol Sci*; 18 (12): 2645.

Cozma-Petruţ A, Loghin F, Miere D, Dumitraşcu DA. (2017) Diet in irritable bowel syndrome: What to recommend, not what to forbid to patients! *World J Gastroenterol*; 23 (21): 3771-3783.

Crohn's and Colitis Foundation

https: //www.crohnscolitisfoundation.org/

Dieli-Crimi R, Cenit MC, Nunez C. (2015) The genetics of celiac disease: a comprehensive review of clinical implications. *J Autoimmun*; 64: 26–41.

Dietitians of Canada (Food Sources of fiber)

https: //www.dietitians.ca/Downloads/Factsheets/Food-Sources-of-Soluble-Fibre.aspx/

Dolezel M et al. (2011). Scrutinizing the current practice of the environmental risk assessment of GM maize applications for cultivation in the EU. *Environmental Sciences Europe*; 23, 33.

Dreher ML. (2018) Whole Fruits and Fruit Fiber Emerging Health Effects. *Nutrients*; 10 (12): 1833.

Drossman DA, McKee DC, Sandler RS, et al. (1988) Psychosocial factors in the irritable bowel syndrome. A multivariate study of patients and nonpatients with irritable bowel syndrome. *Gastroenterology*; 95: 701–708.

Ducrotté P, Sawant P, Jayanthi V. (2012) Clinical trial: Lactobacillus plantarum 299v (DSM 9843) improves symptoms of irritable bowel syndrome. *World J Gastroenterol*; 14;18 (30): 4012–8.

Ducrotté P, Sawant P, Venkataraman J. (2012) Clinical trial: Lactobacillus plantarum *299v* (DSM 9843) improves symptoms of irritable bowel syndrome. *World J Gastroenterol*; 18 (30): 4012–4018.

Dukowicz AC, Lacy BE, Levine GM (2007). Small Intestinal Bacterial Overgrowth (A Comprehensive Review) *Gastroenterol Hepatol*; 3 (2): 112–122.

EFSA (European Food Safety Authority): Scientific Opinion on the substantiation

of health claims related to live yoghurt cultures and improved lactose digestion pursuant to Article 13 (1) of Regulation (EC) No. 1924/2006. *Eur Food
Saf Auth J* 2011.

Emedicine.medscape.com. (2018). Lactose Intolerance: Background, Pathophysiology, Etiology. [online] Available at:
https://emedicine.medscape.com/article/187249-overview#a6 [Accessed 1
Mar. 2018].

Environmental Working Group
http://www.ewg.org/

Eswaran S, Chey WD, Jackson K, Pillai S, Chey SW, Han-Markey T. (2017) A Diet
Low in Fermentable Oligo-, Di-, and Monosaccharides and Polyols Improves
Quality of Life and Reduces Activity Impairment in Patients with Irritable
Bowel Syndrome and Diarrhea. *Clin Gastroenterol Hepatol*; 15 (12): 1890-
1899.

Eswaran S, Muir J, Chey WD. (2013) Fiber and functional gastrointestinal disorders. *Am J Gastroenterol*; 108 (5): 718-727.

Eswaran SL, Chey WD, Han-Markey T, Ball S, Jackson K. (2016) A randomized
controlled trial comparing the low FODMAP diet vs. modified NICE Guidelines in US Adults with IBS-D. *Am J Gastroenterol*; 111: 1824–1832.

European Society of Primary Care Gastroenterology Consensus Guidelines on
Probiotics.

Farmer AD and Oasim A. (2013) Gut pain and visceral hypersensitivity. *Br J Pain*;
7 (1): 39-47.

Fernández M, Hudson JA, Korpela R, de los Reyes-Gavilán CG. (2015) Impact
on human health of microorganisms present in fermented dairy products: an
overview. *Biomed Res Int*; 2015: 412714.

Filippis FD, Pellegrini N, Vannini L, Jeffery IB, Storia A, Laghi L, Serrazanetti
DI, Cagno RD, Ferrocino I, Lazzi C, Turroni S, Cocolin L, Brigidi P, Neviani
E, Gobbetti M, O'Toole PW, Ercolini D. (2016) High-level adherence to a
Mediterranean diet beneficially impacts the gut microbiota and associated
metabolome. *Gut*; 65: 1812–1821.

Filippo Fassio, Maria Sole Facioni and Fabio Guagnini. (2018) Lactose Maldiges-
tion, Malabsorption, and Intolerance: A Comprehensive Review with a Focus
on Current Management and Future Perspectives. *Nutrients*; 10: 1599.

For a Digestive Peace of Mind
https://www.katescarlata.com/

Foran JA, Hites RA, Carpenter DO, Hamilton MC, Mathews-Amos A, Schwager

SJ. (2004) A Survey of Metals in Tissues of Farmed Atlantic and Wild Pacific Salmon. *Environ Toxicol Chem*; 23 (9): 2108-2110.

Ford AC, Talley NJ, Spiegel BMR, Foxx-Orenstein AE, Schiller L, Quigley EMM, et al. (2008) Effect of fibre, antispasmodics, and peppermint oil in the treatment of irritable bowel syndrome: systematic review and meta-analysis. *BMJ*; 337: a2313.

"Free Range' and 'Pasture Raised' officially defined by HFAC for Certified Humane® label", Humane Farm Animal Care (accessed August 19, 2015).

Friesen EN, Ikonomou MG, Higgs DA, Ang KP, Dubetz C. (2008) Use of Terrestial Based Lipids in Aquaculture Feeds and the Effects on Flesh Organohalogen and Fatty Acid Concentrations and Farmed Atlantic Salmon. *Environ Sci Technol*; 42 (10): 3519-3523.

Garcia-Mantrana I, Selma-Royo M, Alcantara C, Collado MC. (2018) Shifts on gut microbiota associated to Mediterranean diet adherence and specific dietary intakes on general adult population. *Front Microbiol*; 9: 890.

Gentile CL, Weir TL. (2018) The gut microbiota at the intersection of diet and human health. *Science*; 362 (6416): 776-780.

Ghoshal UC, Shukla R, Ghoshal U. (2017) Small Intestinal Bacterial Overgrowth and Irritable Bowel Syndrome: A Bridge between Functional Organic Dichotomy. *Gut and Liver*; 11 (2): 196-208.

Gibson GR, Hutkins R, Sanders ME, et al. (2017) Expert consensus document: The International Scientific Association for Probiotics and Prebiotics (ISAPP) consensus statement on the definition and scope of prebiotics. *Nature Reviews Gastroenterology & Hepatology;* 14: 491–502.

Gibson GR, Roberfroid MB. (1995) Dietary modulation of the human colonic microbiota: Introducing the concept of prebiotics. *Journal of Nutrition;* 125 (6): 1401-12.

Gibson PR, Shepherd SJ. (2010) Evidence-based dietary management of functional gastrointestinal symptoms: the FODMAP approach. *J Gastroenterol Hepatol*; 25: 252–258.

Goh KL. (2011) Clinical and epidemiological perspectives of dyspepsia in a multiracial Malaysian population. *J Gastroenterol Hepatol*; 26 (suppl 3): 35–38.

Guglielmetti S, Mora D, Gschwender M, Popp K. (2011) Randomised clinical trial: Bifidobacterium bifidum MIMBb75 significantly alleviates irritable bowel syndrome and improves quality of life - a double blind, placebo-controlled study. *Aliment Pharmacol Ther*; 33 (10): 1123–32.

Hadrich D. (2018). Microbiome research is becoming the key to better understanding health and nutrition. *Front Genet*; 9: 212.

Halmos EP, Power VA, Shepherd SJ, Gibson PR, Muir JG. (2014) A diet low in
FODMAPs reduces symptoms of irritable bowel syndrome. *Gastroenterology;*
146 (1): 67-75.

Hansen M, Thilsted SH, Sandström B, Kongsbak K, Larsen T, Jensen M, Sørensen
SS. (1998) Calcium absorption from small soft-boned fish. *J Trace Elem Med
Biol*; 12 (3): 148-54.

Hayes PA, Fraher MH, Quigley EM. (2014) Irritable bowel syndrome: the role of food
in pathogenesis and management. *Gastroenterol Hepatol (N Y)*; 10 (3): 164-174.

Heiko S,Howard JM. (2005) Yeast metabolic products, yeast antigens and yeasts
as possible triggers for irritable bowel syndrome. *European Journal of Gastroenterology & Hepatology*; 17 (1): 21-26.

Hill C, Guarner F, Reid G, Gibson GR, Merenstein DJ, Pot B, Morelli L, Canani RB,
Flint HJ, Salminen S et al. (2014) Expert consensus document: the International Scientific Association for Probiotics and Prebiotics consensus statement
on the scope and appropriate use of the term probiotic. *Nat Rev Gastroenterol
Hepatol*; 11: 506-514.

Hill P, Muir JG, Gibson PR. (2017) Controversies and Recent Developments of the
Low-FODMAP Diet. *Gastroenterol Hepatol*; 13 (1): 36-45.

Hillilä M, Färkkilä MA, Sipponen T, Rajala J, Koskenpato J. (2015) Does oral
α-galactosidase relieve irritable bowel symptoms? *Scandinavian Journal of
Gastroenterology*; 51: 1, 16-21.

Hites RA, Foran JA, Schwager SJ, Knuth BA, Hamilton MC, Carpenter DO. (2004)
Global Assessment of Polybrominated Diphenyl Ethers in Farmed and Wild
Salmon. *Environ Sci Technol*; 38 (19): 4943-4949.

Ho KY, Kang JY, Seow A. (1998) Prevalence of gastrointestinal symptoms in a
multiracial Asian population, with particular reference to reflux-type symptoms. *Am J Gastroenterol*; 93: 1816–1822.

Hooper B, Spiro A, Stanner S. (2015) 30 g of fibre a day: An achievable recommendation? *Nutrition Bulletin*; 40 (2).

Houghton LA, Whorwell PJ. (2005) Towards a better understanding of abdominal
bloating and distension in functional gastrointestinal disorders. *Neurogastroenterol Motil*; 17: 500–511.

http: //espcg.eu/wpcontent/uploads/2013/

https: //www.kcl.ac.uk/lsm/schools/life-course-sciences/departments/nutritional-
sciences/projects/fodmaps/index/

Hutkins R. Fermented foods. International Scientific Association for Probiotics and Prebiotics website.

Iacovou M. (2017) Adapting the low FODMAP diet to special populations: infants and children. *J Gastroenterol Hepatol*; 32 Suppl 1: 43-45.

Iacovou M, Mulcahy EC, Truby H, Barrett JS, Gibson PR, Muir JG. (2018) Reducing the maternal dietary intake of indigestible and slowly absorbed short-chain carbohydrates is associated with improved infantile colic: a proof-of-concept study. *J Hum Nutr Diet*;31 (2): 256-265.

IBS-Free at Last
https: //www.ibsfree.net/

International Foundation for Gastrointestinal Disorders (IFFGD)
https: //www.iffgd.org/

Iraporda C, Errea A, Romanin DE, Cayet D, Pereyra E, Pignataro O, Sirard JC, Garrote GL, Abraham AG, Rumbo M. (2015) Lactate and short chain fatty acids produced by microbial fermentation downregulate proinflammatory responses in intestinal epithelial cells and myeloid cells. *Immunobiology*; 220: 1161-1169.

Islami F, Ren JS, Taylor PR, Kamangar F. (2009) Pickled vegetables and the risk of oesophageal cancer: a meta-analysis. *Br J Cancer*; 101 (9): 1641-1647.

Iwasa M, Aoi W, Mune K, Yamauchi H, Furuta K, Sasaki S, Takeda K, Harada K, Wada S, Nakamura Y et al. (2013) Fermented milk improves glucose metabolism in exercise-induced muscle damage in young healthy men. *Nutr J*; 12: 83.

Jafari E, Vahedi H, Merat S, Momtahen S, Riahi A. (2014) Therapeutic effects, tolerability and safety of a multi-strain probiotic in Iranian adults with irritable bowel syndrome and bloating. *Arch Iran Med*; 17 (7): 466–70.

James MW, Scott BB. (2000) Endomysial antibody in the diagnosis and management of coeliac disease. *Postgrad Med J*; 76: 466-468.

Jandhyala SM, Talukdar R, Subramanyam C, Vuyyuru H, Sasikala M, Reddy DN. (2015) Role of the normal gut microbiota. *World J Gastroenterol*. 21 (29): 8787-8803.

Junker Y, Zeissig S, Kim SJ, et al. (2012) Wheat amylase trypsin inhibitors drive intestinal inflammation via activation of toll-like receptor 4. *J Exp Med*; 209 (13): 2395-2408.

Karsten HD, Patterson PH, Stout R. (2010) Vitamins A, E and fatty acid composition of the eggs of caged hens and pastured hens. *Renewable Agriculture and Food Systems*; 25 (1): 45-54.

Katz SE. The Art of Fermentation: An In-Depth Exploration of Essential Concepts and Processes from Around the World. Vermont: Chelsea Green Publishing, 2012. Print.

Khanna R, MacDonald JK, Levesque BG. (2014) Peppermint oil for the treatment of irritable bowel syndrome: A systematic review and meta-analysis. *J. Clin. Gastroenterol*; 48: 505-512.

Kings College London – FODMAPs
https://www.kcl.ac.uk/lsm/schools/life-course-sciences/departments/nutritional-sciences/projects/fodmaps/index

Kim B, Hong VM, Yang J, et al. (2016) A review of fermented foods with beneficial effects on brain and cognitive function. *Prev Nutr Food Sci*; 21 (4): 297-309.

Kok CR, Hutkins R. (2018). Yogurt and other fermented foods as sources of health-promoting bacteria. *Nutri Rev*; 76 (Supplement 1): 4-15.

Komericki P, Akkilic-Materna M, Strimitzer T, Weyermair K, Hammer HF, Aberer W. (2012) Oral xylose isomerase decreases breath hydrogen excretion and improves gastrointestinal symptoms in fructose malabsorption – a double-blind, placebo-controlled study. *Aliment Pharmacol Ther*, 36: 980–987.

Kondrashova A, Mustalahti K. (2008) Lower economic status and inferior hygienic environment may protect against celiac disease. *Ann Med*; 40 (3): 223-31.

Krogsgaard LR, Lyngesen M, Bytzer P. (2017) Systematic review: quality of trials on the symptomatic effects of the low FODMAP diet for irritable bowel syndrome. *Aliment Pharmacol Ther*; 45: 1506–1513.

Kühn J, Schutkowski A, Kluge H, Hirche F, Stangl GI. (2014) Free-range farming: a natural alternative to produce vitamin D-enriched eggs. *Nutrition*; 30(4):481-484.

Kurppa K, Paavola A, Collin P, Sievänen H, Laurila K, Huhtala H, Saavalainen P, Mäki M, Kaukinen K. (2014) Benefits of a gluten-free diet for asymptomatic patients with serologic markers of celiac disease. *Gastroenterology*; 147 (3): 610-617.

Lacy BE, Gabbard SL, Crowell MD. (2011) Pathophysiology, Evaluation, and Treatment of Bloating. Hope, Hype or Hot Air? *Gastroenterol Hematol (NY)*; 7 (11): 729-739.

Latham JR, Love M, Hilbeck A. (2017) The distinct properties of natural and GM cry insecticidal proteins. *Biotechnology and Genetic Engineering Reviews*; 33: 1.

Lebwohl B, Cao Y, Zong G, Hu FB, Green PHR, Neugut AI, Rimm EB, Sampson L, Dougherty LW, Giovannucci E, Willett WC, Sun O, Chan AT. (2017) Long term gluten consumption in adults without celiac disease and risk of coronary heart disease: prospective cohort study. *BMJ*; 357.

Lee B, Yin X, Griffey SM, Marco ML. (2015) Attenuation of colitis by Lactobacillus casei BL23 is dependent on the dairy delivery matrix. *Appl Environ Microbiol*; 81: 6425-6435.

Lembo T, Naliboff B, Munakata J, et al. (1999) Symptoms and visceral perception in patients with pain-predominant irritable bowel syndrome. *Am J Gastroenterology*; 94: 1320–1326.

Leroy F, De Vuyst L. (2014) Fermented food in the context of a healthy diet: how to produce novel functional foods? *Curr Opin Clin Nutr Metab Care*; 17 (6): 574-581.

Lewis SJ, Heaton KW. (1997) Stool form scale as a useful guide to intestinal transit time. *Scand J Gastroenterol*; 32 (9): 920-924.

Lorea Baroja M, Kirjavainen PV, Hekmat S, Reid G. (2017) Antiinflammatory effects of probiotic yogurt in inflammatory bowel disease patients. *Clin Exp Immunol*; 149: 470-479.

Love DC, Rodman S., Neff RA, Nachman KE. (2011) Veterinary Drug Residues in Seafood Inspected by the European Union, United States, Canada and Japan from 2000 to 2009. *Environ Sci Technol*; 45 (17): 7232-7240.

Lunder S, Sharp R. (2014) US Seafood Advice Flawed on Mercury, Omega-3s. Environmental Working Group (EWG).

Marco ML, Heeney D, Binda S, Cifelli CJ, Cotter PD, Foligné B, Gänzle M, Kort R, Pasin G, Pihlanto A, Smid EJ, Hutkins R. (2017) Health benefits of fermented foods: microbiota and beyond. *Curr Opin Biotechnol*; 44: 94-102.

Massimo B, Gambaccini D, Usai-Satta P, De Bortoli N, Bertani L, Marchi S, Stasi C. (2015) Irritable bowel syndrome and chronic constipation: Fact and fiction. *World J Gastroenterol*; 21 (40): 11362-11370.

Mast Cells, Mastocytosis, and Related Disorders Theoharides TC, Valent P, Akin C. (2015) *N Engl J Med*; 373: 163-72.

Mayo clinic
https://www.mayoclinic.org/

McIntosh K, Reed DE, Schneider T, et al. (2017) FODMAPs alter symptoms and the metabolome of patients with IBS: a randomised controlled trial. *Gut*; 66 (7): 1241-1251.

McKenzie YA, Thompson J, Gulia P, Lomer MCE. (2016) British Dietetic Association systematic review of systematic reviews and evidence-based practice guidelines for the use of probiotics in the management of irritable bowel syndrome in adults. *J Hum Nutr Diet*; 29 (5): 576-92.

Menees et al. (2012) *Am J Gastroenterol*; 107 (1): 28-35.

Menees S, Chey W. (2018) The gut microbiome and irritable bowel syndrome. *F1000Research 2018, 7 (F1000 Faculty Rev)*: 1029.

Moayyedi P, Ford AC, Talley NJ, Cremonini F, Foxx-Orenstein AE, Brandt LJ, et al. (2010) The efficacy of probiotics in the treatment of irritable bowel syndrome: a systematic review. *Gut*; 59 (3): 325–3.

Monash University The Low FODMAP Diet
https: //www.monashfodmap.com/

Money ME, Walkowiak J, Virgilio C, et al. (2011) Pilot study: a randomised, double blind, placebo controlled trial of pancrealipase for the treatment of postprandial irritable bowel syndrome-diarrhoea, *Frontline Gastroenterology*; 2: 48-56.

Monterey Bay Aquarium Foundation
http: //www.seafoodwatch.org

Moongngarm A. (2013) Chemical compositions and resistant starch content in starchy foods. *Am J Agric Biol Sci*; 8: 107-113.

Mozaffarian D, Rimm EB. (2006) Fish intake, contaminants, and human health: evaluating the risks and the benefits. *JAMA*; 296:1885-1899.

Mozaffarian D, Rimm EB. (2006) Fish intake, contaminants, and human health: evaluating the risks and the benefits. *JAMA*; 296:1885-1899.

Mueller NT, Bakacs E, Combellick J, Grigoryan Z, Dominguez-Bello MG. (2015) The infant microbiome development: mom matters. *Trends Mol Med*; 21 (2): 109-117.

Mullin GE, Shepherd SJ, Chander Roland B, Ireton-Jones C, Matarese LE. (2014) Irritable bowel syndrome: contemporary nutrition management strategies. *JPEN J Parenter Enteral Nutr*; 38: 781-799.

Murphy MM, Douglass JS, Birkett A. (2008) Resistant Starch Intakes in the United States. *J Am Diet Assoc*; 108: 67-78.

Murray K, Wilkinson-Smith V, Hoad C, et al. (2014) Differential effects of FODMAPs (fermentable-oligo-, di-, mono-saccharides and polyols) on small and large intestinal contents in healthy subjects shown by MRI. *Am J Gastroenterol*; 109 (1): 110-119.

My GI Nutrition
http: //www.myginutrition.com/

National Center for Home Food Preservation
http: //nchfp.uga.edu/

Nicklas TA et al. (2009) The role of dairy in meeting the recommendations for shortfall nutrients in the American diet. *J Am Coll Nutr*; 28 (suppl 1): 73S-81S.

NIDDK -Lactose Intolerance
  https://www.niddk.nih.gov/health-information/digestive-diseases/lactose-intolerance/

Nishiyama H, Nagai T, Kudo M, Okazaki Y, Azuma Y, Watanabe T, Goto S, Ogata H, Sakurai T. (2018) Supplementation of pancreatic digestive enzymes alters the composition of intestinal microbiota in mice. *Biochem Biophys Res Commun*; 495(1): 273-279.

O'Grady J, O'Connor EM, Shanahan F. (2019) Review article: dietary fibre in the era of microbiome science. *Aliment Pharmacol Ther*; 49: 506–515.

Pandurangan AK, Divya T, Kumar K, Dineshbabu V, Velavan B, Sudhandiran G. (2018) Colorectal carcinogenesis: Insights into the cell death and signal transduction pathways: A review. *World J Gastrointest Oncol*; 10 (9): 244-259.

Parkman HP, Doma S. (2006) Importance of gastrointestinal motility disorders. *Practical Gastroenterology*; 30 (9): 23-40.

Pedersen N, Ankersen DV, Felding M, Vegh Z, Burisch J, Munkholm P. (2018) Low FODMAP diet reduces irritable bowel symptoms and improves quality of life in patients with inflammatory bowel disease in a randomised controlled trial. (AGA abstracts).

Pedersen N, Ankersen DV, Felding M, Wachmann H, Végh Z, Molzen L, Burisch J, Andersen JR, Munkholm P. (2017) Low FODMAP Diet Reduces Irritable Bowel Symptoms and Improves Quality of Life in Patients with Inflammatory Bowel Disease. *World J Gastroenterol*; 23 (18): 3356-3366.

Peters SL, Yao CK, Philpott H, Yelland GW, Muir JG, Gibson PR. (2016) Randomised clinical trial: the efficacy of gut-directed hypnotherapy is similar to that of the low FODMAP diet for the treatment of irritable bowel syndrome. *Aliment Pharmacol Ther*; 44 (5): 447-59.

Piche T, De Varnnes DB, Sacher-Huvelin S, Holst JJ, Cuber JC, Galmiche JP. (2003) Colonic Fermentation Influences Lower Esophageal Sphincter Function in Gastroesophageal Reflux Disease. *Gastroenterology* 124 (4): 894-902.

Piessevaux H, De Winter B, Louis E, et al. (2009) Dyspeptic symptoms in the general population: a factor and cluster analysis of symptom groupings. *Neurogastroenterol Motil*; 21: 378–388.

Potter MDE, Brienesse SC, Walker MM, Boyle A, Talley NJ. (2018) Effect of the gluten-free diet on cardiovascular risk factors in patients with coeliac disease: A systematic review. *J Gastroenterol Hepatol*; 33 (4): 781-791.

Prince AC, Myers CE, Joyce T, Irving P, Lomer M, Whelan K. (2016) Fermentable

Carbohydrate Restriction (Low FODMAP Diet) in Clinical Practice Improves Functional Gastrointestinal Symptoms in Patients with Inflammatory Bowel Disease. *Inflamm Bowel Dis*; 22 (5): 1129-36.

Raehsler SL, Choung RS, Marietta EV, Murray JA. (2018) Accumulation of Heavy Metals in People on a Gluten-Free Diet. *Clin Gastroenterol Hepatol*; 16 (2): 244-251.

Regueiro M, Greer J, Stigethy E. (2017) *Gastroenterology*; 152 (2): 430-439.

Rej A, Avery A, Ford AC, Holdoway A, Kurien M, McKenzie Y, Thompson J, Trott N, Whelan K, Williams M, Sanders DS. (2018) Clinical Application of Dietary Therapies in Irritable Bowel Syndrome *J Gastrointestin Liver Dis*; 27 (3): 307-316.

Ren JS, Kamangar F, Forman D, Islami F. (2012) Pickled food and risk of gastric cancer — a systematic review and meta-analysis of English and Chinese literature. *Cancer Epidemiol Biomarkers Prev;* 21 (6): 905-915.

Rezaie A, Pimentel M, Rao SS. (2016) How to Test and Treat Small Intestinal Bacterial Overgrowth: an Evidence-Based Approach. *Curr Gastroenterol Rep*; 18 (2): 8.

Ringel Y, Williams RE, Kalilani L, Cook SF. (2009) Prevalence, characteristics, and impact of bloating symptoms in patients with irritable bowel syndrome. *Clin Gastroenterol Hepatol*; 7: 68–72.

Rogha M, Esfahani MZ, Zargarzadeh AH. (2014) The efficacy of a synbiotic containing Bacillus Coagulans in treatment of irritable bowel syndrome: a randomized placebo-controlled trial. *Gastroenterol Hepatol Bed Bench*; 7 (3): 156–63.

S Lunder and R Sharp (2014). US Seafood Advice Flawed on Mercury, Omega-3s. Environmental Working Group (EWG).

Sajilata MG, Singhal R, Kulkarni PR. (2006) Resistant Starch – A Review. *Compr Rev Food Sci Food Saf;* 5: 1-17.

Salas-Salvadó J, Bulló M, Estruch R, Ros E, Covas MI, Ibarrola-Jurado N, Corella D, Arós F, Gómez-Gracia E, Ruiz-Gutiérrez V, Romaguera D, Lapetra J, Lamuela-Raventós RM, Serra-Majem L, Pintó X, Basora J, Muñoz MA, Sorlí JV, Martínez-González MA. (2014) Prevention of diabetes with Mediterranean diets: A subgroup analysis of a randomized trial. *Ann. Intern. Med*; 160: 1–10.

Sandler RS, Drossman DA, Nathan HP, McKee DC. (1984) Symptom complaints and health care seeking behavior in subjects with bowel dysfunction. *Gastroenterology*; 87: 314–318.

Sandler RS, Stewart WF, Liberman JN, Ricci JA, Zorich NL. (2000) Abdominal pain, bloating, and diarrhea in the United States: prevalence and impact. *Dig Dis Sc*; 45: 1166–1171.

Sapone A, Bai JC, Ciacci C, et al. (2012) Spectrum of gluten-related disorders: consensus on new nomenclature and classification. *BMC Med;* 10: 13.

Savaiano DA (2014) Lactose digestion from yogurt: mechanism and relevance. *Am J Clin Nutr*; 99: 1251-1255.

Schmulson M, Chang L. (2011) Review article: the treatment of functional abdominal bloating and distension. *Aliment Pharmacol Ther*; 33: 1071–1086.

Schumann D, Langhorst J, Dobos G, Cramer H. (2018) Randomised clinical trial: yoga vs a low-FODMAP diet in patients with irritable bowel syndrome. *Aliment Pharmacol Ther*; 47 (2): 203-211.

Schuppan D, Pickert G, Ashfaq-Khan M, Zevallos V. (2015) Non-celiac wheat sensitivity: differential diagnosis, triggers and implications. *Best Pract Res Clin Gastroenterol;* 29 (3): 469-476.

Shepherd S and Gibson P. The Complete Low FODMAP Diet. Australia: Penguin, 2011. Print.

Simrén M, Barbara G, Flint HJ, Spiegel BM, Spiller RC, Vanner S, Verdu EF, Whorwell PJ, Zoetendal EG. (2013) Intestinal microbiota in functional bowel disorders: a Rome foundation report. *Gut*; 62 (1): 159-176.

Simren M, Palsson OS, Whitehead WE. (2017) Update on Rome IV Criteria for Colorectal Disorders: Implications for Clinical Practice. *Curr Gastroenterol Rep*; 19 (4): 15.

Sisson G, Ayis S, Sherwood RA, Bjarnason I. (2014) Randomised clinical trial: A liquid multi-strain probiotic vs. placebo in the irritable bowel syndrome - a 12 week double-blind study. *Aliment Pharmacol Therl*; 40 (1): 51–62.

Soedamah-Muthu SS, Masset G, Verberne L, Geleijnse JM, Brunner EJ (2013) Consumption of dairy products and associations with incident diabetes, CHD and mortality in the Whitehall II study. *Br J Nutr*; 109: 718-726.

Sommer F, Backhed F. (2013) The gut microbiota—masters of host development and physiology. *Nat Rev Microbiol*; 11: 227–238.

Staudacher HM, Whelan K, Irving PM, Lomer MC. (2011) Comparison of symptom response following advice for a diet low in fermentable carbohydrates (FODMAPs) versus standard dietary advice in patients with irritable bowel syndrome. *J Hum Nutr Diet*; 24: 487–495.

Staudacher HM, Whelan K. (2017) The low FODMAP diet: recent advances in understanding its mechanisms and efficacy in irritable bowel syndrome. *Gut*; 66: 1517–1527.

Stern EK, Brenner DM. (2018) Gut Microbiota-Based Therapies for Irritable Bowel Syndrome. *Clin Transl Gastroenterol*; 9 (2): e134.

Tack J, Piessevaux H, Coulie B, Caenepeel P, Janssens J. (1998) Role of impaired gastric accommodation to a meal in functional dyspepsia. *Gastroenterology*; 115: 1346–1352.

Talley NJ, Zinsmeister AR, Van Dyke C, Melton LJ. (1991) Epidemiology of colonic symptoms and the irritable bowel syndrome. *Gastroenterology*; 101: 927–934.

Talley NJ. (2008) Functional gastrointestinal disorders as a public health problem. *Neurogastroenterol Motil*;20 Suppl 1: 121-129.

Tapsell LC. (2015) Fermented dairy food and CVD risk. *Br J Nutr*; 113: 131-135.

Teruel C, Garrido EF. (2016) Diagnosis and management of functional symptoms in inflammatory bowel disease in remission. *World J Gastrointest Pharmacol Ther*; 7 (1): 78–90.

Thalheimer JC. (2014) Silent Celiac Disease. *Today's Dietitian*; 16 (5): 22.

The International Scientific Association for Probiotics and Prebiotics (ISAPP) http: //isappscience.org/

The Rome Foundation
http: //theromefoundation.org/about/

Then C, Bauer-Panskus A. (2017) Possible health impacts of Bt toxins and residues from spraying with complementary herbicides in genetically engineered soybeans and risk assessment as performed by the European Food Safety Authority EFSA. *Environ Sci Eur*; 29 (1): 1.

Thiwan S. Abdominal Bloating: A Mysterious Symptom. UNC Center for Functional GI and Motility Disorders.

Tillisch K, Labus J, Kilpatrick L, Jiang Z, Stains J, Ebrat B, Guyonnet D, Legrain-Raspaud S, Trotin B, Naliboff BME. (2014) Consumption of fermented milk product with probiotics modulates brain activity. *Gastroenterology*; 144 (7): 1394-401.

Tortora R, Capone P, De Stefano G, Imperatore N, Gerbino N, Donetto S, Monaco V, Caporaso N, Rispo A. (2015) Metabolic syndrome in patients with coeliac disease on a gluten-free diet. *Aliment Pharmacol Ther*; 41 (4): 352-9.

Tuck C, Barrett J. (2017) Re-challenging FODMAPs: the low FODMAP diet phase two. *J Gastroenterol Hepatol*; 32: 11–15.

Tuck CJ, Taylor KM, Gibson PR, Barrett JB, Muir JG. (2017) Increasing Symptoms in Irritable Bowel Symptoms With Ingestion of Galacto-Oligosaccharides Are Mitigated by [alpha]-Galactosidase Treatment. *Am J Gastroenterol.* 2017.

U.S. Department of Agriculture, USDA: USDA Graded Cage-Free Eggs: All They're Cracked Up To Be.

UEG Journal Research (Research published in the *UEG Journal* in July 2018 revealed some sad statistics.)
http: //www.jnmjournal.org/journal/view.html?doi=10.5056/jnm.2013.19.4.433

USDA Food Composition Databases.

Valdes AM, Walter J, Segal E, Spector TD. (2018) Role of the gut microbiota in nutrition and health. *BMJ*; 361: k2179.

Velasquez MT, Ramezani A, Manal A, Raj DS. (2016) Trimethylamine *N*-Oxide: The Good, the Bad and the Unknown. *Toxins*; 8 (11): 326.

Weaver CM and Heaney RP. (2006) Calcium in human health. Totowa, NJ: *Humana Press.*

Weaver CM and Plawecki KL. (1994) Dietary calcium: Adequacy of a vegetarian diet. *Am J Clin Nutr*; 59 (suppl): 1238S-41S.

Weaver CM et al. (1999) Choices for achieving adequate dietary calcium with a vegetarian diet. *Am J Clin Nutr*; 70 (suppl): 543S-8S.

WGO Practice Guideline - Diet and the Gut 2018/WGO Practice Guideline on Probiotics and Prebiotics
http: //www.worldgastroenterology.org/

Whelan K, Martin LD, Staudacher HM, Lomer MCE. (2018) The low FODMAP diet in the management of irritable bowel syndrome: an evidence-based review of FODMAP restriction, reintroduction and personalisation in clinical practice. *J Hum Nutr Diet*; 31 (2): 239-255.

Whorwell PJ, Altringer L, Morel J, Bond Y, Charbonneau D, O'Mahony L, et al. (2006) Efficacy of an encapsulated probiotic Bifidobacterium infantis 35624 in women with irritable bowel syndrome. *Am J Gastroenterol*; 101 (7): 1581–90.

Wilkins T, Sequoia J. (2017) Probiotics for Gastrointestinal Conditions: A Summary of the Evidence *Am Fam Physician*; 96 (3): 170-178.

World Gastroenterology Organization (WGO) Global Guidelines -Diet and Gut p.26.

Yano JM, Yu K., Donaldson GP, Shastri GG, Ann P, Ma L., Nagler CR, Ismagilov RF, Mazmanian SK, Hsiao EY. (2015) Indigenous bacteria from the gut microbiota regulate host serotonin biosynthesis. *Cell*; 161 (2): 264–276.

Yu and Rao. (2014) *Therap Adv Gastroenterol*; 7 (5): 193-205.

Zevallos VF, Raker V, Tenzer S, et al. (2017) Nutritional wheat amylase-trypsin inhibitors promote intestinal inflammation via activation of myeloid cells. *Gastroenterology*; 152 (5): 1100-1113.e12.

Zhan Y, Zhan Y, Dai S. (2017) Is a low FODMAP diet beneficial for patients with inflammatory bowel disease? A meta-analysis and systematic review. *Clin Nutr*; 37 (1): 123-129.

Acknowledgements

This book couldn't have been completed without the priceless help of some very important people. Natalie Keenan for creating and testing various recipes with us and lending us her excellent eye for presenting food in beautiful ways. Our photographer Kyriaki Leventi for her great work, input, vision and sense of humor during the many hours of photo shooting. Patsy Catsos, MS, RDN, LD, Kate Scarlata, MPH, RDN and Susan M. Hazarvartian, MS, RDN, LDN for taking the time to read our book and provide us with a recommendation. We are truly honored to have their seal of approval. Also, Elena Christoforou Petsa, MD, PhD and author Thalia Kounouni for helping us navigate through the world of publishing. A huge thank you to all of you.

Finally, we'd like to thank our families for their willingness to be our guinea pigs, repeatedly tasting our various creations and testing the recipes in this book with boundless enthusiasm. Also, for their love, support and patience during this long but utterly fulfilling process. We couldn't have done this without you.

Index

B

C

D

E

F

G

H

I

J

K

L

M

N

O

P

Q

R

S

T

U

V

W

Whole roasted fish, 293
Wine, 42, 79, 87, 94, 148
    Dessert wine, 108
World Gastroenterology Organization (WGO), 86

X

Xylose isomerase, 96

Y

Yeast, 41, 45–46, 87, 165
Yersinia, 37
Yoga, 97
Yogurt, 87–89, 91, 107, 111, 114–116
    Low FODMAP raita, 359
    Low FODMAP tzatziki, 358
    Steamed fish with fennel and leeks with yogurt dressing, 299
    Yogurt dressing, 299

Z

Zesting, 166

A

B